PRAISE FOR *TAPPING*

"Who would guess from its unassuming title that this work is destined to become one of the most consequential books of our era! . . . It is a stunning call to action at a time of desperate personal and collective need."

JEAN HOUSTON, PhD
cultural historian, from the foreword to *Tapping*

"Based on shifting internal states of bodily experience, *Tapping* provides a lucid guide to energy psychology that demonstrates techniques and procedures that can bring about remarkably rapid changes in the way people feel and move through the world."

BESSEL VAN DER KOLK, MD
#1 *New York Times* nonfiction bestselling author of *The Body Keeps the Score*

"David Feinstein and Donna Eden masterfully blend the extraordinary power of energy psychology with the best of contemporary mental health practices. Their rigorous research, coupled with real-world testing, provides a framework that is as innovative as it is transformative. A beacon of hope and healing, this book is an essential companion for anyone seeking profound personal evolution."

TONY ROBBINS
New York Times bestselling author of *Awaken the Giant Within*

"*Tapping* places into your hands a profound tool for manifesting the health and life you desire. It is a practical and scientifically informed guide for psychological transformation. With simple, step-by-step instructions, it empowers individuals to move beyond personal limitations and write new, empowering stories for themselves, their children, and, in that process, the world."

BRUCE H. LIPTON, PhD
bestselling author of *The Biology of Belief*, coauthor of *Spontaneous Evolution*

"Energy psychology is a powerful tool for reprogramming your subconscious mind to help overcome limiting beliefs. *Tapping* is a beautifully crafted book that guides you to your own personal transformation. It gives you the practical, hands-on tools to live a better life."

DR. JOE DISPENZA
New York Times bestselling author of *You Are the Placebo* and *Becoming Supernatural*

"In *Tapping*, David Feinstein and Donna Eden meticulously merge ancient wisdom with contemporary science, crafting an invaluable resource for both novices and seasoned professionals. Their extensive research, integration of best mental health practices, and feedback-driven approach deliver a master class on energy psychology. This book is not just a guide— it's a revolution. An absolute must-read for anyone on a journey to emotional and spiritual well-being."

NICK ORTNER
New York Times bestselling author of *The Tapping Solution*

"*Tapping* is a comprehensive guide that explores the benefits of energy psychology and its application in various aspects of life. I can't stress enough how this book will offer readers a deep understanding of the transformative power of tapping and how it can be used to address common challenges and enhance overall well-being. David and Donna not only bring their years of clinical skill and research experience to this book, but share real-life examples, making *Tapping* accessible to both beginners and those already skilled and familiar with this life-changing modality."

PETA STAPLETON, PhD
Australia's 2019 Psychologist of the Year, author of the groundbreaking *The Science Behind Tapping*

"Tapping is a tour de force for the field of psychology. Eden and Feinstein's heartfelt, practical, and scientific approach to energy psychology simultaneously demystifies and celebrates the connection between spirit, mind, energy, and body for healing so that all can benefit. This book gives incredible insight and guidance on self-healing, which gives hope to clinicians, patients, and scientists alike. A highly enjoyable and inspirational read!"

SHAMINI JAIN, PhD
author of *Healing Ourselves: Biofield Science and the Future of Health*
and CEO of the Consciousness and Healing Initiative

Tapping

Tapping

Self-Healing with the Transformative Power of Energy Psychology

DAVID FEINSTEIN PhD
& DONNA EDEN

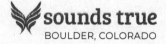

sounds true
BOULDER, COLORADO

Sounds True
Boulder, CO

Published 2024

Cover design by Charli Barnes
Book design by Meredith Jarrett

Printed in the United States of America

BK06528

Library of Congress Cataloging-in-Publication Data

Names: Feinstein, David, author. | Eden, Donna, author.
Title: Tapping : self-healing with the transformative power of energy psychology /
    David Feinstein, Ph.D., Donna Eden.
Description: Boulder, CO : Sounds True, 2024. | Includes bibliographical references
    and index.
Identifiers: LCCN 2023027447 (print) | LCCN 2023027448 (ebook) | ISBN
    9781683649960 (trade paperback) | ISBN 9781683649977 (epub)
Subjects: LCSH: Energy psychology. | Acupuncture points.
Classification: LCC RC489.E53 F4584 2024 (print) | LCC RC489.E53 (ebook) |
    DDC 616.8914--dc23/eng/20231222
LC record available at https://lccn.loc.gov/2023027447
LC ebook record available at https://lccn.loc.gov/2023027448

FSC
www.fsc.org
MIX
Paper | Supporting
responsible forestry
FSC® C103098

For our grandchildren, Tiernan Ray Devenyns and Sequoia Rayne Richards Dahlin, that they and their generation may thrive as they move into an unwritten future.

Contents

List of Illustrations

Gratitude

AS WE EACH LOOK back on our full and adventurous lives, we are well aware that the people who have contributed to our well-being and evolution comprise a long line, extending from our infancies up to this moment. They have each, in their own unique ways, left their mark on our approach to life and ultimately to our approach to writing this book, and we are taking a moment to bathe in gratitude.

Our visionary publisher and longtime friend Tami Simon; our brilliant editorial team of Jaime Schwalb, Jessica Carew Kraft, Angela Wix, and Emily Wichland; our amazing staff at Innersource; the people who served as the chapter-by-chapter "test drivers"; and the numerous colleagues who reviewed sections of the book that were in their areas of expertise have been joys to work with, and they have also made this a far stronger presentation.

And of course, our families, friends, teachers, students, clients, and close colleagues all deserve special mention. If we attempt to properly acknowledge each of their contributions, however (we started), we would be on our way to another book. So, we will take a shortcut and get right into *Tapping*. Meanwhile, if you are one of the above intimates, please know you are precious to us and accept, from the bottom of our hearts, our profound gratitude!

David Feinstein
Donna Eden

Foreword

WHO WOULD GUESS FROM its unassuming title that this work is destined to become one of the most consequential books of our era! *Tapping* provides no less than a framework for navigating the gap between humanity's past wisdom and its shared hopes for the future. It invites you to take a deep dive into the boundless expanse of your personal consciousness and summon the vast potentials that reside within. It is a stunning call to action at a time of desperate personal and collective need.

With the emergence of these urgent needs, a world of possibilities also unfolds, inviting us to explore and embrace new ways of understanding. From these possibilities a remarkable synthesis has appeared, merging the timeless practices of ancient healing traditions with the cutting-edge insights and methods of contemporary psychotherapy. Within the rapidly growing field of energy psychology, the focus of this tour de force, lies a potent technology, a synergy that surpasses the individual strengths of its predecessors, unleashing new transformative forces.

At the heart of energy psychology is a simple yet profound technique—one that echoes the wisdom of ages. It involves stimulating specific energy points on the skin, a practice known as tapping. This ancient art, harnessed and refined by modern psychological science, serves as a gateway to unlock the hidden potential within us. As these energy points are gently tapped while memories, fears, or aspirations are vividly engaged, a cascade of subtle yet powerful shifts occur, allowing the release of energetic blockages and a restoration of balance within the human psyche.

With energy psychology, the boundaries that once constrained our understanding of healing and development are transcended. The procedures invite us to explore the depths of our own being, to unearth the hidden layers of our psyche, and to embrace the power within us to effect profound change. It is a modality that invites us to become active participants in our own transformation, harnessing the combined power of ancient and modern wisdom to unlock our fullest potential.

You will see in the following pages marital strife turn into harmony via techniques you'd not expect to have such impact. You'll learn of a woman whose fast-progressing throat cancer was reversed, to her oncologist's amazement, by a series of tapping sessions. You will read of a man who had become hateful and vicious after his village was destroyed during civil warfare—with neighbors brutally murdered in front of him—transformed into a force for "peace and mercy." You will hear about athletic teams that soared to win national championships after being introduced to tapping. You will share in the details of a police officer —a man who had been an entrenched alcoholic—becoming a resource, turned to by his department when other officers have drinking problems. You will be brought behind the scenes, following the massacre of 20 six- and seven-year-olds at Sandy Hook, as family members and first responders found that tapping sessions were able to bring them peace and healing "when nothing else does." You will tune in to a girl who had been emotionally paralyzed for the decade after witnessing her father's death by machete during the Rwanda genocide as she finds peace with all the symptoms of her severe PTSD erased and the benefits maintained on follow-up psychological testing a year later. The book's provocative stories are poised to inspire you.

The practice of tapping sets in motion an activation and deactivation within the intricate landscape of the human brain. As you tap on specific energy points, deactivating signals are sent to brain areas that typically come online in the face of anger, fear, threat, and distress. These ancient evolutionary responses, deeply ingrained within our neural circuitry, are momentarily soothed and calmed. The calming effects of the tapping invite these distress signals to recede, allowing you to loosen the grip of negative emotions and access the expansive realms of possibility that reside within you.

Simultaneously, the stimulating effects of tapping send activating signals to executive brain areas—those regions responsible for problem-solving, stress management, and creativity. They come alive, ready to engage with the topic at hand, igniting the fires of cognitive prowess and inventive solutions.

In this exquisite interplay of activation and deactivation, acupoint tapping brings you into a state of balance and flow. It allows you to transcend the limitations of past wounds and narratives, ushering you into a space where deep healing becomes possible. As the deactivating signals quiet the storms of distress and the activating signals turn on your evolution-honed capacities for problem-solving and creative thought, you find yourself equipped with the tools to move through the complexities of life with greater resilience and clarity.

As you delve into the realm of energy psychology, you also embark on a journey that blurs the boundaries of the tangible and intangible. It is a voyage that takes you beyond the limits of the electromagnetic spectrum and invites you to explore the domain of subtle energies—a terrain that carries profound implications for modern physics and our understanding of the universe.

These subtle energies, although not yet fully embraced by conventional science, hold the key to unlocking hidden dimensions of our existence. They are not limited by the constraints of our current understanding, for they carry information and exhibit a form of intelligence that expands the frontiers of our knowledge.

Probing deeper into the mysteries of subtle energy, we uncover a pathway that leads us to the next emergent stage of our evolution. It is a time of profound opportunity —a chance to weave together the wisdom of the ages with the innovative spirit of the present and glimpses into the aspirations of generations yet to come. As we find our way through this maelstrom, we must summon the resilience within, for it is in times of challenge that our greatest potential is often revealed.

But beyond the personal struggles lies a broader, more profound concern. The world's shifting tides jeopardize the very future of our existence. The challenges we face today—the ecological crises, social upheavals, and existential uncertainties—call for fundamental transformations in our collective consciousness. Humanity stands at the precipice, poised to make an evolutionary leap that is not only necessary but imperative for our survival and flourishing. By working with these energies and developing our capacity to engage with them, we tap into deep potentials that lie dormant within us, waiting to be actualized. It is a call to action, a do-or-die challenge that humanity faces in the critical decades ahead.

It is within the individual, the unit of our collective consciousness, that the seeds of this cultural makeover must take root. To navigate the currents of change, we must cultivate a deep sense of self-awareness—a profound understanding of our unique gifts, talents, and purpose. By diving into the depths of our own consciousness, we access the wellspring of creativity, resilience, and vision that can propel us forward. Through this inward journey we discover the interconnectedness of all beings, recognizing that our individual growth is intricately woven into the fabric of the collective human experience.

As we engage the invisible powers of subtle energies, we encounter fascinating properties that defy conventional notions of space and distance. These energies possess the remarkable ability to transcend the limitations of physical proximity, opening us to our potential to become catalysts for global change. It is within this framework that we discover our capacity to shift the vibration even in crime-torn areas, transforming environments plagued by violence and despair into harbors of greater peace and harmony. Through focused attention and intention, we can harness the potency of these subtle energies to enhance the common good, fostering a collective shift toward a more awakened and compassionate humanity. The time to usher in a new era of expanded consciousness, interconnectedness, and harmonious coexistence is now.

So, let us embark on this extraordinary path of energy psychology, where the ancient echoes of shamans and priests mingle with the wisdom of contemporary science. Let us tap into the wellspring of healing and growth, accessing the limitless reservoir of our own inner resources. Through this fusion of traditions we stand poised to embrace a journey of profound personal evolution, guided by the light of ancient wisdom and the pioneering spirit we bring to an unknown future.

Jean Houston, PhD

Introduction

IMAGINE THIS: YOU ARE sleeping peacefully in your home when you are abruptly awakened by the bullhorn of a fire officer blaring two words: "Evacuate! Now!" You and your partner groggily register the words and look out the window. You are jolted into full alert when you see the red glow of a wildfire filling the width of your window as it rapidly heads toward your semirural neighborhood. You quickly put on some clothes and rush outside to assess the situation. Other neighbors are already driving away from the direction of the approaching flames. You can't find your beloved cat but feel the urgency to get into your car. As you speed away, the fire is following you.

You escape its path and head into safety. But by the next morning, you learn that many of your neighbors didn't. Your home is in ashes. Your cat is never found again. You can't fall asleep the first night, ruminating about the experience. Or on the second night. Or the third.

A month later, you are still unable to get a good night's rest. In your brain, new neural pathways have been formed. Simply being in bed activates the experience of terror when you woke up to a living nightmare. Other neural pathways have also formed, leaving you dwelling in guilt about having left your cat behind, grieving the horrible deaths of your neighbors, and suffering from the loss of your family photos, treasured pieces of art, literally everything you own. Worry centers are also activated. Where will you live? How will you deal with the financial loss?

How do we survive such a psychological assault that may befall any of us without notice? Your brain is able to meet dire circumstances with resilience, but it can also be overwhelmed. It may need assistance. What if you could send signals to your brain that disrupt the extreme emotional aftermath of a trauma? You would still know the impact of the fire, but you would be able to sleep at night. You would still cherish the memories of your cat and feel the loss without being plunged into unreasonable guilt. You would still need to address the problems of where to live and the unanticipated financial difficulties but without being mired in excessive worry. And what if you could also send signals to your brain that help you think more clearly and creatively as you confront these challenges? All of this was the experience of two of our dearest friends who sought our help following a fire in Northern California that almost claimed their lives.

Energy psychology is a relatively new development within psychology that can show you how to accomplish all of this. It generates signals that directly impact your brain's reactions to the trying events of daily life as well as memories of past difficulties that haven't been adequately processed. It is not confined to dealing with traumas such as escaping a wildfire, though it is very effective even in horrendous situations. Stimulating acupuncture points (acupoints) by tapping on them while activating pertinent thoughts and feelings puts you at the keyboard as you reprogram the neural pathways that impact the quality of your life.

Acupoint tapping, combined with well-chosen words and images, can eliminate unfounded fears, reduce irrational anger, and counter jealousy. It can be the catalyst for creating positive changes in the beliefs that guide your actions. It can

help you overcome self-defeating patterns of behavior. It can keep you calm as you face triggers that had previously produced distress. It can be a force in healing an illness. It can help you overcome emotional obstacles that were preventing you from reaching a desired goal and bring clarity at times of overwhelm or confusion. It can support you in new and more life-affirming directions and connect you with intuitive sources of wisdom that transcend your usual day-to-day awareness.

NEW METHODS, NEW POSSIBILITIES

Tapping: Self-Healing with the Transformative Power of Energy Psychology provides an authoritative overview of one of the most effective and increasingly well-researched approaches for supporting your personal evolution.[2] The combination of contemporary therapeutic methods, ancient healing practices such as acupressure, and contemplative techniques such as mindfulness and guided imagery has produced a remarkably accessible and potent procedure that can be applied to virtually any area of your life. The approach allows you to gently rearrange your psychological makeup in ways that will help you bring out the best version of yourself. It has many applications. You can use it for:

- Addressing emotional wounds you may carry from the past

- Changing patterns of behavior that get in your way

- Navigating more freely through the challenges life presents

- Meeting with greater peace and dexterity the worries, angers, jealousies, losses, and irritations provoked by the situations you encounter

- Improving your relationships with friends, colleagues, and intimates

- Building skills that will increase your success in whatever matters to you

We know this is a bold list of promises. Rather than them being *our* promises, however, we are merely emissaries of recent advances within the behavioral sciences that demonstrate how each possibility can be accomplished on a self-help basis. And these developments come at a time when we all need such abilities as we move through a world whose challenges have become ever more dangerous and demanding.

CAN TAPPING DO ALL THAT?

As innocuous as it may look, tapping on selected acupuncture points sends tiny but potent electrical signals to your brain that can change the way you think, feel, and act. The emergence of psychoanalysis in the West, along with enormous refinements over the past century in showing people how to take charge of their inner lives in empowering ways, has been a soul-enriching development. Combining it with ancient systems for healing and spiritual evolution, as presented in this book, is a step into a richer future built on a new embrace of the past.

WHY WE HAVE WRITTEN *TAPPING*

Because energy psychology is proving beneficial with such a wide range of situations, its practice has been expanding exponentially in the past few years. In addition to striking increases in its use in mainstream treatment settings,[3] a recent paper in the prestigious journal *Frontiers in Psychology* estimated that acupoint tapping is "used as self-help by tens of millions of people each year," noting that one tapping app alone has more than two million documented subscribers.[4]

However, since tapping just a few acupuncture points can be at least somewhat helpful in reducing anxiety, sadness, and other difficult emotions, and can be learned in minutes, it's a reasonable guess that most of these millions of people have only a superficial understanding of the method. They likely have little idea of how to use it to reap benefits far beyond what they imagine is possible for a self-help approach. Providing a comprehensive and up-to-date resource for acquiring deeper understanding and expanded skills with this trailblazing method is a primary purpose for this book.

Tapping is a tutorial for learning or deepening your knowledge about energy psychology, designed for both newcomers and experienced practitioners. It won't make you a therapist if you aren't one already, but it will put powerful self-help tools into your hands. If you are a therapist, it will increase your effectiveness. This book integrates essential concepts, how-to instructions, and scientific understanding in applying energy psychology to a range of issues, including worry, sadness, anxiety, depression, stress, trauma, habits, addictions, and relationships.

Psychotherapists have identified "best practices" for helping people in each of these areas. Illustrating ways of integrating tapping protocols with these best practices has been a major objective for us in writing *Tapping*. Beyond working with everyday concerns such as worry, sadness, and relationships, all the way up to clinical issues such as anxiety, depression, and addictions, the book also shows you how to use tapping to reach goals that have been eluding you; improve your performance in sports, on the stage, or at work; and unfold your finest potentials.

INTRODUCING OURSELVES

The two of us enjoy the immense privilege of being a couple whose professional aspirations converge into a single, shared, passionate purpose. Whether it is David in his role as a psychologist or Donna serving as an energy medicine practitioner, our deepest motivations are to reduce suffering and empower each person we work with so that their lives become happier and more fulfilling. For as long as you stay with this book, *you* are the person on whom these intentions are focused!

Donna has brought an energy perspective into David's understanding of the human psyche. David has brought a more coherent scientific framework into Donna's energy healing system. An offspring of this merger is our passion for this book's topic, the rapidly growing field of *energy psychology*. Energy psychology is the application of energy healing tools for overcoming emotional wounds and promoting psychological and spiritual growth. This development has provided us a rich arena for expanding one another's horizons, and we believe it to be one of the most exciting and significant advances ever in the art of guiding people toward more fulfilling lives.

David's Reflections

I received my doctorate in clinical psychology in 1972, and I have worked as a licensed psychologist in a variety of contexts for five decades. When I first heard about tapping, in the late 1990s, I was as skeptical as anyone. One of the therapists in a clinical consultation group I was leading had stumbled onto the technique, began to study it, and was describing it to the group. I was dismissive, if not derisive, on first hearing about the approach.

How in the world was tapping on the skin going to impact serious psychological conditions? Worse than that, wordings used in its practice, such as *"Even though I get furious at my son for no good reason, I deeply love and accept myself,"* seemed to affirm rather than challenge the very responses and behaviors the person was trying to overcome. "If ever there was a bogus therapy based on frivolous procedures," I thought, "this has to be it!" In retrospect, I was probably more flippant and closed-minded about this new approach than I'd been about any other clinical innovation I had ever encountered. I had no inkling that within a few years I would become a spokesperson for the method! Life has a way of bringing us face to face with our arrogance.

At the time, no credible peer-reviewed research had been published about tapping therapies. There were only passionate claims from a small number of therapists enthusiastically championing it. I doubted that this tapping technique could have anything to do with personal evolution and wondered why anyone would be claiming that it is more effective than established therapies, which even with their limitations, enjoy both acceptance and empirical support.

What I never anticipated is that a series of circumstances would lead me into a training program for clinicians learning to incorporate energy psychology into their practices. Despite my strong skepticism, I kept hearing about energy psychology in workshops I was coleading for therapists and other healers. Then I received an invitation to attend, as a guest, a meeting of psychologists in a city where I was teaching a workshop. A demonstration of acupoint tapping was to be the theme of the meeting that evening. Because there seemed to be a growing buzz about the method, I attended, skepticism in hand.

One of the psychologists who had recently introduced energy psychology into his practice was going to demonstrate the method with a woman being treated for severe claustrophobia by another of the group's therapists. Having done research on "new psychotherapies" while on the faculty of the Johns Hopkins Department of Psychiatry and Behavioral Sciences early in my career, I was keenly attuned to influences on therapeutic outcomes that have nothing to do with the therapy's distinctive techniques. Called "nonspecific therapeutic factors," these include placebo effects expectation, suggestion, and the healing power of a therapist's caring. My suspicions only mounted as I watched the treatment unfold.

What occurred during the first few minutes was actually familiar and comfortable for me—taking a brief history of the problem (which had not responded to treatments from several therapists) and having the client imagine being in an elevator and giving her discomfort a rating on a standard 0-to-10 Subjective Units of Distress (SUD) scale. She said it was a 10. The next part, however, seemed implausible. The client mimicked the therapist's lead in tapping on about a dozen points on the skin while saying out loud, *"Fear of elevators."* This was followed by a brief "Integration Procedure" that included a set of odd physical incantations and then another round of tapping. When the client next rated her discomfort being in an elevator, her SUD had diminished from 10 to 7. She said her heart wasn't pounding as fast.

I was surprised to see any decrease in her sense of distress. I was at the time using systematic desensitization, a behavioral therapy method for calming the nervous system. Systematic desensitization can be effective, but not so rapidly. This new procedure had required only a couple of minutes from the first rating to the second. I wondered if the woman had developed some affection or loyalty to the therapist and didn't want to embarrass him in front of his colleagues. Another round of the procedure brought the SUD down to 5. After another round, however, it was back up to 7. I was thinking, "See, just superficial fluctuations caused by the set and setting. I knew it wouldn't work!"

When the therapist inquired about the increase in her sense of distress, the woman reported that a long-forgotten memory had come to her of being about eight and playing with her brother and some of his friends. They had created a fort out of a cardboard appliance box. When she was in it, the boys pushed the open end of the box against a wall so she was trapped. They then left her there amid derision and laughter. She didn't know how long it was until she was found and freed, but it seemed to her to be a very long time, and she screamed until she was exhausted. She had not recalled this incident for years, and as she focused on it, she now rated her discomfort related to the memory as a 10.

I thought, "Okay, so something was accomplished! A formative childhood event has been identified that some good talk therapy will be able to resolve over the next month or so. However strange the method, it has led to an important discovery that will give the treating therapist a new direction. It has been a useful case consultation." I did, however, wonder why her previous therapists hadn't worked with this memory. Only after I was studying the method did I come to realize that reducing the emotional charge on an issue through tapping often unearths long-buried memories into awareness, as I had just witnessed.

Anyway, recovering this memory is not where it ended. The therapist doing the demonstration started having the woman tap using phrases related to the childhood experience that focused on her shock, terror, sense of betrayal, and resentment. Within 15 minutes, she was able to recall the incident with no subjective sense of distress (SUD at 0). They then returned to elevators and quickly had that down to 0 as well. I looked on with my skepticism, fighting what my eyes and ears were registering. One of the group members suggested that it would be easy to test this (psychologists like to test things), and the woman agreed to step into a coat closet and shut the door.

The therapist was careful to make it clear to the woman that she was to open the door at any point she felt even slightly uncomfortable. The door closed. We waited. And waited. And waited. After about three long minutes—imagine a dozen psychologists quietly peering at a closet door—the therapist knocked and asked if she was okay. She opened the door and triumphantly announced that for the first time she could remember, she was comfortable in a small, enclosed space. Meanwhile I was thinking, "Okay, I'm onto them now! This is a social psychology experiment. We are about to be informed that we have been subjects in a study of how gullible therapists can be!" But that announcement never came, and my career was about to shift forever.

Even after that demonstration, however, I was still doubtful that it would work for me. Because procedures like tapping on your body while repeating short phrases look so strange, and it seems so counterintuitive that they would have a therapeutic effect, I'm not sure that anyone *really* believes tapping is going to do much before they experience it. However, the demonstration was convincing enough that I enrolled in the psychologist Fred Gallo's four-weekend training program for mental health professionals wanting to learn the approach. The training involved, in part, applying the method to our own issues. I found and have continued to find over the past two decades that whatever the emotional challenge I would focus on—whether my own or a client's—its intensity would be reduced after a bit of tapping, and this would open a path to rapid progress on the challenges being addressed.

By 2023, the number of published clinical trials demonstrating the effectiveness of the method had gone from zero to some 250, including 90 in non-English-speaking journals. As a tech geek, I love being able to demonstrate to conference audiences how a person's brain wave patterns become disturbed when the person focuses on stressful thoughts. Sometimes I work with EEG specialists Gary Groesbeck and Donna Bach. They are able to describe how, as the session progresses, the changes on the screen correspond with reduced distress, improved left-right brain hemisphere synchronization, and an overall optimization of brain wave ratios (see Figure I.1).

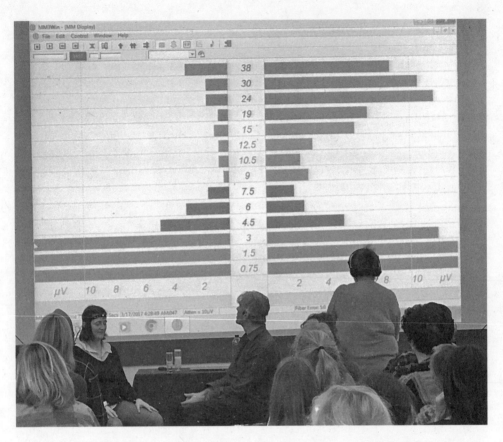

Figure I.1. A demonstration subject (left) wearing EEG sensors as David (right) conducts a tapping session with real-time EEG changes projected for a conference audience.

While I'm now devoting most of my professional time to teaching, research, and helping run Donna's and my organization, I still work with a limited number of clients. I recently finished treating a woman who had just been diagnosed with cancer. She arranged for a series of energy psychology sessions with me, concurrent with scheduled radiation for malignant masses in her lymph nodes and at the base of her tongue, just above

her vocal cords. The diagnosis was a rude surprise as she had no history of smoking or other exposures that are known to contribute to this type of cancer.

Focusing at first on her fears and the physical discomfort caused by the radiation treatments, it soon emerged that she was blaming herself for having gotten cancer. On questioning, she didn't believe that this was a particularly rational belief, but she nonetheless felt it strongly. I asked if she could remember other times that she felt unfairly blamed. A powerful incident from her childhood immediately came to her mind. At age 10 she was held responsible for something terrible, but she was unable to defend herself because it would implicate others in her family. She was the active target of this unfounded blame for years, and she felt she had to swallow the truth.

Once the tapping eliminated the emotional charge carried about these experiences, we explored a lifelong pattern of her not being able to tell her truths and linked them to these formative experiences. The therapy then examined possible connections between her suppressed verbal expression ("shoving my truths down my throat"; "keeping what I need to say under my tongue") and the subsequent cancer in the area of her throat, tongue, and vocal cords.

After each round of tapping, I asked her to imagine what was happening in her throat area as a quick gauge of the effects of that round. Then she would do another round of tapping, focusing on the images she was seeing in her throat at that point. She continued this tapping and imagery as homework. At first she saw heavy black tar and cobwebs. I noticed during the sessions that her self-blame about having "given" herself cancer was transforming into self-compassion as she recognized the possible connections between her childhood situation and her current illness.

As the emotional charges on various aspects of the associated issues were lifted during the next two therapy sessions, the imagery changed until she had a sense of spaciousness and light moving through the area. The tar and cobwebs were gone. This corresponded with improvements in her CT scans that far exceeded her oncologist's expectations, particularly since she had discontinued radiation against his advice due to the grueling side effects of the first couple of radiation sessions, and she also refused a recommended course of chemotherapy. Rather than increasing in size, all the masses had shrunk, some up to 50 percent.

Three months later, she went in for another round of CT scans. When her oncologist told her she was completely cancer-free, she enthusiastically went to high-five him, but he uncomfortably said, "I didn't do anything . . . I don't know what happened!" But she felt she knew. She believed the tapping work was instrumental. Along with her enhanced ability to express difficult truths rather than "shoving them down my throat," her biochemistry had shifted dramatically, as reflected in the cancer-free diagnosis. Her most recent CT scan as of this writing, two years later, still showed her to be cancer free.[5] While you should never assume that tapping alone can cure a serious physical illness, tapping has often been a powerful adjunct to other treatments.

Now more than 20 years into using acupoint tapping, I am still amazed yet somehow no longer surprised by the results that can be produced. While I've always found it deeply satisfying to provide psychotherapy services, tapping adds jet fuel to the process. It heightens the ability to reduce emotional intensity, heal childhood wounds, and change guiding models that keep people stuck in self-defeating life patterns. And it opens new vistas for creative choices and spiritual attunement.

Donna's Reflections

I've never defined myself as a psychotherapist, yet over the decades I've worked intimately with more than ten thousand people, in 90-minute sessions, on their personal problems and emotional challenges. While I am always happy to share my thoughts about their situation, what has been most helpful was working with their *energies*, which told me at least as much about their story as did their words.

I've always been able to see the body's energies. It was as normal for me and my mother, brother, and sister as seeing the color of the sky. The energies surrounding a person—known in many traditions as the "aura"—may have many colors and shades. By talking about what she saw, Mama kept this ability alive in us, which I believe is a potential for all children.

These colors may be relatively stable or quickly shifting, and I see such colors not only in the energies surrounding a person but also in the energies that flow *within* each of us. Energies moving through your liver look different from the energies moving through your kidneys. I can also see a conflict when a person's energies don't match what their words are saying or when the energies are revealing information that isn't even known to the person. And I can work with those energies using various methods to help resolve inner turmoil that may be compromising the person's health and playing havoc with their emotional life.

If I, for instance, hold points on the forehead (called "neurovasculars") of someone who is in distress, blood will return to their brain in a way that interrupts the fight-or-flight response and helps them think more clearly. Even when a physical threat isn't occurring, many people live almost constantly within at least a low level of fight or flight. I can hold these points until the person's energy systems are no longer in distress. The physical intervention changes the emotional response.

Each emotion interacts with a different energy pathway, known as a meridian; ongoing work might shift to another meridian, to the aura, or to the chakras. The chakras are energy pools that hold information about people's past as well as themes that shape their perceptions and choices. Each chakra tells a story. Clearing blockages in these pools and flows of energy and bringing them into better harmony helps the person on a physical level, but it can also bring greater clarity and balance to their thoughts and emotions. This often leads to new insights and shifts in their habits and behaviors in addition to improving their mood and promoting their physical healing.

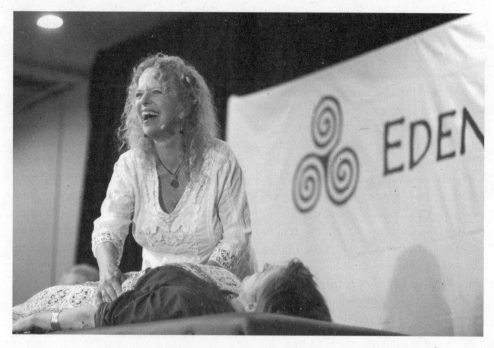

Figure I.2. Donna doing a demonstration session for a class.

Not everyone is conversant with terms like *meridians* and *chakras*, or even convinced that they exist. But just like the way the physical body has many complex systems—circulatory, respiratory, immune, reproductive, and so forth—the energies that govern and support those systems are very real and every bit as complex as the body's anatomy. In my specialty—energy medicine—we work with nine major independent yet always interacting energy systems that orchestrate the body's physical structures. Over 1,000 studies show that energy healing is effective for a wide range of conditions.[6]

When David began to study energy psychology more than two decades ago, I was one of his first practice clients. Being accustomed to working with so many energy systems all at once, I was surprised to see that David's training was teaching him how to work with only one of them—the meridians. And he was only learning one way to activate them, which was through the stimulation of the acupuncture points that fall along the meridian lines, by tapping on them. This is just one of the many ways the acupuncture points can be stimulated, with others including holding them lightly, massaging them deeply, or using acupuncture needles or electrical stimulation. When I experienced the more limited range of techniques used in the sessions with David, however, I was impressed by how quickly the issues I was focusing on shifted in ways I welcomed.

I discovered from my own experience that some words, when combined with tapping, were profoundly calming. Others were energizing. Still others sharpened my thinking and helped me to see how past difficulties played into current problems. Whatever the effect, the simple wordings combined with tapping produced an experience that had meaning, and that meaning went deep into me. I could feel it kind of like a wave traveling along my meridians and pulsing into my brain. This was new for me. I usually experience energy as a flow or a spiral. But tapping created a pulsing. I had in the past used tapping to work with pain and self-defeating habits, so it wasn't entirely new, but what was new was how the pulses going up to my brain were affecting my thoughts and emotions. My entire body was being connected in an energetic flow with my consciousness. It was exciting to experience energy in a different way than I usually did.

As I watched David get more and more involved with tapping, I was pleased to see him become a leader within the professional energy psychology community. With his focus on the mind and my focus on the body, our professions had seemed quite separate from each other, but "energy" was becoming a bridge. Because energy medicine is the wider field from which energy psychology draws, I was invited to speak at some of the energy psychology conferences where David was also presenting.

I found that with my background in energy medicine, which considers all the body's energies, I was able to broaden the scope for these psychotherapists. For instance, if a person is struggling with depression, you can correct a particular pattern in the energies through a set of physical movements that are quite different from tapping. If you do that correction first, the tapping will bring about improvements more rapidly and thoroughly. This type of information was eagerly absorbed by these therapists who were so fervently invested in helping alleviate their clients' suffering.

Although tapping protocols have proven to be powerful and effective, I learned that many of these therapists went on to study the broader field of energy medicine. An in-house survey of 115 energy psychology practitioners conducted by the Association for Comprehensive Energy Psychology (ACEP) in 2012 found that, by that time, 76 percent of those responding to a question about the energy methods they use most frequently said that Eden Energy Medicine, the system I developed, is one of their top three modalities. This surprised everyone, but me, since my approach is known primarily for working with physical rather than psychological issues. But I recognize that the energies of mind and body are in an exquisite dance and believe that energy medicine can be of great value to anyone in a healing profession, including mental health specialists.

What I brought to the energy psychology conferences is the type of contribution I bring to this book. While David is the primary author, I have provided a broad perspective of the body's energy systems as well as insights based on my clinical experiences and my ability to see how the energies move in relation to the various topics covered in the book.

A TOOL FOR THE TIMES

We are all navigating unprecedented changes in the world that surrounds us—in how to earn a living, in the ways we can spend our free time, in how to guide our children or grandchildren, in the ways information technology changes our consciousness and relationships, in the multiple crises impacting the environment, in the ways people of different races and genders relate to one another, even in the meaning of "gender." Throughout human history, new needs and possibilities have spawned new tools. Amid the dizzying array of changes and challenges in today's world, the culture has developed a variety of ways to help people cope and adapt. The one we are highlighting here uses energy-oriented procedures that can be applied for emotional healing and psychological growth. Mapping this possibility in a practical and compelling manner is the overriding purpose of this book.

Energy psychology interventions, at their core, align your body with your psyche's impulse toward your greatest potentials. Coded into your psyche is not only the design for your highest possibilities but also the deep motivation, the call, for actualizing them. Tapping protocols help bring your potentials into being. These protocols have two components:

1. They stimulate selected acupuncture points by tapping on them.

2. They include the simultaneous use of words or imagery.

Talk, See, Tap

The words and imagery, as you will see throughout this book, can map new ways of constructing the deep guiding models that orchestrate your life. Language, imagination, and tapping form a powerful triad for orchestrating self-improvement. Your words can describe and explore every aspect of your life. Your imagination allows you to experience and move among the past, present, and future at will. It empowers you to practice what you've never attempted and can be used to alleviate stress, reduce anxiety, boost confidence, and enhance performance. Adding acupoint tapping engages the nervous system to increase the beneficial impact of carefully chosen words and imagery.

Is It Fringe or Is It Fact?

Energy psychology draws upon a variety of techniques derived from ancient healing and spiritual traditions and combines them with contemporary methods for psychological change. Peta Stapleton, a psychologist at Bond University who was Australia's Psychologist of the Year in 2019 and is one of the leading researchers in energy psychology, noted that while early explanations focused on the body's energies, subsequent research demonstrates that the approach has profound effects on the nervous system, brain activity, DNA regulation, and the production of stress hormones.[7]

A recent review of more than 100 published investigations of acupoint tapping treatments found that virtually every study showed positive outcomes based on standard research methods, often with surprising speed and strong durability on follow-up.[8] Comparisons with established treatments for anxiety, depression, and post-traumatic stress disorder (PTSD), summarized in that review, found that therapies that use tapping on acupuncture points are simply more effective than approaches that rely primarily on talk. At the physiological level, the approach has consistently shown statistically significant improvements in cortisol levels, gene expression, cardiovascular measures, and brain wave patterns after a single session.[9]

Growing Popularity

Although tapping protocols emerged in the psychotherapist's office, their use on a self-help basis has become enormously popular. Traffic on the top five energy psychology websites was tracked using a statistical tool that showed more than six million visits during a randomly selected month.[10] The annual online Tapping World Summit has had more than half a million people register every year for many of the 15 years it has been held. A sophisticated smartphone app that guides users in applying acupoint tapping protocols was investigated in a large-scale study that included 270,461 app users.[11] Symptom reduction after using the app was robust enough to attain the scientific benchmark of "strong statistical significance for anxiety and subjective distress."[12]

The distinguishing feature of the energy psychology approach used throughout this book is the stimulation of acupuncture points by tapping on them. Other variations of energy psychology focus on energy systems that are known in ancient healing disciplines as *chi*, *qi*, and *chakras*; or in scientific circles as the *biofield*, the modern equivalent for the aura. Because acupoint tapping is by far the approach that is in the widest use within energy psychology, we use the terms *tapping* and *energy psychology* somewhat interchangeably. The approach builds on a scientifically informed neurological framework,[13] and its speed and effectiveness are being validated by a growing body of research.

Introduced in the 1980s, the most popular and well-researched energy psychology formats include the Emotional Freedom Techniques (EFT) and Thought Field Therapy (TFT), both of which teach clients how to stimulate acupoints by tapping on them. The approach is sometimes referred to simply as "tapping," the title we've chosen for this book. The original EFT manual, written by Gary Craig in 1995, has had over a million downloads. Since then, more than 100 books have been published on energy psychology or one of its variations. Recently learning about the extent of this abundant output was inspiring in the sense that *we knew* the book we are writing had *better be good*!

A credible estimate by the Harvard psychiatrist Eric Leskowitz, published in *Medical Acupuncture*, suggests that "tens of thousands" of psychotherapists, representing a wide range of theoretical orientations, have incorporated acupoint tapping into their practices.[14] Most of this has occurred in the past decade as the popularity of the method has been filtering into the clinical community.

WHAT DOES *ENERGY* HAVE TO DO WITH ENERGY PSYCHOLOGY?

Energy psychology is an umbrella term for personal development approaches that combine contemporary psychotherapeutic procedures with techniques that claim to have a special facility for working with the body's energies. In the most basic sense, atomic particles with continuously changing energies are at the foundation of the chemical reactions in every cell of the body. The science writer Sally Adee summarizes what is well established about the electrical properties of the cell:

Every one of the 40 trillion cells in your body is its own little battery with its own little voltage. . . . When a nerve impulse comes roaring down a nerve fiber, channels open in the neuron, and millions of ions get instantly sucked through them. . . . The electrical field generated by this mass migration of charge works out to about a million volts per meter.[15]

Electromagnetic fields surround every organ. The nervous system uses electrical signals to control not only breathing, walking, speaking, swallowing, digesting, and sleeping but also thinking and learning. With approximately 86 billion neurons in the human brain, each connected to up to 10,000 other neurons, the nervous system is an incomprehensibly complex electromagnetic and electrochemical network. Diagnostic procedures in modern medicine such as MRIs, EKGs, EEGs, and PET scans are based on assessments of the body's shifting electromagnetic activities. Researchers at major universities are experimenting with ways to manipulate the body's energy fields to treat medical and psychological conditions.[16]

In fact, using electrical impulses to support the body's health is not new. Beyond the familiar pacemakers, a surgically implanted device that sends electrical signals to the brain has helped more than 160,000 patients with advanced Parkinson's disease improve motor function while reducing symptoms such as tremors, sluggishness, and rigidity.[17] The procedure is now being tested for epilepsy, anxiety, obsessive-compulsive disorders, and obesity. Surgical implants the size of a grain of rice, which emit tiny electrical signals, clamped around targeted nerves, have helped paralyzed people walk again and severely depressed people get out of bed.[18] Transcranial direct current stimulation, which sends a few milliamps of electricity through the brain, has produced a range of benefits from reducing treatment-resistant depression to heightening concentration and improving math skills. This last procedure uses electrodes that are placed on the scalp rather than surgical implants.[19]

In each of these interventions, the curative electrical signals these devices generate to enhance brain function are minuscule compared to the electrical output of, say, your TV remote. Is it possible for these tiny signals to be generated by your body's own electricity?

That is precisely what acupoint tapping does! Imaging studies have shown that acupuncture can produce signals that, for example, instantly reduce arousal in the brain's emotional centers and increase arousal in areas involved with planning and emotional regulation.[20]

All psychological remedies, whether deliberately or not, impact the electromagnetic energies that literally animate the physical body. Energy psychology, however, uses techniques for targeting these energies directly, with deliberation and in a manner that shifts them for greater emotional stability and well-being. Tapping generates an electrical charge that can decrease activities in brain regions involved with excessive fear, anger, jealousy, or other problematic emotions and increase activity in brain regions involved with reasoning and creativity.

Energy psychology also works with so-called "subtle energies,"[21] energies that can't be detected by existing scientific instruments but are known by their effects. Such energies are recognized in the healing traditions of dozens of cultures around the world, from chi in China to prana in India to Wakan Tanka for the Lakota Sioux in the Great Plains of the US.[22] The Hungarian physician Albert Szent-Györgyi, who was the 1937 Nobel Laureate in Medicine, observed, "In every culture and in every medical tradition before ours, healing was accomplished by moving energy."[23]

IS IT SPIRITUALITY?

While working with the body's subtle energies can be a bridge into the realm of spirituality—to a sense of connection with forces larger than yourself—this book focuses on taking charge of the more psychological planes of your life: your emotions, thoughts, and behavior. Although it happens often enough that acupoint tapping sessions spontaneously bring people to a higher vantage point and deeper levels of meaning, providing you with tools for thriving in the everyday tangible domain is our ambitious enough objective here.

Meanwhile, many people find ways to combine acupoint tapping with more explicitly spiritual practices, such as meditation, prayer, or sacred rituals. The two pursuits can complement one another beautifully, as illustrated in Dawson Church's scientifically informed volume, *Bliss Brain*.[24] Even the recent upsurge in the use of psychedelics for spiritual exploration can utilize tapping for integrating the changes in perception and inspiring implications once the person has come down from the experience.

REPORTS FROM THE BOOK'S TEST DRIVERS

While we have used the methods presented in this book extensively with our clients and in our classes and workshops, it was new territory for us to present some of them in a book format, which doesn't allow interaction. So, in developing the program, we enlisted about a dozen "test drivers" to go through each chapter as we completed its first draft. These test drivers provided us with feedback about the chapter's clarity and what else was needed to more successfully work through the process when guided only by a book. Their experiences also served as additional case material for the next draft of that chapter. Most of the test drivers were new to energy psychology so we could be sure that preexisting knowledge about the approach was not needed, but we also enlisted a few skilled practitioners so their critiques would reflect a more experienced perspective. Names and identifying information of the test drivers and others described in case reports have been changed to protect privacy.

An interesting observation from several of our test drivers is that they experienced gains not only in the topics covered in the chapters but also in broader areas of their lives. One wrote to us,

Outside of the issues I'm using during the book readings and deep dives, I have been able to implement so much more tapping and protocols from the book in day-to-day life, knocking out a lot of the fears and phobias I have had for decades.

For example, I had a *severe* fear of flying, to the point of having to be sedated every time before walking onto a plane to go anywhere. Recently I took a trip to Argentina with three flights there and three flights back with no fear, no sedatives, not even herbal supplements to help me deal with flying. Although I could imagine things that *might* go wrong, they did not trigger me or cause any gripping fear as I've experienced in the past.

Many other issues have also been helped or dissipated due to the protocols you have brought to light in the program.

Another wrote,

After I finished Chapter 3, I was driving down a busy freeway, hurrying to an appointment, when I suddenly realized I was not stressed about traffic, time, or the appointment itself! That just never happened.

Then over the next few days, getting ready for houseguests, I was also struck to realize that I was not stressed or panicked about that either! It was always, everything in the house had to be perfect. I've been fighting against these reactions all my life, never very successfully. But now!! I don't even feel the stress anymore!

It's like someone took a laser scalpel and carved out my mother's imprint on some deep layer of my personality, a place where her stress style and her concerns became embedded and reinforced in my own expression into the world. I am amazed!

You will hear more from the other test drivers throughout the book.

HOW TO USE THIS BOOK

Tapping is written for everyone. It's for all of us living and navigating the human experience in these demanding times. It teaches the methods of energy psychology and how to apply them to a myriad of issues and challenges. It is framed within current scientific understanding of how and why it works.[25] Whether the emotional issue at hand is caused by stress or anxiety, physical ailments, aging, the pressures of parenting, work, or the challenges of staying centered and grounded in this world, we offer a framework and a set of tools to help you show up at your best. An equally important goal of this book is to offer authoritative commentary and guidance for psychotherapists who use or are considering using energy psychology.

A Personally Tailored Approach

"One-size-fits-all" scripts—the primary format in the hundreds of books, articles, and websites presenting a self-help tapping approach—fall far short of what we believe is possible. When using a "tapping script," you tap along as you say the words that are written or repeat the script as it plays from an audio or video recording. For instance, *"I am attracting everything I need to succeed"*; *"My fear of heights is softening and releasing"*; *"I notice the beautiful moments this day offers."* Tapping scripts can focus on virtually any issue imaginable, from blocks to success, to financial abundance, to anxiety, depression, or PTSD.

While these one-size-fits-all approaches bring the power of tapping to the issue of concern, they are not customized to who you are, your history, or the unique way the issue manifests in you. When everyone is given the same wording, individual differences are not factored into the procedure. Tapping scripts cannot orchestrate the detective work that ensures the procedure will be aligned with your character, learning style, and deeper needs. They are rarely able to heal long-standing problems at their roots. Nonetheless, what they offer can be impressive. You may be able to sleep better, feel more confident before giving a talk, reduce anxiety, or take the edge off an uncomfortable interaction after a few minutes of tapping. We do not object to tapping scripts, and you will see that we use them in the "Quick Fix" boxes in Part II of the book. But our intention is to also offer tools that take you far beyond them, teaching you how to think like a practitioner when applying the methods to yourself.

This is not to say that this book replaces the need for well-trained professionals. It doesn't. In addition to the greater skills of proficient practitioners, we all have our blind spots. Experienced therapists who use acupoint tapping can take you to places that it would not occur to you to go. They can provide support as you grapple with difficult issues. They are well practiced with the tools you may just be learning.

But with or without professional guidance, a great deal can be accomplished using self-tapping if you put in the effort to learn the method. Of course, reasonable cautions also apply. If you need psychotherapy, please work with a competent therapist in conjunction with this program. Adapt the methods in whatever ways are right for you. We are all on a path of personal evolution, and this book is the best resource we know how to craft to support you on that journey.

The Technique and Its Applications

Tapping takes you on a journey that changes your relationship to your interior mental and emotional landscape as well as to how you relate to your external surroundings. The tools it offers can guide in healing emotional wounds or outdated learnings that limit you and help you move forward to a life that is healthier and happier.

Part I ("How to Do It") teaches a basic tapping protocol that you can apply to any issue you wish. Part II ("Ways to Apply It") guides you in focusing these tools on everyday issues such as worry, sadness, habits, peak performance, relationships, and in the face of disaster. It also instructs therapists and their clients on how to apply acupoint tapping protocols with clinical conditions such as anxiety, depression, addictions, and PTSD.

A final note here on using these tools is that while your desire to quickly resolve emotionally challenging issues may be strong, please pace yourself kindly as you move through the program. You will also see that the instructions provide guidance if you begin to feel overwhelmed.

Working with a Partner

Most people will use the program in this book for a solo journey. That is how it is written. You might, however, find it valuable to share and discuss some of your experiences with someone who is close to you or with an intimate group. Like sharing your dreams, you could read a passage from the journal we will encourage you to keep or describe your inner experience with a particular procedure. You and a tapping partner could even go through the process at the same time, sitting next to one another. Two of the test drivers, who were already friends, coordinated their work with the program so they could share their progress after completing each chapter. They found that these reflections deepened their experiences. Setting a regular time dedicated to the program and making a mutual commitment to complete the exercises also helped keep them on track.

What If I'm Already Trained in a Different Energy Psychology Approach?

If you already know and use a different set of acupoint tapping points, feel free to stay with them instead of those taught in Chapter 1 and used throughout the book. Either set will send the needed signals to your brain. Any number of the hundreds of acupuncture points on the body could produce comparable benefits. Different practitioners and instructors have experimented and identified the combination of points they find to be most effective. If you are an experienced EFT or TFT practitioner, you can skip Chapters 2 and 3 and go directly to the application chapters in Part II. You might, however, still want to skim Chapters 2 and 3. They contain the best guidance we have to offer for the essential procedures when using an acupoint tapping approach, and you can refer back to these instructions at any point as you move through the book.

For a Quick Overview

There are many ways to move into a book like this. You could go directly to Part I and start reading. You could begin with a chapter whose theme is of particular interest to you. Some people, however, like to start with an overview of what is to come. If you thumb through and read the quote under each chapter title, you will have given yourself a brief but informative tour. We want to tell you where we got those quotes. Their authors represent many of energy psychology's most influential pioneers. We hold immense respect and appreciation for their contributions to the field and are pleased to be able to call attention to them in this book!

AN INTIMATE MOMENT

With writing the book we are envisioning still ahead of us, we pause, eyes meet, hands join, and hearts open as we enter deeply into our intention that our highest wisdom may emerge to create a resource that calls to your highest wisdom and potentials.

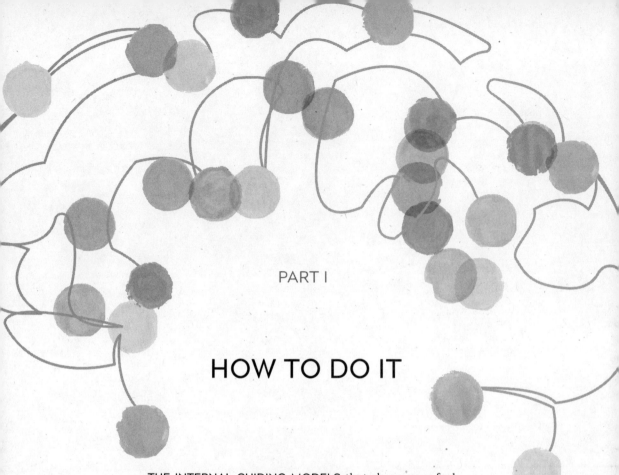

PART I

HOW TO DO IT

THE INTERNAL GUIDING MODELS that shape your feelings, motivation, and choices—and how energy psychology can modify them for your benefit—are the central themes of this book. They receive the full focus of Chapter 1.

Chapter 2 is a tutorial that teaches you a basic protocol for using tapping to reprogram guiding models that aren't serving you and to cultivate new ones that help you make yourself the best possible you.

Chapter 3 shows you how to do the detective work that will let you customize the approach to your unique needs and circumstances if the basic protocol isn't producing the benefits you wish.

CHAPTER 1

The Guiding Models That Move You Forward or Hold You Back

Energy psychology is a ground-breaking approach for upgrading
your guiding models to support you in overcoming what has limited
you and stepping more fully into your highest possibilities.[1]

—**David Gruder, PhD**

Founding President, Association for Comprehensive Energy Psychology

THE SCOPE OF THE human mind is dazzling. Out of it came the logic of Aristotle, the plays of Shakespeare, the music of Mozart, the sculptures of Michelangelo, and the nonviolent revolutionary actions of Mahatma Gandhi and Martin Luther King Jr. Such achievements are possible because of our ability to construct extraordinarily sophisticated internal models of reality, to rely on them as maps for navigating our way through the world, to use them as springboards for our imagination, and to continually update them.

For an example of how guiding models work culturally, you may have noticed that the above examples are all men. Not so fast. A compelling argument has been set forth that Emilia Bassano, a trailblazing Elizabethan-era poet, penned the Shakespeare plays but didn't receive credit because women couldn't be identified as playwrights in England's 1600s.[2] How many extraordinary contributions by unsung women do we not know about? Apropos of that little thought experiment, we move into our discussion of the models of reality we tend to assume to be accurate and reliable and how to change them when they are proven to be outdated or otherwise flawed.

Guiding models contain lessons from your past, strategies for the present, and anticipations about the future. They shape the way you view your life, the way you feel about what you see, and what you do about it. They use your capacities for abstraction, symbolism, and inner vision to fashion a dynamic understanding of your circumstances and novel expressions of who you are. And they are extraordinarily flexible. One of the great strengths of your mind is its ability to reflect on itself and to make changes based on new information as well as on faults you are able to discern.[3]

You can shift your guiding models in ways your dog or cat can't. It's not that Fido and Felix don't have guiding models or an internal logic that is a product of their inherited brain structures modified by their experiences. They do. To illustrate with a somewhat tongue-in-cheek example, the British journalist Christopher Hitchens, reflecting on the eternal debate about cats or dogs, observed,

> Owners of dogs will have noticed that, if you provide them with food and water and shelter and affection, they will think you are god. Whereas owners of cats are compelled to realize that, if you provide them with food and water and shelter and affection, they draw the conclusion that they are god.[4]

Fido and Felix live according to their guiding models without a lot of internal debate. They don't question whether what they are doing makes sense or could be done better. They don't wonder if they have blind spots. They simply update their internal realities based upon how the world reinforces or punishes them for the behaviors that emerge from their existing internal models. We, however, not only respond to environmental and social feedback, but we also use our critical faculties to purposively modify the guiding models that govern our choices and worldview. "We may not be responsible for the world that created our minds," observed the Hungarian-Canadian physician Gabor Maté, "but we can take responsibility for the mind with which we create our world."[5]

A SINGLE CONCEPT WITH MANY NAMES

Examining how these invisible guiding models develop and function has been, not surprisingly, of great interest to psychologists.[6] Guiding models are known variously as cognitive structures, cognitive schema, cognitive maps, internal representations, private constructs, knowledge structures, life scripts, personal mythologies, interpretive frameworks, mindsets, or inner theories of reality. Different psychologists have different takes on these models and how they work, but they share some common features:

- Guiding models are internal representations of reality that provide understanding and direction.

- Your psyche constructs them based on a mix of your temperament, culture, and unique life experiences, usually outside your conscious awareness.

- They direct your thinking, feeling, and behavior.

- They provide the mechanism by which you filter and store new information.

- They are generally quite stable but can be revised or updated throughout your life, sometimes spontaneously, sometimes with deliberation.[7]

You will be working with your guiding models throughout the book. Because guiding models operate largely beneath the surface of consciousness, they are not always easy to recognize. In fact, you might not be able to name a single one, even one that plays a central role in your life. Try that now. Based on what you've read so far, name three guiding models that shape your thoughts, feelings, and actions. Here are six examples, three with empowering guidance and three with corresponding but disempowering guidance:

"I'm great in emergencies."

"I buckle in emergencies."

"My kids respect me for my firm and fair rules."

"My kids walk all over me."

"People naturally trust me."

"People are suspicious of me."

It may be sobering to realize that such underlying models are often calling the shots, even when you think you are operating out of free will.

HOW ENERGY PSYCHOLOGY CAN HELP YOU CHANGE GUIDING MODELS THAT GET IN YOUR WAY

We embark on this self-guided journey of personal evolution by focusing on the inherent power of acupoint tapping to transform obsolete or otherwise harmful guiding models so they may better serve you. Your guiding models are keys for understanding what acupoint tapping protocols, or any therapy or personal development approach for that matter, attempt to change.

Guiding models map the complex realities that make up the human experience. Like a GPS, if you make a wrong turn and are going in a different direction than your original plan, your guiding models help you recalibrate to get you to your destination from the unexpected route. Sometimes, however, finding yourself in familiar territory causes you to rethink a guiding model and reprogram your internal GPS. That's where this book comes in.

You will be discovering more about your guiding models throughout the program. They are at the core of your most intimate experiences with yourself. The acupoint tapping protocols you will be applying will help them evolve. We will illustrate this with two scenarios. If you are interested in a more theoretical discussion about guiding models, you can find it at models.energytapping.com.

TRANSFORMING A GUIDING MODEL

We will begin by showing how this might work in your life with a hypothetical example (though it is based on an actual case). Imagine that you are Paul. You work in a midsize business and manage a team of eight employees. *Your* issues and guiding models will, of course, be different from Paul's, but the *process* for changing a guiding model has common elements. Lately, you (as Paul) have been finding that you are not eager to go to work, and you have been feeling especially anxious about the team meetings you lead. You decide to guide yourself through a tapping session to explore this unease.

You begin by recognizing and accepting that something is wrong, despite not knowing its cause. You stimulate some energy points as you acknowledge and accept the current situation: *"Even though something isn't right at work, I am recognizing and accepting this discomfort."* Then you tune in to your anxiety and notice that the feelings seem to be tied to some tightness in your throat. You rate this tightness as a 6 on the 0-to-10 SUD (Subjective Units of Distress) scale of how much discomfort it evokes. After a round of acupoint tapping, it goes down to 4. Following another round, it is down to 1. But with the tightness almost gone, you

realize that the constriction was keeping down feelings of sadness and preventing you from recognizing that it has something to do with one of your team members, Johanna.

Johanna is a very effective employee. She is eager and full of good spirit. Everyone likes her. You, however, are starting to feel that she is challenging your authority. You close your eyes and search within while keeping the feeling of being challenged mentally active. The tightness in your throat is no longer noticeable, but you now sense a kind of emptiness in your chest. You ask yourself, "When in the past have I had a similar feeling?" You immediately recall your first job. You were exceeding everyone's expectations and headed for a big promotion. But an employee who hadn't been there as long as you received the promotion you were expecting. This was both painful and humiliating. You tap while focusing on the physical sensation, which is the same sense of emptiness in your chest that had been evoked by Johanna.

As the sensation of emptiness subsides with the tapping, you recall how you didn't understand the company's choice not to promote you and how sad and disillusioned it left you. You are reminded of the basic but elusive truth that while feelings flow through you, they are temporary. They do not define you. You tap on the sadness. As the tapping sends deactivating signals to the emotional areas of your brain, the sadness also diminishes. Next, you realize that you have been holding anger toward your former boss. You tap that down.

It's not that feelings are wrong and need to be eradicated. Your feelings are like radar that provides you with vital information as you navigate your experiences. But once you've registered that information, staying caught in old emotional reactions rooted in painful experiences can keep you from moving forward as life presents new challenges. When you identify emotional triggers from your past and defuse them with tapping, you stop them from creeping into the present. In this instance, you (as Paul) uncovered a guiding model that tells you that even when you are succeeding, an unexpected situation with a fellow employee will suddenly emerge to unfairly derail you. You have been projecting that anticipated scenario onto Johanna. This is the insight that allows a new model to be built, one that isn't threatened by someone else excelling.

Now when you (as Paul) scan within, you can find nothing else that remains emotionally unresolved about your loss of that promotion. You might further embed these shifts by tapping on and affirming something like *"That old betrayal doesn't predict the future."* You are only half an hour into the session, and you bring your attention back to Johanna. The sense of threat is still there, but it's not as strong. You tap on it, first focusing on a few remaining physical sensations in your throat and chest and then on your thoughts about Johanna. Finally, you imagine seeing her shine in a meeting while you feel no sense of threat or discomfort, only appreciation for what she is contributing to your team. You tap on that response to embed it into your nervous system.

You have dismantled the model that expects you to be sabotaged in your job. The next morning you notice that you feel your accustomed enthusiasm about going to work. Rather than having an underlying sense that the office is full of traps that can take you down, you are feeling confident about your leadership role and your next team meeting.

While this may seem like a mere fairy tale, it accurately illustrates how transformative the practice can be for a *day-to-day* concern. It can also be applied to transforming *long-standing* self-defeating patterns. This book will provide you with detailed instructions for bringing about shifts in your guiding models that can address immediate concerns as well as issues that have been with you for many years.

OVERCOMING AN AUTOMATIC REACTION ROOTED IN A DYSFUNCTIONAL GUIDING MODEL

Paul first recognized that something was wrong by focusing on his growing discomfort about going to work. Many emotional issues show up in visceral responses before you can even think about them. Irrational fears, anger, and jealousy are common examples. If you have a phobia, for instance, you *experience* it as an automatic reaction beyond your conscious control. These experiences are so tangible that it may be hard to imagine that they have anything to do with something as amorphous as an internal guiding model. However, old models and automatic responses are intimately entwined. Consider this use of tapping to help a woman overcome her long-standing fear of heights.

Nancy is a nurse, successful in her work and happy in her marriage. Anyone who knows her would consider her well-adjusted, even flourishing. But she had a fear of heights that was at times debilitating. The thought of having to climb a flight of stairs to get to an appointment filled her with apprehension. She couldn't join friends on hikes in nearby hills. And forget about getting near the edge of a balcony. Following a tapping session of about half an hour, however, she was comfortably leaning over a balcony on the top floor of a high-rise hotel.

The internal model that was governing Nancy's fear of heights had several components. Foremost in her awareness was her sense of panic when encountering or even anticipating a height and her overpowering belief that she was or would be in serious danger. This was accompanied by sweating, dizziness, heart palpitations, and sometimes shaking. Her internal model about heights not only predicted these physical reactions but also triggered them when she was in situations that involved heights or even brought up thoughts about heights.

Nancy's guiding model about heights included strategies for avoiding situations where heights were involved. It also challenged her well-earned sense of herself as a strong woman. This seemingly irrational model was built around a very real experience from her teenage years. She had been standing at the edge of a cliff when a trusted adult came up from behind her and playfully grabbed her shoulders and pushed forward. While he of course held on to her so she wouldn't fall, the incident initiated a terror of heights that had, by the time of the tapping session, plagued her for more than two decades. That, however, was not in her awareness when she would encounter a height. She would only feel fear and aversion.

After the first round of tapping, Nancy reported a change in her physical sensations when she imagined facing a height. This is how an internal model that grew out of traumatic events often begins to change. After a few rounds of tapping while mentally focusing on various aspects of her fear of heights, such as the dizziness and embarrassment, it was clear that something was shifting. For instance, on the 0-to-10 SUD scale, she had initially rated her internal distress and anger about being pushed as "an 11."

After tapping while reflecting on her fear, when she revisited her memory of being pushed, she simply said, "That was a long time ago," with no troubling physical or emotional reactions whatsoever. By the end of the session, Nancy could imagine being in a situation that involved a height with no sense of panic. The surprise on her face and her tears of relief were palpable as she tuned in to her feelings and said with astonishment, "It's gone!" She then demonstrated this by calmly and confidently leaning over the balcony of a 17-floor hotel room.

At a follow-up interview two and a half years after this session, Nancy reported that her fear of heights not only hadn't returned but she had also developed greater confidence in other areas of her life since she was able to overcome that fear of heights. She even sought situations that challenged her new relationship with heights, such as taking the opportunity, while vacationing in Ireland, to ascend a wall of the Blarney Castle. According to legend, a magical stone in this wall bestows the power of eloquence to anyone brave enough to kiss it. To accomplish this feat, Nancy had to complete a steep climb of 127 steps on spiral staircases, lie on her back, hold on to an iron railing to avoid falling, and lean way back to kiss the stone, all the while managing the riveting sight of the ground from 85 feet up. This is challenging even for someone who doesn't have a fear of heights.

Triumphantly announcing, "I bent over and I kissed that stone," was a declaration of the way her inner model about heights had been completely transformed. You can view excerpts from her treatment and the follow-up interview in a 12-minute video available at phobiacase1 .energytapping.com.

ROOTS IN ANCIENT HEALING PRACTICES

Energy psychology is a relatively new practice within psychotherapy, but stimulating acupuncture points to produce health benefits goes back thousands of years. Texts based on the principles of classical Chinese medicine offer explanations for the effects of each of the acupuncture points that are used in the tapping protocol you will be learning.[8] At least 361 acupuncture points are distributed primarily along 14 major energy pathways, which we have already referred to as meridians (see Figure 1.1). These acupuncture points are recognized for special electrochemical properties compared with nearby areas of the skin.[9] Stimulating an acupuncture point generates an electrical charge that is transported along the body's connective tissue to sites that may be located at a distance from the point being activated.[10]

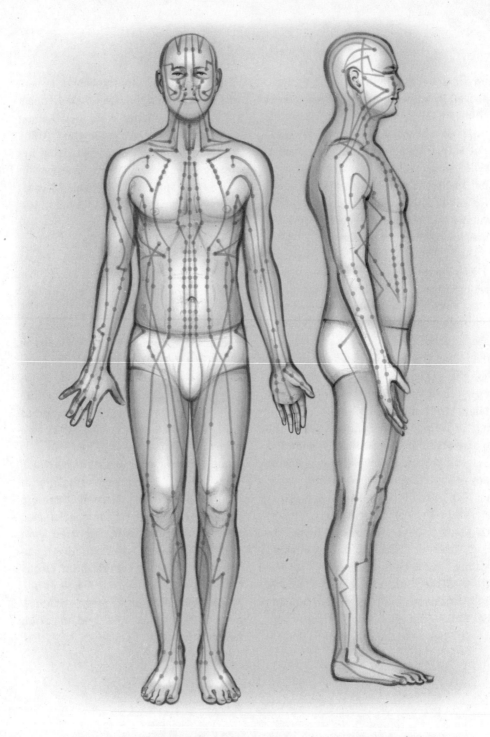

Figure 1.1. The meridian lines represent the body's major energy pathways.

Most energy psychology protocols use between seven and 12 of the acupuncture points. The procedure you will be learning in this book uses 12 points, which activate nine of the 14 meridians (some meridians are more connected to emotional issues than others). Our selection of points is similar but not identical to those in the *EFT Manual* that has become a standard for the field.[11] Many practitioners, based on their observations and experience, come to use a somewhat different set of points from those they were shown in their original training. Our sense is that the general approach allows various acupoint combinations to produce approximately equivalent results. This is interesting in itself, though this question has not to our knowledge been submitted to research that systematically compares one tapping protocol with another.

Table 1 contains a list of the 12 points you will be learning and a little bit about each. A round of tapping on this set of points, combined with a short phrase or imagined sequence, requires about a minute. Even if you are not working on an issue, if the anticipated benefits from acupuncture theory shown in Table 1 are accurate, you can see the potential physical and mental health–related advantages. Even without the use of words or images, stimulating points that "reduce stress," "improve judgment," "strengthen resolve," and "invigorate mental faculties" —among the other outcomes listed in Table 1—will have considerable benefits.

But these benefits are usually in the background rather than being the focus of energy psychology protocols. In fact, tapping practitioners don't need to know the functions that the ancient Chinese physicians attributed to the specific points. It is the collective influence of the points stimulated during a round of tapping, perhaps through some type of resonance with the body, that captures one's attention when watching a session.[12] The changes in emotions and understanding happen in front of your eyes, generally far more quickly than in talk-oriented therapies. It is not a fluke that the use of tapping is the primary difference between conventional psychotherapy and most energy psychology protocols.

LEARNING THE TAPPING POINTS BY EXPERIMENTING WITH YOUR BREATHING

We want to introduce you to the tapping points you will be using throughout the book with a technique that is designed to help your breathing become freer and clearer.[13] Most people in developed industrial societies do not breathe fully, and we all tend to constrict our breathing when under stress or experiencing a difficult emotion. As restricted breathing becomes habitual, we tend not to give ourselves the amount of oxygen we need to function at optimal levels, physically and emotionally.

Table 1: The Tapping Points

MERIDIAN & POINT #	LOCATION	TRANSLATION OF CHINESE NAME	HELPS WITH
Governor Vessel 20	Top of head: use three or four fingers to be sure to hit it	Meeting of the 100 Spirits	Receives heavenly influxes, nourishes the brain, counters frustration and depression
Bladder 2	Inside beginning of eyebrow	Collect Bamboo	Refreshes body and mind, calms nervous system, releases trauma, promotes peace, manages fear
Gall Bladder 1	Side of eye	Pupil Crevice	Improves clarity, vision, and decision-making; releases resentment; strengthens resolve
Stomach 1	Under eye	Weeping Support	Provides grounding; helps digest feelings; releases fear; promotes calmness and moving on when stuck
Governor Vessel 26	Under nose	Ghost Palace	Calms the spirit, restores yin/yang balance within, regulates fluctuations of emotion
Conception Vessel 24	Under lip	Heavenly Pond	Coordinates all parts of body and mind; cleanses, bathes, and washes away impurities
Kidney 27	Collar bone points	Treasury	Restores physical, mental, and spiritual reserves; promotes ease in moving forward
Conception Vessel 17	Middle of chest (Heart Chakra)	Central Hall	Brings support and vitality to the heart and lungs, promotes clarity and self-acceptance
Spleen 21	Under arms	Great Enveloping	Brings care and harmony to all the body's energies, promotes relaxation and compassion
Gall Bladder 32	Side of leg	Central River	Promotes decisiveness, improves judgment, releases anger
Small Intestine 3	Side of hand	Back Stream	Invigorates mental faculties, decision-making, and letting go; counters emotional instability
Triple Warmer 3	On ridge beneath ring and little finger	Central Islet	Fights destructive forces; reduces stress; maintains balance and harmony; releases worry

The Experiment

Take three slow deep breaths, stretching your lungs as far as they will expand without forcing yourself. (If you have asthma or other respiratory difficulties, use discretion about proceeding with this technique.) On the third breath, rate the depth of your breathing with a percentage, where 100 percent is your estimate of your maximum capacity. For most people, this number is between 30 and 90 percent. If yours is 100 percent, do the exercise anyway to see if it expands beyond your estimate. In our experience, this often happens.

The Tapping Points

You will be tapping on the 12 acupoints (or left/right pairs of acupoints) while you say, *"Even though it's possible to breathe more fully, I accept myself just as I am."* Tap on each point or pair of points for the amount of time it takes to say the statement out loud and deliberately. Most people use the fingertips of their index and middle fingers to tap (see Figure 1.2). Tap firmly but not aggressively, about three beats per second, for as long as it takes to say the statement.

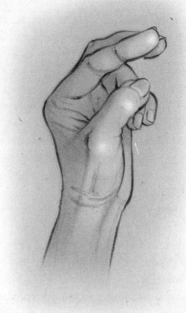

Figure 1.2. Tap firmly but never so hard as to bruise yourself.

While tapping is the method we prefer and teach for stimulating the points, a small percentage of people are uncomfortable with or do not respond to *tapping* on acupoints. If that is the case for you, experiment with massaging or simply touching each acupoint. This last variation, called "Touch and Breathe,"[14] is preferred by some practitioners as a more meditative approach. You make the statement and then take an easy, relaxed, moderately deep breath before going on to the next acupoint.

Whichever method you decide upon, here are the 12 points in the Protocol we use. Do not be concerned about memorizing them. By the end of Part I of this book, they will have become automatic, and you will have a technique you can use whenever you are feeling stressed or experiencing a difficult emotional reaction. Again, for this experiment, as you tap on each point, say out loud, *"Even though it's possible to breathe more fully, I accept myself just as I am."* The following descriptions of the points are illustrated in Figure 1.3.

1. **Top-of-Head Point (Crown Chakra).** Tap on the top center of your head with either hand. For this point, if you use all five fingers, you will be sure to hit the right spot.

2. **Inside-Eyebrow Points.** The points where your eyebrows end; near the bridge of your nose.

3. **Side-of-Eye Points.** Outside edges of your eye sockets.

4. **Under-Eye Points.** The bony ridge of your eye sockets centered under your eyes.

5. **Under-the-Nose Point.** Slightly closer to the bottom of your nose than the top of your lip.

6. **Under-the-Lip Point.** In the middle of the groove beneath your lower lip.

7. **Collarbone Points.** Find the inside corners of your collarbone and drop into the hollows that are just beneath them.

8. **Thymus Point.** Center of your chest, also known as the Heart Chakra.

9. **Side-of-Chest Points.** About four inches below your armpits. These are the "imitate a monkey" points.

10. **Outside-of-Leg Points.** Between your hips and knees where a pant seam would be. Tap where your middle finger gravitates.

11. **Side-of-Hand Points.** Clap together the outside edges of your hands (little finger sides); also known as the Karate-Chop Point.

12. **Back-of-Hand Points.** With two, three, or four fingers of one hand, tap on the back of your other hand on the *valley* leading to the "V" between your little finger and fourth finger. This is the only pair of points that can't be tapped simultaneously on the left and right sides. It is also known as the Gamut Point.

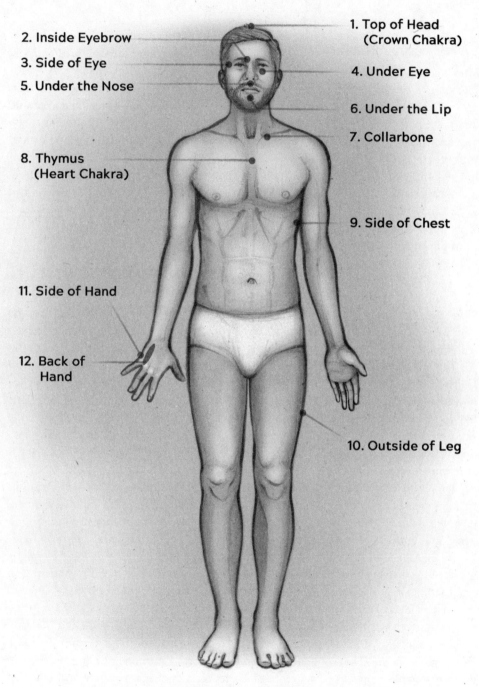

2. Inside Eyebrow

3. Side of Eye

5. Under the Nose

8. Thymus
   (Heart Chakra)

11. Side of Hand

12. Back of
    Hand

1. Top of Head
   (Crown Chakra)

4. Under Eye

6. Under the Lip

7. Collarbone

9. Side of Chest

10. Outside of Leg

Figure 1.3. The numbers indicate the order in which the points are usually tapped. For points not in the center of the body (numbers 2, 3, 4, 7, 9, 10, 11, and 12), tap on the corresponding points on both sides of the body.

Evaluating Your Results

After you have tapped on each point while repeating *"Even though I'm not breathing my full capacity, I accept myself just as I am,"* take another deep breath. Repeat the sequence. Then, again rate the depth of your breathing with a percentage, where 100 percent is your estimate of your maximum capacity.

You may notice a big improvement, a slight improvement, or no improvement at all. Most people are surprised to experience a perceptible improvement after doing this tapping sequence one or two times.

If you don't notice any improvement after two or three rounds, it usually indicates an issue with a memory, an emotion, or a belief regarding breathing. You can tap on whatever comes up. For instance, if the exercise leads to a realization that constriction is a theme in your life, you might do another round, saying as you tap on each point, *"Even though my constricted breathing reflects other constrictions in my life, I accept myself just as I am."* If the exercise brings up a stressful memory, such as feeling suffocated or nearly drowning, you might select that as your focus in the following chapter.

One person, who started at 30 percent and wound up at 99 percent, explained, "At first I felt like my ribs were the prison for my lungs and my lungs could not expand through them, as if they were walls. Then, after the tapping, my chest area felt so much more elastic and flexible." For another person, the exercise brought up memories of holding her breath as a child to try to make

herself appear "invisible" in threatening situations. She tapped on "Holding my breath" while bringing to mind one of the times this occurred, and her breathing improved by 30 percentage points. For another, as she focused on her breathing, she had a memory of how her breath would become shallow when her parents would argue and yell. She tapped on *"Breathing shallow when Mom would scream at Dad"* and went from 40 to 75 percent.

USING GRATITUDE TO "LIFT YOUR BOAT"

Many of the procedures throughout the book will address a specific guiding model. You just challenged the model that guides the way you breathe. You will, in the following chapter, focus on an experience that left you with unresolved emotions you still carry. Processing it changes the related guiding models. As you move into subsequent chapters, you will focus on the guiding models that underlie specific fears, worries, and anxieties. You will also shift other internal models to improve your relationships and advance specific goals.

Besides these specifics, you can focus on thought patterns that have a generic impact on all your guiding models. One such thought pattern is the degree to which you are oriented toward meeting new experiences with gratitude. We want to show you how to "grow your gratitude" as a way of introducing you to the use of tapping for changing a guiding model that will have a broad influence on your life.

Regularly tuning in to what you can be thankful for is high up on the list of actions that will improve your outlook and boost your overall happiness and well-being.[15] Our minds are programmed more for solving problems than dwelling on what is going right. While all manner of self-help approaches and relationship books will encourage you to feel appreciation, few help you shift the ancient programming that gives primary focus to what needs to be fixed. Having the experience of sinking into a deep sense of gratitude begins to change this deeply ingrained thought pattern.

The more you use the following procedure to recognize your blessings and dwell in their emotional glow, the more you will train your mind to go there spontaneously. To guide yourself through the following ten steps: Read an instruction. Close your eyes and carry out the instruction. Open your eyes and read the next instruction. Continue through all ten steps. This will probably require only five to ten minutes.

1. Make a mental list of a few things that you appreciate.

2. Select one of them.

3. Focus on this aspect of your life. Describe it in a few words that you can easily remember while you are doing the tapping, such as *"My comfortable bed," "My husband's smile," "A job I love," "My family's good health."* This will be your "Appreciation Phrase."

4. Once you have your Appreciation Phrase, sink into your appreciation and give a rating, from 0 to 100 percent, of how fully you have entered a state of gratitude. To what degree does gratitude fill you?

5. Now visualize a cell in your heart. Imagine it as feeling happy, looking happy, being happy about the source of your gratitude.

6. The happiness starts to spread to the cells around it. Those cells start to vibrate and glow. Soon your entire heart is pulsing with happiness and gratitude.

7. As you breathe into your heart, state your Appreciation Phrase.

8. Tap on the point at the top of your head as you again state your Appreciation Phrase.

9. Move through all 12 tapping points, stating your Appreciation Phrase as you tap on each point. This will take only about a minute once you have internalized the 12 tapping points.

10. Repeat the same tapping routine and Appreciation Phrase one or more times, and end by placing your hands over your heart as you tune in again to your gratitude. When you are finished, take a deep breath, focus on your appreciation, and again rate how fully you have entered into a state of gratitude, from 0 to 100 percent.

Most people find that their gratitude becomes more palpable based on the appreciation phrase combined with the tapping and repetition. Some find the imagery to be particularly vivid. For instance, one of our test drivers saw her first heart cell as the Pillsbury Doughboy reaching out with an infectious smile to the other heart cells. Another saw a blue light emanating from the cell, filling her heart. Another tapped to the jingle, *"Every little cell in my body is happy; every little cell in my body is well."*

Besides giving you a procedure you can use any time you wish to focus in on and deeply register what is right in your world, this tapping exercise gives you a preview of how *words, visualization,* and *tapping* will be combined throughout the book.

WHAT HAPPENS IN THE BRAIN

Combining acupoint stimulation with procedures from conventional psychology supercharges both approaches. Here are five principles that we believe account for the brain changes following acupoint tapping sessions:[16]

1. **Acupoints Have Less Electrical Resistance.** Every spot on your skin can conduct electricity, but acupoints are better conductors than adjacent areas. They have less electrical resistance.[17] Most acupuncture points are also located in areas with a high density of free nerve endings.[18]

2. **Tapping on an Acupuncture Point Generates Electricity.** Certain large proteins within the membranes of cells convert mechanical pressure into electrical impulses called "piezoelectricity" (literally, "electricity caused by pressure"). The process is scientifically established[19] and can be produced by tapping, massaging, or inserting a needle into the acupoint.

3. **The Electrical Signals Can Reach Anywhere in the Body Almost Instantly.** The path traveled by the electrical impulses produced by tapping on the skin is embedded in the body's connective tissue.[20] The majority of acupoints are located above aggregates of connective tissue, which is composed largely of collagen. Because collagen conducts electricity, signals can quickly reach specific areas of the body with minimal distortion rather than having to travel neuron to synapse to neuron through the nervous system.[21]

4. **The Words and Images Accompanying the Tapping Tell the Signals Where to Go.** For instance, if you bring a threatening situation to mind, which activates your amygdala and prefrontal cortex, the electrical signals generated by the tapping will be attracted to those areas of your brain. In an imaging study investigating the

acupoint tapping treatment of a flying phobia, thinking about flying initially evoked arousal in brain areas involved with fear, as would be expected. Following the tapping treatment, thinking about flying no longer activated fear areas but it did activate "executive regions" of the brain that are involved with managing fear.[22]

5. **The Signals Are Oriented Toward Bringing Balance.** Acupuncture points may increase or decrease activation of specific areas of your brain or body, inherently seeking to create a state of balance or homeostasis.[23]

In brief, by what you bring to mind while you are tapping, you are able to *target* which brain regions will attract the electrical impulses generated by the tapping. Some of these electrical signals will decrease problematic emotions. Others will increase adaptive thoughts and behavior. The process seems to follow an internal logic that is oriented toward well-being. As the acupuncturist Beth Kearns explains, working with an acupuncture point in a healing context "has a built-in safety mechanism. The point will do what is needed."[24]

ON TO CHAPTER 2

Guiding models that cause people to repeatedly think, feel, and act in ways that are self-defeating are often rooted in childhood experiences that were psychologically harmful. You can use acupoint tapping protocols to transform your guiding models. The following chapter will walk you through the steps of applying a basic energy psychology protocol to bring healing to an emotional injury from your past.

CHAPTER 2

A Basic Tapping Protocol

There is nothing more satisfying than helping a suicidal
teenager shed her self-hatred and confusion—and hearing her
whisper "I love and accept myself" through her tears.

There is nothing more fulfilling than tapping with a battle-
scarred veteran as he frees himself from the flashbacks
of PTSD—and seeing his eyes shining with peace.

There is nothing more rewarding than helping a grieving widow
overcome her unbearable sorrow—and watching her smile again.[1]

—Dawson Church, PhD
Leading EFT Trainer and Researcher

WHILE TAPPING PROTOCOLS LIKE EFT are deceptively simple, they are also surprisingly potent. They build upon the complex processes by which your brain manages emotion and revises the internal models that guide your every choice. This chapter introduces you to the basic skill set you will use for the remainder of the book. It will systematically lead you to develop the ability to go through 12 steps that are organized around the four phases of a tapping session:

Phase 1   Preparation

Phase 2   The Tapping Cycle

Phase 3   Adjusting the Protocol

Phase 4   Testing Your Results

We encourage you to treat this chapter as you would approach an ambitious but self-paced training program rather than just reading a book. You will gain more from it if you go through the steps and apply them to a meaningful issue as you read the chapter. Like anything worth learning, this will require allocating dedicated time and exerting the effort that is needed for internal transformation. If this leads to a greater capacity to defuse painful emotions and increase your success and happiness, as we believe it can, it will have been a wise investment. Before leading you through the four phases, we would like to provide some additional background.

THE VERY FIRST TAPPING TREATMENT

In 1980, the clinical psychologist Roger Callahan was baffled after more than a year of using various psychotherapeutic methods without success to treat "Mary" for a severe phobia.[2] Mary, a mother of two in her late 30s, was unable to carry out even the most basic activities if they involved water or getting near water. If it rained, she would feel compelled to retreat to an inner room of her house. She couldn't drive along the beach because the sight of the ocean terrified her. She couldn't bring herself to bathe in anything more than a few centimeters of water. Despite cognitive and behavioral therapy treatments, her intense fear was unchanged. She also continued to have terrifying nightmares of water "getting her."

Her bodily reactions to the thought of water included nausea. Dr. Callahan had studied the health-promoting effects of stimulating certain acupuncture points and decided there was nothing to lose. During one of their sessions while Mary was feeling nauseous as they talked about her fear of water, Callahan asked her to tap on a spot directly beneath the orbit of her eye, an acupuncture point on the Stomach Meridian. He hoped it would at least reduce her nausea. While he wasn't thinking about it at the time, this point also happens to be associated with obsessive fear and worry. After tapping on it, Mary exclaimed in astonishment, "It's gone. . . . That awful feeling in the pit of my stomach. It's completely gone."

The treatment took place at Callahan's home office, and his home had a pool. Callahan recounts how Mary "sprang from her chair and began running toward the swimming pool . . . gazed briefly at her reflection, then bent down and splashed water on her face." To Callahan's amazement, she had no fear. That evening Mary decided to further test her apparent cure by driving to the ocean during a rainstorm and wading in up to her waist. She was completely free of fear. This held on follow-up sessions and continued through her last report more than a decade later. Her long-standing, deeply embedded, self-limiting guiding model in relation to water had been radically transformed in an instant at the psychological level of her thoughts and fears as well as at the level of her bodily responses.

That was the birth of "Thought Field Therapy" (TFT), the initial formulation of energy psychology. Trying to make sense of what had happened, Callahan began having his patients tap on various acupuncture combinations during their therapy sessions. The procedure seemed to accelerate their progress. Callahan developed a set of treatment formulas that he found to be effective with a wide range of ailments. Within a few years, he was teaching his new method to other psychotherapists.

THE RAPID RISE OF TAPPING THERAPIES

The *first* wave of modern psychotherapy was Sigmund Freud's psychoanalysis in the early twentieth century. The *second* wave was behavioral therapy, which appeared in the 1940s and pioneered ways of rearranging "contingencies" (rewards and punishments) to support desired behaviors and discourage undesired behaviors. The *third* wave, emerging in the 1960s, added a *cognitive* dimension to *behavioral* therapy. This "cognitive behavioral therapy" (CBT) incorporated the realization that as well as behavioral therapy's focus on shifting the reinforcements in the environment, focusing on patterns of thought could also change behavior. The *fourth* wave of psychotherapy adds somatic components, such as movement, sensory stimulation, or the activation of areas of the skin, as is done with tapping. In her book *The Science Behind Tapping*, Dr. Peta Stapleton asserts that she considers acupoint tapping protocols "to be the most promising of the fourth-wave psychotherapies I've investigated."[3]

By 2000, more than 30 variations of TFT or related energy psychotherapy approaches had emerged, each with its own name, procedures, and explanatory frameworks. One of Callahan's early students, Gary Craig, a Stanford graduate with a degree in engineering, had long been interested in personal improvement techniques such as self-hypnosis. Craig felt that Callahan's approach could be simplified, streamlined, and put into the hands of anyone, not just psychotherapists. He called his approach "the Emotional Freedom Techniques," or EFT.

By the time Craig announced his retirement in January 2010, more than 1.2 million people had downloaded his free EFT Manual,

30,000 to 40,000 more were downloading it each month, and EFT had become not only the most popular form of energy psychology but possibly the most widely practiced psychological self-help approach in history.

While acupoint tapping is powerful enough to change tenacious guiding models, the approach appears at first to be too simple. Steve Wells and David Lake, two pioneers of energy psychology, describe EFT as "the simple process of tapping on acupressure points on the body as you focus on your issue or problem."[4] Of course they realize that beyond this basic procedure, there is much more to it. A total of 48 "core techniques" are taught in one of the most well-regarded tapping certification programs (EFTUniverse.com). Among these, in addition to physical interventions such as the tapping, are:

- Techniques for tuning in to core issues

- Examining specific events linked to the origin of psychological difficulties

- Handling excessive emotional intensity

- The difference between working with physical symptoms and psychological symptoms[5]

EFT practitioners often modify the Protocol based on their personal and professional preferences. What does not change are the two essential elements underlined by Wells and Lake:

1. various aspects of a psychological difficulty or other desired change are vividly brought to mind while

2. a group of acupuncture points is stimulated, usually by tapping on them.

The tapping protocol we use in this book is based on *The Promise of Energy Psychology*, a volume we coauthored with Gary Craig in 2005.[6] *Tapping* reflects the further evolution of our thinking and covers much more than the 2005 volume. It is also backed by the substantial research on tapping therapies that has been conducted in the past two decades.

WHAT A TAPPING SESSION WITH A THERAPIST LOOKS LIKE

This book teaches you how to *self-apply* a tapping protocol. We want to begin, however, by giving you a sense of what a *therapist-guided* session looks like, since the steps you will be following are similar.

Rosa had been having a difficult go of parenting since her teenage daughter, Carmen, hit adolescence. Rosa's anger and impatience with Carmen seemed excessive, even to Rosa in her more reflective moments, yet her reactions were also feeling out of her control. While Rosa wasn't thinking in terms of "guiding models," you will see that her guiding model for parenting was about to be put under the microscope.

After developing rapport and discussing her reasons for seeking help, the therapist asked Rosa to bring to mind one of the many trying incidents with Carmen and to rate the amount of anger it evoked in her. This initial SUD rating was 8 out of 10.

Rosa then formulated a "Reminder Phrase" that succinctly went to the heart of the issue. Her Reminder Phrase was simply *"My anger toward Carmen."* This kept Rosa emotionally engaged with the issue as she repeated the Reminder Phrase while doing the tapping.

She then created an "Acceptance Statement." Acceptance Statements are built on the Reminder Phrase. They are constructed, however, in a manner that supports self-acceptance and a compassionate, affirming understanding of the person's situation. Rosa's initial Acceptance Statement was:

> *"Even though I have difficulty controlling my anger toward Carmen, I love and accept myself anyway."*

Rosa was then shown how to stimulate certain energy points on her body that enhance the suggestive effects of a repeated affirmation. She did this while repeating her Acceptance Statement several times.

Then the tapping began, with Rosa restating her Reminder Phrase, *"My anger toward Carmen,"* as she tapped on the 12 acupoints for a few seconds each. This tapping sequence took less than a minute to complete. A brief set of physical and mental procedures, called the "Integration Procedure," was then carried out, followed by another round of tapping, again accompanied by her Reminder Phrase.

Rosa then gave another 0-to-10 rating on the earlier scene. It was down to 6. This led to a discussion that revealed that Rosa's anger had several layers, extending back to her own mother's way of expressing anger. You can see how the guiding model about parenting that Rosa had unconsciously developed is slowly revealing itself. At this point, Rosa's Acceptance Statement evolved into one that was more discerning:

"Even though I have difficulty controlling my anger toward Carmen, I recognize that I am managing it in ways my own mother never could."

The phrases that accompanied the tapping were also expanded. In addition to *"My anger toward Carmen,"* the statements the therapist directed Rosa to say included:

"Mama wouldn't let Carmen get away with that."

"The heat I feel in my face when Carmen talks back to me."

"Mama slapped me for crying when Grandma died."

"Expecting Carmen to respect me."

"I'm embarrassed that I let Carmen talk back to me."

"I'm not Mama!"

"Feeling powerless with Carmen."

Each of these statements addresses an *aspect* of Rosa's responses to Carmen's anger, and each traces to Rosa's guiding model about a child's anger and how to respond to it. While energy psychology is by no means unique in its ability to identify multiple aspects of a personal challenge, a special strength of the technique is in its ability to rapidly tap down the emotional charge of each aspect. Along with each of the statements, the tapping lowers the distress involved with the issue that is brought to mind. As this occurs, shifts in perceiving and understanding the situation unfold organically and the guiding model is reshaped.

Each layer of Rosa's anger received attention during the tapping until the amount of anger or upset evoked by that aspect was down to 0 or near 0. After a dozen cycles of tapping on various aspects of the situation, Rosa was able to vividly bring each issue to mind with no negative emotional charge. In the process, aspects of Rosa's guiding model about how to handle Carmen's behavior that were causing problems were being dismantled, one piece at a time.

This opened the way for envisioning more creative and effective strategies for responding to Carmen's provocations, a transformed guiding model. Rosa tapped on these imagined scenarios to reinforce them and embed them into her guiding model about parenting. After this single session, Rosa was no longer easily triggered into anger by what she now recognized as typical teenage behavior, even the defiance. Meanwhile, Rosa had sorted out unresolved feelings toward her own mother and brought about a substantial shift in her guiding model as a parent.

BEFORE YOU BEGIN

The Basic Tapping Protocol you will learn in this chapter is quite straightforward, yet it can be surprisingly effective. It can make a difference when you want to address elusive goals, excessive emotional reactions, long-standing patterns that have been resistant to change, or getting past a specific problem or challenge.

We all have areas where we are unwittingly operating from old programming that keeps us from accessing greater joy, love, peace, or success. Updating your understanding of yourself, your relationships, and your views about how the world works can be as challenging as it is empowering. The first step is to recognize guiding models that are no longer serving you. The Basic Tapping Protocol tends to bring such outmoded models into your awareness. Any substantial shifts in your guiding models can, however, temporarily disrupt your equilibrium. We want to address a few points about going through the program.

Does Tapping Replace Therapy?

Any self-help approach has its limitations. While tapping on a self-directed basis has been shown to be an effective tool for relieving painful emotions such as anxiety, anger, and disproportionate fear,[7] as well as for shifting self-defeating behavioral patterns,[8] it does not necessarily replace the need for therapy. Particularly if you are:

- Experiencing serious mental health problems or persistent post-traumatic reactions

- Struggling with an addiction to alcohol, drugs, or harmful behaviors

- Currently in an emotionally or physically abusive relationship

If any of these apply to you, we strongly encourage you to seek professional help and support. The methods taught here can, in fact, be a potent supplement to psychotherapy.

Sensitive Territory

Whether used with the support of a professional or—as will probably be the case for most readers—solely on a self-help basis, the Basic Tapping Protocol can have an impact with a wide range of concerns. It is also designed to bring you face to face with uncomfortable issues—unresolved traumas from your past, emotional wounds in need of healing, confining beliefs, or languishing potentials.

While tapping is one of the safest self-help tools you can hope to find,[9] tapping on a tough issue may in some cases increase the intensity of the related emotions *before* it begins to reduce it. This is not a sign that the approach isn't working or that it is exacerbating the problem but rather that it *is* working. Tapping provides a way to more fully connect with inner processes at an emotional level. This creates space for repressed emotions to rise to the surface.

In short, accessing bad feelings isn't necessarily a bad thing. Rather, it usually means that you have uncovered significant emotional material that may be maintaining outdated guiding models, and you now have a chance to process them in new and more effective ways. In our experience, when tapping causes previously forgotten painful memories to arise into conscious awareness, they are often unprocessed experiences that are calling out to be healed at a time in your life when you are ready to heal them.

When they come into your awareness, you don't need to push them away. Meet them with interest. Know that their very appearance is an invitation for their healing and surround them with that intention. Working with memories that still need to be processed emotionally is often a necessary step in transforming guiding models that are limiting you.

If It Gets to Be Too Much

The Basic Tapping Protocol is designed so that even when you come to unpleasant bumps in what you are exploring, you will move through them mindfully and productively by simply continuing with the steps that have been outlined. But any activity that thrusts you deep into your inner world can bring up painful material. Again, that's not a bad thing. The usual outcome after working with such memories is to have greater compassion for your earlier self and, in the process, change your relationship to that piece of your history. Tapping as you go through this process helps heal old emotional wounds and updates outmoded guiding models. However, at any time the experience becomes too uncomfortable (something only you can judge), please stop. Nothing is wrong. You're in the midst of meaningful self-examination. It may occur in this chapter or anytime after.

If you reach such a point, it is more important to rebalance your body's energies than to proceed with the program. We show you how to do this with some simple exercises in the book's Appendix: "If the Program Becomes Unsettling." In fact, please look that over now so you know it is there if or when you need it.

Can You/Should You Tap Away Your Emotions?

We asked Mai, a highly educated woman who had faced enormous traumas during her early years, to go through the program as one of our test drivers. She raised a question that is pertinent to everyone: Should you "tap away" your emotions? Here is what she wrote:

> I felt a great deal of resistance to the idea of tapping as a way to remove the emotional charge behind disturbing memories. Throughout my tumultuous childhood and young adulthood, I've taught myself to recall painful and distressing memories.

This reminds me of my strength and resilience. I felt skepticism and resistance about the idea of tapping away my feelings. I think it is important to validate our emotions as a necessary part of the healing experience rather than something to be detected and then tapped away.

What we explained to Mai is that tapping doesn't eliminate the *memory* of the situation that produced the emotion. You can "tap away" the reactivation of an emotional response to a past trauma *without forgetting* what happened, what you felt, and how you handled it. It does *not mean* that your initial response was somehow wrong or that it is now wrong to recall the emotion. It means, rather, that if accessing the memory continues to cause you to relive the original pain and terror, your psyche and energy system are carrying a burden that interferes with your ability to heal from the trauma and move forward free from the restraints it has placed on you. With energy psychology, *tapping away* long-standing emotional reactions requires that you first acknowledge, engage, and accept them.

Tracking Your Progress

We encourage you to keep a pen and paper close at hand (or use a laptop or other digital device) as you read through this book so you can journal your experiences and note insights. This will help you stay focused as you do the procedures and record the outcomes. It will also become a log of the guiding models you will be exploring throughout the book. A journal allows you to strengthen a deep-seated resource that spiritual traditions refer to as the "Inner Witness." Your journal can also become a kind of "surrogate therapist" as you go through the program—one that can be an exquisitely patient and inviting listener to your experiences, thoughts, and feelings. Describing your experiences with the techniques will also help further anchor them into your memory.

By reflecting on what is happening in your life in the sanctuary of your journal or laptop, you can discover what is going on beneath the surface. And by naming these deeper dynamics, even patterns that have been keeping you trapped start to lose their power over you.

The downside of keeping a journal is that it can cause you to "overthink" or to keep dwelling on what is negative and painful. Tapping can help even with this. Rather than becoming stuck in such loops, you can simply identify the loop and tap on the emotion that is driving it.

Making the Time

One of our test drivers, who had benefited in the past from psychotherapy, described his dilemma with the program:

> With a demanding job and limited personal time, I found it difficult to devote the time it takes to utilize the program. I found I needed two hours to really sink into a chapter and make significant

headway with it. I wound up making appointments in my calendar and treating them as serious time commitments, just as I did when going to my therapist. Now at the end of the program, I feel the rewards have been worth the effort many times over, but it took me a while to figure out how much time needed to be committed and to carve out that time.

Changing lifelong psychological and behavioral patterns that interfere with your well-being and fulfillment requires more than a casual read through a book. So sorry!

Enlisting Others to Partner with You

While the instructions are written for going through the program alone, they can—as mentioned in the Introduction—also be applied to working with a partner or in a group. Among other benefits, this can get your work with each subsequent section of the book "onto your calendar," so to speak. Each week you could read an agreed-upon section of the book at home, do the procedures, and share your experiences with your partner or group. Or you could read everything but the "Your Turn" instructions for the meeting that is coming up and do those together.

So many men's groups, women's groups, addiction recovery groups, grief and other support groups help people deal more constructively with their life challenges. Such groups could dedicate a given number of weeks to the program in this book. This approach could also be adapted for working in partnership with one other person or for online groups. Joining forces with a partner or a group can provide a forum for reflecting on your experiences, drawing on mutual support, and receiving inspiration from one another.

Other Resources

Additional resources—such as how to find a tapping practitioner or training program—might have been included at the end of the book, but because available information about energy psychology is expanding so rapidly, we maintain an up-to-date list you can access at any time. To find a tapping practitioner, training program, or other resources, visit resources.energytapping .com.

THE BASIC TAPPING PROTOCOL

The Basic Tapping Protocol consists of 12 steps. While you are learning it, we suggest that you follow the sequence as it is laid out in this chapter. Once the Protocol has become familiar to you, you can adapt it to your pace, your preference, and the situation you are confronting. In this chapter, we will limit your focus to processing a single unpleasant memory. After learning the Protocol while working with this memory, you will be able to apply it to a wide range of issues—any type of problem or situation that involves unwanted emotional responses, behavior patterns, or unmet goals.

The 12 steps are organized into four phases. As mentioned before, you will be moving back and forth among them:

Phase 1: Preparation—Four Steps

Phase 2: The Tapping Cycle—Five Steps

Phase 3: Adjusting the Protocol—Two Steps

Phase 4: Testing Your Results—One Step

PHASE 1: PREPARATION

The Protocol typically begins with a preparation phase. For this chapter, you will begin by selecting an uncomfortable memory that will be your focus. In this opening phase, you will be going through four steps, each of which helps you develop a basic skill:

Preparation, Step 1: Choose your initial focus

Preparation, Step 2: Rate your discomfort about it

Preparation, Step 3: Create a *Reminder Phrase* to keep it psychologically active

Preparation, Step 4: Formulate an *Acceptance Statement* about the issue and the feelings it triggers

Preparation, Step 1: Choose Your Initial Focus

You might use a tapping session to address:

- A challenge you are facing at the point you are doing the tapping session

- A longstanding problem in your relationships, work, or other area

- An emotional or behavioral pattern that is getting in your way

- A desired goal, such as doing your best at an upcoming competition or performance

The initial focus is usually defined on its own terms:

"I am furious with my neighbor."

"I can't keep getting to work late."

"I am thrown off by my mother-in-law's constant judgments."

"I want to beat my previous best time at the Boston Marathon."

Frequently the work quickly moves into earlier experiences that shaped the guiding models underlying the current concern. So for this initial session, we'll begin with an incident from your past.

Everyone has lived through some difficult experiences, and your first task here will be to select an uncomfortable memory. For instance, you might recall when:

- You lost a beloved pet.

- Your family moved to a new city and you got lost coming home after your first day of school.

- You landed a major role in the school play and you forgot your lines on opening night.

- Your best friend shared one of your deepest secrets on social media.

- You took your boss and her husband out to dinner but forgot your wallet.

The memory can be from your childhood or a more recent time. The memory you select may evoke strong emotions, but for this first cycle, please do not choose a memory that involved physical injury or any kind of abuse—physical, sexual, or emotional. While tapping is among the most effective approaches for resolving such trauma, your focus right now should be on learning the method with a memory that isn't overwhelming.

Why Revisit a Disturbing Memory?
Memories that trigger a distressing emotion in the present have, generally, not been fully processed. We all have them. Some just never emerge into awareness until you are ready. Processing a disturbing memory involves the following:

bringing it into a *reflective awareness*

that allows the difficult sensory and emotional components to be *recognized*

and systematically *soothed*

until they are *no longer reactivated* when the memory is brought to mind.

You will find that the Basic Tapping Protocol is very good at helping you accomplish this.

Working with a traumatic memory using the Protocol won't erase it, yet it can modify neural pathways that make recalling it retraumatizing and that maintain self-limiting guiding models tracing to the original incident. This allows the memory to be reintegrated so it is no longer a source of pain. Instead, difficult memories that have been psychologically processed become a source of resilience and greater emotional freedom. Gary Craig focused on this possibility when he named the tapping approach that has gained the greatest popularity: the Emotional *Freedom* Techniques.

Some of the memories that enter your mind as you think about where to concentrate your attention might seem unsuitable for this exercise because you don't think about them much, if at all. You might be tempted to dismiss them. But as long as painful experiences remain unresolved, even memories that you don't think about can impact your emotional equilibrium, like a slow energetic leak.

You may also be unwittingly shaping your day-to-day choices, actions, and behaviors to avoid circumstances that would recreate the original feeling. For example, if you had the humiliating experience of forgetting your lines during the school play, it might be the underlying reason (knowingly or not) that you pass up the opportunity to give the opening toast at the annual company dinner.

Focusing on a *Specific* Scene. Once you have selected a memory, choose a specific scene within that memory for the tapping. If you decide to focus on the day that you lost a beloved pet, you would identify a particular moment (such as *when you learned of the loss* or *crying yourself to sleep that night*) rather than general thoughts or themes (such as a series of memories about your pet or the theme of losing what you love). If your memory was starting school in the middle of the year due to a move to a new city, a specific event might be *the moment you walked into the classroom and someone made a comment that caused the whole class to laugh at you.*

Introducing Emma

Most of the test drivers we recruited to go through the instructions presented in this and subsequent chapters were new to tapping. One of these was Emma, a high school teacher in rural Texas. In this first exercise, Emma returned to a scene from when she was seven years old. She had been cast as a model on a live television morning show. She was wearing a Cinderella costume and had to hold hands with a boy who was dressed as Prince Charming. They had to face TV cameras that looked gigantic. The director kept telling her to look up at the camera. Emma reflected, "I couldn't. I felt terrified, humiliated, exposed, unprepared, and I froze staring at the floor."

Your Turn to Choose Your Focus

Jot down in your journal the memory you selected and the specific scene you will focus upon. If you wish, describe your feelings and thoughts about the memory.

Preparation, Step 2: Rate the Amount of Discomfort the Memory Causes

Next, you will rate your memory, giving it an SUD (Subjective Units of Distress) score. As you've already seen, SUD scores range from 0, indicating a total absence of distress, to 10, indicating extreme distress. The rating will be based on what you feel in your mind and/or body as you recall the memory (rather than what you *imagine* you felt back then). Before you do this, here are a few nuances about taking an SUD rating.

Dialing Down If Necessary. An important principle to keep in mind throughout the book is that all you have to do is "enter lightly" into a memory to make it neurologically active. This is enough to give it an SUD score and to create a positive outcome as you tap. It is not necessary or even desirable to recreate a past traumatic experience in such vivid detail that you become emotionally flooded by it. In fact, one of the strengths of energy psychology is its ability to work with traumatic experiences without retraumatizing the person. If an emotion becomes overwhelming, shift your focus so you are tapping on the overwhelming feeling that is occurring in the moment rather than continuing to focus on the memory or situation that brought up the feeling. This immediately sends calming signals to your limbic system.

For Overwhelming Memories or Experiences. During this preliminary step, while you are establishing your initial SUD rating, you can also counter the rise of overwhelming feelings by shifting *the way* you focus on the memory. For instance, if you are concerned that the feelings brought up by the memory will be too painful or intense, you could imagine that you are seeing the experience through a long tunnel or the wrong end of a telescope so it appears farther away. For a particularly difficult memory, it is not even necessary to bring the specifics to mind. You can, instead, ask yourself, "If I *were* to focus on [the remembered incident] and give it an SUD rating, what would that number be?" The number that comes to mind in the "Tearless Trauma" technique, as it is called in EFT, has proven to be a good baseline as the person moves through the Protocol. This principle of moderating the intensity of your experience applies anywhere in the Protocol you feel it is needed. Again, for the Basic Tapping Protocol to be effective, it is not necessary to fully immerse yourself in a deeply troubling memory. Just hold the memory lightly in your mind.

If You Can't Come Up with a Feeling. Sometimes the memory you selected may seem too distant, and you can barely recall anything about the experience. Or you may remember it but not recall the emotions evoked by that experience. Or you may recall the incident but not identify with it, as if it happened to someone else. If you have difficulty accessing your feelings or really "getting into" the memory, you can use your imagination to vividly step into the scene. Fantasize what you *might* have seen, heard, smelled, tasted, felt, or thought during the incident and create as vibrant an experience as you can for reliving the memory. This blend of biography and fantasy will bring you into the emotional zone that will allow the tapping to have the desired effects.

If *Discomfort* or *Distress* Doesn't Fit the Situation. Rating the amount of discomfort or distress you feel in your mind and/or body usually applies. But other wording might be more appropriate. What you are looking for is a problematic feeling. For instance, resistance to doing a task might be measured in the amount of aversion you have to it rather than a term like *distress*. Difficulties with a person or a situation might be measured in the amount of aversion you are feeling when bringing the person or situation to mind. These can all be reduced by tapping. At any point in the book that *discomfort* or *distress* aren't quite the right words, find what fits.

Alternatives to the Numerical Rating. The 0-to-10 SUD rating is convenient for making comparisons at different points in time as you move through the Protocol, but it is not the only way to assess how emotionally problematic the memory or issue is. In our experience, a relatively small percentage of people are uncomfortable with numbers or for other reasons find it difficult to come to an SUD score. If you are one of them, any other way of registering your sense of distress about the issue that can be contrasted with your sense of distress after each round of tapping will do. Some people use

descriptive words like *intense*, *large*, or *little*. When using the Basic Tapping Protocol with children, rather than a number rating, they might be asked to indicate the amount of discomfort they are feeling by showing the distance between their hands, palms facing, with their arms outstretched (meaning "this much").

Emma's Rating

"My memory at the television studio feels like a 6. Of course, back when it was happening, I'm relatively sure it would have been a full-blown 10. I couldn't get myself to do what the director was asking me to do. I was also terribly embarrassed."

Your Turn

Now bring your memory to mind, guided by the above instructions, and give it a 0-to-10 SUD rating. Write the number in your journal next to your description of the memory. If you wish, also reflect on the experience of focusing on the memory and any insights you had about it or the guiding models that may be based upon it.

Preparation, Step 3: Create Your Initial Reminder Phrase

The Reminder Phrase is a word or short description of the memory or situation you identified in Step 1. While it will change as you move through the Protocol, the initial Reminder Phrase gives you a baseline. It also provides the initial wording as you begin to tap. The purpose of the Reminder Phrase is to keep the situation you are focusing upon psychologically and neurologically active. The Reminder Phrase doesn't need to be a complete description, only a brief statement whose meaning is clear to you. This is enough to activate the neural pathways the tapping will impact. If you are processing the time you forgot your lines on the opening night of the school play, your Reminder Phrase might be as simple as *"The school play"*; *"Forgot my lines"*; or *"The panic on my costar's face."* Others tied to the earlier examples might be:

"Fido died."

"My first day at school in Chicago."

"I was humiliated on Facebook."

"My boss' husband made fun of me."

Emma's Reminder Phrase

"My Reminder Phrase is *'Freezing up in front of the TV camera.'* Further reflections: I was only seven. I had no idea how scary the HUGE television cameras would be. My mother should have helped me feel safe. I had just recently moved with my immediate family from Oregon to Atlanta, leaving all my relatives. I wish I could have been helped to handle it better, to have enjoyed it, even to have made my mother proud."

Your Turn

Write your Reminder Phrase in your journal. Also, if you wish, describe any thoughts, insights, or questions that occur to you about the original experience.

Preparation, Step 4: Formulate Your Initial Acceptance Statement

Among the greatest ironies of self-initiated change is the importance of self-acceptance —embracing the very parts of yourself that you wish to alter. A more general way to state this is that *not* accepting the realities you face is among the largest blocks to coping effectively.

Carl Rogers, among the most well-regarded psychologists of the twentieth century, observed the "curious paradox [that] when I can accept myself just as I am, then can I change."[10] This is a principle that is emphasized in energy psychology and an attitude we will keep spotlighting throughout the book. You don't need to make the "problem" your *enemy*. Rather, accepting and understanding the forces that brought about the difficult experience allows you to process it with self-compassion.

Built into the Basic Tapping Protocol is the formulation of an "Acceptance Statement" that reinforces an accepting, compassionate attitude. Your initial Acceptance Statement will follow a simple formula that builds on your Reminder Phrase (for example, *"Even though I got lost coming home from school and my parents called the police, I accept that little girl who was doing the best she knew how"*).

The Acceptance Statement pairs the painful emotion, memory, problem, or unmet goal that is embodied in the Reminder Phrase with a phrase that surrounds it with self-acceptance or another positive feeling. For instance, a frequently used phrase is *"I love and completely accept myself."* The one you used in the breathing exercise in Chapter 1 was simply *"I accept myself just as I am."* You don't have to fully believe it for it to become meaningfully associated with your Reminder Phrase. Once this association has been established, every time you bring the problem to mind you are also activating your acceptance of it.

If, however, saying that you love yourself or accept yourself is such a stretch that it brings up resistance, you can address the related issues later and adjust the wording for now. Most people can, without too much internal resistance, make a statement such as *"I'm learning to love/accept myself,"* *"I'm doing the best I know how,"* or *"I know deep down that I am a good and worthy human being."*

To create your Acceptance Statement, you weave the Reminder Phrase together with the affirming Acceptance Phrase. Then begin with the words "Even though":

> *"Even though [Reminder Phrase], I deeply and completely accept myself."*

You may need to slightly modify the Reminder Phrase to fit this format. Some examples from the earlier scenarios might be:

> *"Even though my breathing is constricted, I accept myself just as I am."*

> *"Even though my first day at school after we moved was terrifying, I deeply love and accept myself."*

> *"Even though my boss' husband made fun of me, I'm learning to love myself."*

> *"Even though I still have all this anger toward Carmen, I love and accept myself anyway."*

If you are familiar with using positive affirmations as a personal development tool, or if you're trained in the use of self-hypnosis, you might be puzzled that the Acceptance Statement emphasizes what is wrong. The first part of the statement typically elicits unwanted or negative feelings. "What kind of affirmation is that!" we've been asked by colleagues. "Aren't you reinforcing what you are trying to change?" No! The Acceptance Statement associates a positive affirmation with the difficult memory whenever it arises.

Emma's Acceptance Statement

"Even though I froze up in front of the TV cameras, I love and deeply accept myself." Reflection: "This feels a little strange. Having fallen apart in front of all those adults is a dark memory, so 'I love and deeply accept myself' seems inconsistent. But it also feels comforting."

Your Turn

Now craft your own Acceptance Statement as described above, building upon your Reminder Phrase. Write it in your journal, along with any reflections. The following step will involve saying it out loud, with feeling and emphasis, while stimulating energy points that further embed the statement into your psyche and nervous system.

PHASE 2: THE TAPPING CYCLE

The second phase is the core of the Basic Tapping Protocol. Called "the tapping cycle," it includes five steps:

The Tapping Cycle, Step 1: Anchoring your Acceptance Statement

The Tapping Cycle, Step 2: Tapping on the 12 acupoints while saying your Reminder Phrase at each point (called a "round of tapping")

The Tapping Cycle, Step 3: An "Integration Procedure"

The Tapping Cycle, Step 4: Another round of tapping while saying your Reminder Phrase

The Tapping Cycle, Step 5: Taking a new SUD rating

We'll detail each step.

The Tapping Cycle, Step 1: Energetically Anchor Your Acceptance Statement

First some background. Simply placing your fingers on acupuncture points ("the light touch") is the most familiar form of acupressure. Tapping the points, as you have been learning to do, is a variation that we believe is even more powerful for certain outcomes, including those involved with psychological issues. Another procedure used in acupressure is to firmly massage the points ("the hard rub").

The "light touch" and the "hard rub" are used when anchoring the Acceptance Statement. In addition, two energy systems that are different from the acupoint system are used. One involves the chakras—energy centers located in various regions of the body. The chakras hold emotions and carry information about your history. We will be using the Heart Chakra. The other system, known as the "neurolymphatic reflexes," are linked to the body's lymph system and, when rubbed fairly hard, can help optimize the flow within that system.[11]

Finding Your "Chest Sore Spots." In the daily use of our bodies, energies simply become congested, not entirely unlike the way that you need to reboot your computer every now and again to clear it of the residue of previous use. Massaging congested neurolymphatic reflex points is like rebooting the flow of the lymph system and the energies associated with it.

Each neurolymphatic reflex point is connected to a specific meridian. By massaging a point that is congested, you are not only reviving the *physical flow* within your lymph system but also getting the *energies* of the associated meridian into harmony. This will reverberate through your entire body. Doing this while saying your Acceptance Statement gives an energetic boost to the statement, embedding it more deeply into your nervous system.

A set of neurolymphatic reflex points that accumulate considerable excess energy for most people are at the sides of the chest, near the area where your arms attach. Let's see if you have a sore spot

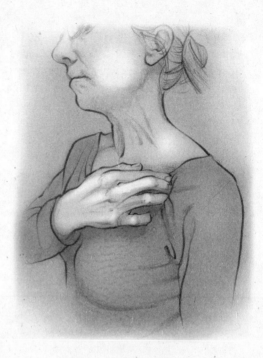

Figure 2.1. With your middle finger—or your second, third, and fourth fingers—rub firmly along the seam where your arms connect to your chest (or find other points on your chest that feel a bit sore when you press on them).

that falls along this curved line on each side of your body (see Figure 2.1). Reach up to those points and rub hard with your middle finger or your second, third, and fourth fingers (but never so hard as to bruise yourself). You may find that it feels good, even vitalizing, or you may find that the spot is uncomfortably sore. If no physical injury accounts for the soreness, you have probably located a clogged neurolymphatic reflex point.

If Your "Sore Spots" Aren't Sore. If you were unable to find any sore spots, an alternative is to "clap" the sides of your hands together (the Side-of-the-Hands Points). This stimulates three acupoints that are on the fleshy outside of each hand. All three are on the Small Intestine Meridian, which is involved with discernment and incorporating information. Whether or not you have found chest sore spots, you are now ready for the next steps in the protocol:

1. Memorize your Acceptance Statement.

2. See if you have any soreness on the points where your arms meet your chest (Figure 2.1). These are the neurolymphatic reflex points on the Central Meridian and often accumulate excess energy. Rubbing them releases the excess and stimulates one of your most important energy pathways.

3. Firmly rub these points (but not so hard as to risk bruising yourself) as you say the first half of your Acceptance Statement out loud, with focus: *"Even though [insert a variation of your Reminder Phrase]."* For instance, *"Even though I forgot my lines during the play . . ."* Alternatives if these points aren't sore or if they are sore due to an injury or overexertion are to find other points on your chest that are sore or to clap the sides of your hands together (see Figure 2.2) while saying the first half of your Acceptance Statement.

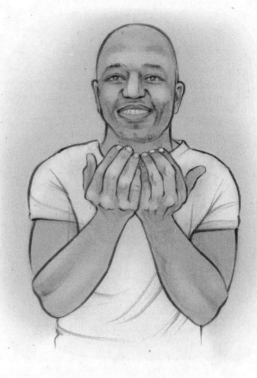

Figure 2.2. Clapping the sides of your hands together.

4. Then place both hands over the center of your chest (your Heart Chakra) and state the positive affirmation: *"I love and deeply accept myself," "I love myself and accept my feelings," "I accept myself just as I am," "I'm learning to love myself," "I know that deep down I am a good and worthy person,"* or any other variation you choose.

5. Repeat until you have said your Acceptance Statement three times while massaging any chest sore spots or clapping the sides of your hands together during the *"Even though"* part and with your hands over your Heart Chakra during the positive affirmation part. You can modify your Acceptance Statement on the second or third tapping cycle for a better fit or to make it more complete.

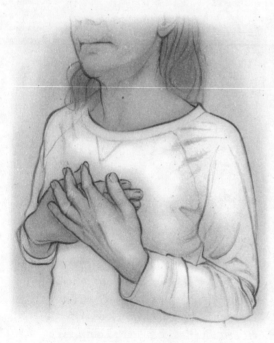

Figure 2.3. Placing both hands over the center of your chest as you state your affirmation.

Emma's Anchoring

"I didn't want to push in real hard, but with the amount of pressure I was comfortable using, I couldn't find any points that were particularly sore, so I used the Side-of-the-Hands Points."

Your Turn

After completing the five steps for anchoring your Acceptance Statement, consider describing any thoughts, insights, or questions in your journal.

The Tapping Cycle, Step 2: The First Round of Tapping

Now you are ready to begin tapping. This isn't an entirely new skill since you used it in the breathing exercise. You will be tapping on the same 12 acupoints (or left/right pairs of points) shown in Figure 1.3. Tap on each point or pair of points for the amount of time it takes to say your Reminder Phrase out loud and deliberately. Follow the instructions given during the breathing exercise in Chapter 1 for the speed and firmness of the tapping and the fingers to use, as well as alternatives to tapping. You will find that it will become automatic to go through the tapping points, and you will be able to do a round of tapping (assuming you are using the same brief Reminder Phrase at each point) within a minute.

Your Turn: First Round of Tapping

As you tap on each point, state your Reminder Phrase. You don't need to shout it, but do say it with some feeling rather than falling into rote repetition. From the previous examples:

"I forgot my lines during the school play."

"That terrifying first day at school."

"My boss' husband laughed at me."

After stating your Reminder Phrase out loud as you tap on each of the points, the next step in the Protocol is a brief routine that we call the "Integration Procedure."

The Tapping Cycle, Step 3: The Integration Procedure

The Integration Procedure was first introduced by Thought Field Therapy developer Roger Callahan. He called it the "Nine-Gamut Procedure" for reasons no one has ever been able to fully explain to us. Whatever you call it, it is a quick, simple, effective sequence of physical activities for balancing the energies in your brain. It can be done independently of a tapping session, and it is a good tool to have in your back pocket. We've noticed that doing it in the middle of a tapping session helps the thoughts and feelings evoked by the Reminder Phrase to be updated and reintegrated.

However, if you are like most people, you may initially find the Integration Procedure rather strange. While we agree, we also encourage you to set aside any initial doubts or unfavorable first impressions. We find it to be an effective procedure for activating specific areas of the brain through a combination of tapping, eye movements, humming, and counting.

The last acupuncture point you tapped during the first tapping sequence was the Back-of-the-Hand Points, the valley leading to the V where your ring finger and little finger meet (see Figure 2.4). You continue tapping on this valley as you do the Integration Procedure. Use the same speed and pressure you were already applying—firm tapping at about three beats per second. Switch hands as often as you like.

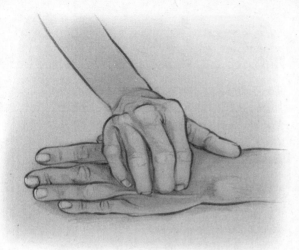

Figure 2.4. Tapping with two, three, or four fingers along the entire ridge beneath the V of your fourth and fifth fingers.

Next, close your eyes, then open them. Move them down to the right and then down to the left. Then circle them (rotate 360 degrees in one direction and then the opposite direction). Hum the first few bars of a familiar song, such as "Twinkle Twinkle Little Star" or "Row Row Your Boat." Count slowly and deliberately from one to five. Then hum again. Keep tapping on the valley leading to your ring finger and little finger while you carry out each element in the sequence (summarized in the following "Integration Procedure" exercise).

The sequence ends with what is called the "Eye Sweep." Begin by keeping your face straight ahead, eyes looking down. Consciously send the energy involved in your issue out your eyes and into the floor. Then, again keeping your face straight ahead, slowly and deliberately move your eyes across the floor, up the wall or background, and up to the ceiling or sky, continually sending the energies involved in your issue out your eyes. Once you have learned the steps, the entire sequence can be done within half a minute. Try the Integration Procedure now.

Your Turn: The Integration Procedure

While tapping on the valley leading to the spot where your ring finger and little finger meet, do the following:

1. Close your eyes.

2. Open your eyes.

3. Move your eyes down to the right.

4. Move your eyes down to the left.

5. Circle your eyes, rotating them 360 degrees in one direction.

6. Circle your eyes, rotating them 360 degrees in the opposite direction.

7. Hum the first few bars of a familiar song.

8. Count slowly and deliberately from one to five.

9. Hum again (the end of the traditional "Nine-Gamut" Procedure).

End with the Eye Sweep.

The Tapping Cycle, Step 4: The Second Round of Tapping

This next round is straightforward. Follow the brief "Your Turn" instructions below.

Your Turn: Second Round of Tapping

After completing the Integration Procedure, do another round of tapping. It will follow the same pattern as the first round from Step 2. Same points. Same Reminder Phrase. Same pace.

The Tapping Cycle, Step 5: Reassessing the SUD

Now give your original memory another SUD rating. Bring to mind the scene from the memory that you focused on earlier and sense the amount of distress, on the 0-to-10 SUD scale, it triggers in your mind and/or body now. You may be able to quickly assign a number to the intensity. Usually the number just comes to people without a lot of thought.

If you aren't sure, one way to get your rating gears going is to ask yourself if you feel better bringing the scene to mind now than you did before the tapping sequence you just completed, or about the same, or worse. The SUD score will indicate the degree of any change. Even if you're not sure, work with whatever number comes into your mind. If a number isn't appearing, don't fret. Just notice whether you feel better, worse, or about the same.

Emma's New SUD

Emma's SUD went from the original 6 down to 4. She wrote, "I was still embarrassed and confused, but I didn't have that frozen feeling."

Your Turn

Even if you've been following along with each instruction, again apply the core procedure on yourself, step by step:

1. Acceptance Statement while rubbing your chest sore spots and holding your Heart Chakra

2. First round of tapping

3. Integration Procedure

4. Second round of tapping

5. Reassessing the SUD

If other memories, thoughts, or feelings have arisen, note them, but for now focus on the scene you selected from your initial memory. Then reflect on the experience and speculate on the reasons your SUD rating changed or didn't change.

PHASE 3: ADJUSTING THE PROTOCOL

EFT practitioners refer to the above sequence as "the Basic Recipe." It is a formula that can be carried out by following the steps with a minimum amount of decisions or even insight. Yet it works. Most readers will have found that the SUD rating on their memory went down by following the formula.

If your SUD has decreased to 0 and your memory no longer evokes feelings of distress—that memory has been emotionally processed. The neural pathways triggering the uncomfortable feelings have been altered. You are able to recognize an injury, injustice, or dangerous situation from your past, but the stress response in your autonomic nervous system that was previously attached to that memory is no longer activated.

Usually, however, it takes more than one tapping cycle to neutralize a disturbing memory. If your SUD for the memory did go down to 0, that's great! To continue with this chapter, find another memory, perhaps with a stronger emotional charge this time, and go through the steps again.

If your SUD level has not gone down to 0, or even if it has gone up (this usually means that a previously buried emotional component of the situation has emerged, such as being trapped in the appliance box during the claustrophobia treatment described in the Introduction), the next phase of the Basic Tapping Protocol will be tailored to what is unique about you and the way your memory lives within

you. This might include the guiding model that developed out of this experience and others like it, the emotions it evokes, and the rules for living contained in that guiding model. This phase involves two basic steps that you may run through as many times as is needed, making further adjustments each time:

Adjusting the Protocol, Step 1: Modifying your Acceptance Statement

Adjusting the Protocol, Step 2: Addressing specific aspects of the situation by going beyond your Reminder Phrase

Adjusting the Protocol, Step 1: Modifying Your Acceptance Statement

The first step in adjusting the Basic Tapping Protocol focuses on your Acceptance Statement. The Acceptance Statement is like a letter you send to give instructions to your unconscious mind—the pool of emotions, thoughts, urges, and memories that are outside your conscious awareness yet that drive much of your feelings and behavior. Your guiding models reside largely in this nether region of your psyche, the ever-mysterious realm where your nighttime dreams are also authored. When we use the term *unconscious*, we are referring to both the subconscious mind (available to your consciousness by shifting your attention) and the realms that are usually beyond your reach.

Opening communication channels between your conscious intentions and this vast but submerged reservoir of your memories, emotions, and motivations is a goal of any sophisticated program for personal development. Tapping sessions are always riding the line between conscious experience and the creative working of the deep psyche.

Your Acceptance Statement is formulated to use your focused awareness *in the service of influencing* your unconscious mind. Specifically, it surrounds the problem, emotional reaction, or unmet goal you want to change with an atmosphere of acceptance and self-affirmation. It is like a wise person saying, "Nothing wrong with *having* a deeply embedded pattern needing your attention," at the very moment you are working to *change* that pattern. It puts a positive slant on your efforts, smoothing the way for desired outcomes.

Your initial Acceptance Statement was based on your Reminder Phrase, keeping your uncomfortable memory emotionally active while adding the positive affirmation. Because the unconscious mind is quite literal, if your SUD rating went down, even a little bit, you will want your Acceptance Statement to also stay congruent with the change.

This can be easily accomplished by adding the words *still* and *some*, such as, "Even though, I **still** have **some** of this mortification . . ." If you made some progress but still have some residue, the modified Acceptance Statement recognizes this with your wording. Also, if possible, have your modified Acceptance Statement *name the emotion* that is embedded in the memory. Not just *"Even though I* **still** *have* **some** *of . . ."* but also **"mortification** *since the cheating incident."* Building on the earlier examples:

> *"Even though I* **still** *have* **some** **shame** *about having forgotten my lines during the school play, I . . ."*

> *"Even though I* **still** *feel* **some** **terror** *when thinking about that first day of school, I . . ."*

> *"Even though I* **still** *go into* **some** **humiliation** *about my boss' husband having laughed at me, I . . ."*

The words following "I" can be any of those suggested earlier:

> *"I love and deeply accept myself."*

> *"I love myself and accept my feelings."*

> *"I accept myself just as I am."*

> *"I'm learning to love myself."*

> *"I accept myself anyway."*

> *"I'm doing the best I know how."*

> *"Deep down, I know I am a good and worthy human being."*

Or they can be any variation you come to that expresses self-acceptance and acceptance of the very qualities or responses you are trying to change.

Emma's Revised Acceptance Statement

Emma's original statement began *"Even though I froze up in front of the TV cameras."* She added feeling and modified it to: *"Even though I **still** feel **some** shame about freezing up in front of the TV camera, I deeply love and accept myself."* She reflected: "It feels good to recognize this progress. Not feeling so frozen gives the whole memory a different texture. It still wasn't any fun, but that sense that I couldn't move had been the worst part."

Your Turn

Now revise your initial Acceptance Statement so that it includes a feeling and adds the words *still* and *some*. Write it in your journal. Repeat it three times, rubbing your chest sore spots with the first phrase and placing your hands over your Heart Chakra with the second phrase. You can also reflect on any insights that came to you as you recrafted the statement and took yourself through the routine.

Adjusting the Protocol, Step 2: Going Beyond Your Reminder Phrase

Identifying and resolving the remaining aspects of your issue is where much of the transformative work is accomplished during a tapping session. Because the skills involved are so fundamental and need to be applied with flexibility, we will go into greater detail here than with the other steps.

Recall that a guiding model is a constellation with many parts. Deep emotional learnings interact with your biological dispositions to create inner models that include *beliefs, memories, images, sensations, emotions, values, intentions, programs for your behavior,* and *filters that shape your perceptions.* Any of these "parts" might become the focus for tapping.

What starts with difficulties in managing your finances, for instance, might bring up a memory of your parents arguing about whether they can afford to buy you a saxophone so you could try out for your high school band. This leads to recalling a scene from a year later: Your parents are proudly watching your first solo performance for a group of their friends during a party celebrating their twentieth wedding anniversary. They've made the financial sacrifice, you've practiced like mad, but you misplay several notes, get flustered, and can't finish. As you recall all of this, you are feeling a tightness in your throat and tears of embarrassment welling up behind your eyes.

As you tap on these sensations, they diminish, but now an image comes into your mind that occurred a few years after the humiliating anniversary performance. You see your father's face looking disappointed as you tell him you are switching your college major from business to art history. Your parents have been paying your tuition, and you sense your father's doubt that you will ever find gainful employment as an art historian. Once more he has made a major investment in you, and you have, in his eyes at least, let him down. And once more, you feel tears behind your eyes. After tapping on the tears and the memory, you become aware of a belief you've never before put into words: that you don't deserve to have much money because look what happened when your parents put their faith in you.

This belief has shaped some key choices throughout your adult life. You have filtered out of your consciousness opportunities to invest in your future and instead made penny-wise but dollar-foolish decisions that keep you financially challenged. Had you simply been tapping on "managing my finances," these guiding beliefs would likely still have their hold on you. But after reducing the tightness in your throat, the welling tears, the intensity of each of the memories, and the beliefs that grew out of these experiences, the old model that has been keeping you in economic distress begins to unravel. Let's look at how this might work in a tapping session on another issue.

Case Illustration: Tapping on Previously Hidden Aspects

An "aspect" in EFT refers to a facet of a larger issue that may require individual attention. The following case was provided by Dawson Church, PhD, a dear friend and one of the most prominent teachers and researchers in the energy psychology community. It describes a demonstration session he did during one of his training programs:

A woman in her late 30s volunteered as a subject. She'd had neck pain and a limited range of motion since an automobile accident six years before. She could turn her head to the right most of the time but had only a few degrees of movement to the left. The accident had been a minor one, and why she still suffered six years later was something of a mystery to her.

I asked her to sense where in her body she felt the most intensity. When recalling the accident, she said it was in her upper chest. I then asked her about the first time she'd ever felt that way, and she said it was when she'd been involved in a more serious auto accident at the age of eight. Her older sister had been driving the car. We worked on each aspect of the early accident. The two girls hit another car while driving around a bend on a country road. One emotionally triggering aspect was the moment she realized that a collision was unavoidable, and we tapped till that lost its force. We tapped on the sound of the crash, another aspect. She had been taken to a neighbor's house, bleeding from a cut on her head, and we tapped on that. We tapped on aspect after aspect. Still her pain level didn't go down much, and her range of motion didn't improve.

Then she gasped and said, "I just remembered. My sister was only 15 years old. She was underage. That day, I dared her to drive the family car, and we totaled it." Her guilt turned out to be the aspect that held the greatest emotional charge. After we tapped on that, her pain disappeared, and she regained full range of motion in her neck.[12]

Aspects of Larger Issues

If Dr. Church had focused only on the more recent accident or failed to uncover the aspects involved with the earlier accident, it is not likely that the session would have led to the dramatic outcome. For you, this first time around, your focus is on a memory. Drawing on the earlier examples involving memories, aspects that might have needed attention included:

Based on having forgotten your lines during the school play:

The feeling of panic.
Can't catch my breath.
Mind went blank.
Not knowing where to look.

Based on getting lost on the way home after the first day of school:

Seeing the intersection and not knowing which way to turn.
Screaming "Mommy" but no one comes.
Running and falling.
Your mother and the policeman looking angry when they finally find you.

Based on your boss' husband having made fun of you:

The feeling of panic when you realize you don't have your wallet.
The heat of embarrassment on your face.
The moment your boss' husband said, "Well, that explains a lot!"
The sinking feeling in the pit of your stomach.

Aspects may be physical or psychological. Physical aspects in the earlier scenarios include seeing that a collision was unavoidable, the sound of the crash, the cut on her head, an inability to catch a breath, falling, the bruised knee, the heat of embarrassment in face, the stab in the heart, seeing the reactions of others. The psychological aspects include guilt, mind going blank, not knowing where to look, panic, mother looking angry. Neutralizing physical aspects often results in unrecognized psychological aspects emerging, and vice versa, as you will see in the following account.

Physical Aspects. Physical aspects that are playing into an issue are not always apparent, especially when you first start to tap. But they may become prominent as the tapping starts to reduce the strength of your emotional reaction.

For instance, the woman being treated for claustrophobia (p. 5) was bringing to mind, while she was tapping, the experience of being in an elevator. Once her distress about being in an elevator was down to 0, the outcome was tested by having her step into a hallway coat closet and closing the door. She was able to remain calm. However, if *darkness* was an aspect of her phobia, and if the only situation she brought to mind during the tapping was a well-lit elevator, darkness would not have been identified as being relevant and would not have been tapped down. In her case, however, the initial experience of being trapped in the appliance box involved darkness. In fact, she specifically tapped on the total darkness during the session, so darkness was no longer a major issue by the time she stepped into the closet.

A classic example of a physical aspect, first described by Gary Craig and frequently retold, is of a woman's fear of mice, which she often saw in her workplace. The tapping reduced her fear to 0. But the next time she saw a mouse, she was terrified. As they explored why the treatment hadn't held, they realized that the image she had in her mind while tapping was of a static mouse. It wasn't moving. The real mouse she saw after the session was moving very fast. Movement was the physical aspect they had missed. After generating and tapping on images of a moving mouse, and getting that down to 0, seeing a mouse scurry by no longer triggered her fear.

Many events that have an emotional impact have strong physical components. A car accident may include sounds, such as screeching brakes, screams of another passenger, or a loud crash. A damaging encounter with a loved one may include the *expression* on a face, the *tone* of voice, the *smell* of alcohol on an abuser's breath, or the *pain* of a physical assault.

Bodily sensations such as shortness of breath, tightness in a particular area, or other types of discomfort frequently emerge at some point during a tapping session. While many people will just ignore them and move on, we encourage you to be alert for them and to shift the focus of your session to address them with tapping: *"The queasiness in my stomach." "The tingling in my hands." "The heaviness in my chest."* These are the physiological components of your emotions. Addressing them at this body level is a potent way to begin to shift the emotional response.

Psychological Aspects. Psychological aspects often involve incidents that are precursors to the current issue. These may be memories you've thought of often or memories that have been repressed. They can also include emotional reactions, thoughts, and impulses toward action that are connected to cues or triggers rather than specific memories.

Many painful experiences and issues involve unresolved psychological aspects that go far deeper than the current problem. The woman with claustrophobia traced her irrational fears to being trapped in an appliance box. Nancy's fear of heights started when she was nearly pushed over while standing by a cliff. Simply tapping on *"Fear of closed spaces"* or *"Terror of heights"* was not likely to resolve the phobia for either woman.

Unresolved psychological aspects often reveal themselves when the tapping treatment has softened the edge of a problem but isn't resolving it. We saw this when the appliance box entered the woman's awareness while she was tapping on her fear of elevators. Often a recent incident—an accident, a loss, an intense argument, an embarrassing situation—will trigger a reaction that is out of proportion to the situation, as seen with the woman whose more recent automobile accident stirred up unresolved feelings and bodily memories from the accident when she was eight. It may also become a source of obsessing, with endless ruminations or even intrusive emotions such as unprovoked fear, anger, jealousy, sadness, or physical symptoms. Exploration will usually reveal that an unprocessed psychological aspect, specifically an earlier

experience, is at play in such situations. These will often enter awareness while you are neutralizing the negative charge on the original situation.

In addition to emotional reactions that aren't fully responding to tapping, forgotten incidents from your past may be the root cause of, for instance, a sudden fear of flying that starts at, say, age 45. After witnessing television images of people falling from a plane during the August 2021 Afghanistan evacuation, a woman found herself shaking with fear when she would think about getting on a plane. Up to this point, she had always been comfortable flying. Tapping on *"Fear of flying"* reduced her distress somewhat, but it didn't eliminate the fear. It did, however, clear the way for a memory to come into her mind of having fallen off a porch as a toddler and being injured. Processing this memory with tapping was a required step before overcoming her newly acquired fear of flying. While inconvenient, the emergence of out-of-proportion reactions to a recent event is one of your psyche's ways of "cleaning house."

Working with Aspects

During the first tapping cycle, the instructions were to simply restate your Reminder Phrase at each tapping point. In this adjustment phase, that restriction is lifted. While you can still use your Reminder Phrase, and repeating it at least occasionally will keep bringing you back to your initial focus, being able to change the words allows you to explore the territory in all its facets. Here are some issues you might be asking about as the session proceeds:

How Do I Know If an Unresolved Aspect Is Needing My Attention? You can be reasonably sure that an unresolved aspect of your issue is at play if the intensity of your discomfort won't go down to 0 or near 0, if it increases, or if it returns as you shift to other topics or over time. Generally, once you have eliminated the intensity of an aspect in a situation that was triggering you, the next aspect needing attention will present itself. Working with aspects is like peeling the layers of an onion. As you resolve the issues involved with one layer, it will no longer feel important, but the next layer will be there just beneath it. However, unlike an onion's layers, there is no "right order." Focus on whatever comes into your mind as still contributing to your discomfort about the situation: *beliefs, sensations, emotions, behaviors, values,* or *intentions.*

When Should I Look for Aspects? Aspects needing attention may come into your awareness at any point during the tapping, but you are most likely to notice them each time you take an SUD rating. In fact, a way to identify the next aspect to tap on is to ask yourself how you know the SUD is where it is. For instance, if you are tapping on your jealousy toward your sister, and it has gone down from an 8 to a 3, you might ask yourself, "How do I know it is still at 3? What's left?" Scan for sensations, emotions, beliefs, or images. This tells you where to focus next.

Should I Tap on Physical Aspects First or Psychological Aspects? Again, the order doesn't matter. Go with whatever comes most strongly into your awareness. If you aren't sure where to focus, gravitate toward the most concrete aspects, which are the physical ones. Scan your body for physical sensations. Or ask yourself, "What did I see, hear, touch, smell, or taste during the earlier event?" Physical sensations are often the building blocks for the emotions associated with a situation, and tapping on them can clear a great deal.

Should My Wording Be More General or More Detailed? In most cases, the wording should be as specific as possible. A department store clerk who is dealing with being oversensitive about criticism could simply say, *"My oversensitivity to criticism."* But the tapping will be more effective if he identifies specific incidents: *"I felt criticized when my boss didn't implement the idea I proposed." "I felt criticized when the couple bought a different TV than the one I recommended." "I felt criticized when no one replied to my Facebook post."* Even physical sensations can be divided into many aspects. Gary Craig points out that a headache may be an umbrella term for a combination of sensations, such as a sharp pain behind the left eye, a throbbing in the left temple, and a heaviness in the forehead. Tap on the one that is most intense. As it subsides, the next one needing attention will become evident.

Are There Times to Be Less Specific? An exception to the suggestion that you be as specific as possible involves working with severe trauma. For memories that may be "too hot to handle," in order not to risk retraumatizing yourself, you can use extremely general wordings such as *"That terrible thing that happened"* without naming what happened or who was involved. Or name the place, such as *"The basement."* Or name the theme, such as *"Alone"* or *"Injured."* Again, you don't need to fully immerse yourself in a traumatic memory to make it psychologically and physiologically active enough for the tapping to be effective.

Do I Have to Tap on Every Aspect of the Situation? For an intense experience, you may be surprised by how many aspects it contains. However, you may also be surprised by how quickly you can neutralize them as you tap on them one by one. Also, as you neutralize some of them, the intensity of others you haven't yet gotten to may simultaneously decrease. In addition, if many incidents had a similar theme, such as abuse or abandonment, fully processing several of the memories may have a "generalization effect," so the others lose their emotional charge. Your SUD ratings will let you know what still needs attention.

Do I Have to Do an Entire Tapping Cycle on Each Aspect? At this point, we suggest you go through an entire tapping cycle, focusing on only one aspect at a time. In fact, try to get the SUD for that aspect down to 0 or near 0, even if it means multiple rounds of tapping on it. However, if another aspect emerges, you may need to shift the focus of your tapping to that one and later return to the one you were originally working with. If you watch a skilled tapping practitioner, you may see the wording change at each acupoint during a single round of tapping. The phrases may approach the same aspect from different angles or you may see multiple aspects being addressed. You will find yourself becoming much more fluid in your use of words, but while you are learning the Protocol, we suggest that your tapping cycles focus on one aspect at a time.

What Is the Most Obvious Aspect That May Be Missed? A persistent problem often has roots in an earlier experience, though this might not occur to you spontaneously. Unprocessed experiences from your past may impede progress until they are addressed. To get at these earlier experiences, you might step back and ask yourself, "What does this situation [or image, feeling, thought, or memory] remind me of?" Tightness in your chest or feelings of anger are aspects that may lead you back to a pivotal memory. If your SUD won't go down, you can follow the strongest feeling or sensation back to one of the first times you had that feeling or sensation. You will learn more about this technique, called the "Affect Bridge," in the following chapter.

Aspects of Emma's Memory

Emma identified these aspects as she worked with her memory, and she tapped on each of them. By this point, they were already in the range of 2 to 4, and each went down to 0.

"The giant TV cameras."

"Having to hold hands with the boy in the Prince Charming costume."

"Feeling humiliated and ashamed."

"The director getting impatient with me."

"The design on the carpet as I stared down at the floor."

"Feeling judged and unsafe."

"Feeling inadequate."

Emma also identified two other memories that came up while working with the TV studio. In one, also at age seven, she was going to be in a ballet recital but had been ill with bronchitis and missed most of the rehearsals. At the time of the recital, she was well enough to perform, and her mother made her go to it. She felt scared, unprepared, and afraid of making mistakes because she didn't know the dance routine. In the other, she was nine and her entire class laughed at her when she flubbed a line during a video recording. The next day, the class was going to watch the video. She felt so embarrassed and fearful about being teased by her classmates that she didn't want to go to school. She told her mother she was sick. Her mother wasn't very sympathetic but let her stay home nonetheless. As each memory emerged, she shifted the focus of her tapping to that incident. This was the path to getting her memory about the TV studio down to 0, with no unpleasant charge mentally, emotionally, or physically.

Your Turn

Return to your memory and give it another SUD rating. Assuming it still has some emotional charge, focus on any aspect that comes up around the SUD not being at 0. If you're not sure, scan your body for sensations that may be related to the memory. Or go back into the memory and ask yourself, "What did I see, hear, touch, smell, or taste?" In addition to these physical aspects, related memories may come to mind; or emotions, beliefs, or images that don't necessarily seem directly connected to the memory. Tap on whatever arises. Be patient as you tap on each aspect you can identify. Remember, each round of tapping can usually be done within a minute.

See if you can get the SUD rating for your initial memory down to 0 by addressing all of its aspects. If you can't, skip the next section, "Testing Your Results," jump ahead to the following chapter on doing the "detective work," and then return to the remainder of this chapter when your SUD is down to 0.

PHASE 4: TESTING YOUR RESULTS

If the SUD for your memory is down to 0, terrific. This final step is to verify that the issue has indeed been fully resolved. We do this by mentally intensifying the scene or the issue.

As you replay it in your mind, let the colors be brighter, the sounds crisper, the interactions more real, the stakes higher—whatever makes the experience more vivid. If after this you are unable to reproduce any trace of the initial emotional response, the probability is strong that you have succeeded in deactivating your nervous system's autonomic response to the memory. But if you don't pass this test, simply tap on whatever came up. There will likely be some back-and-forth between this phase and working with aspects in the previous phase.

The other way of testing your results is to see what happens after the session when you are actually confronted with the challenges you were tapping on instead of imagining them. Because you have been working on your emotional response to a memory, this doesn't apply right now. You can't make the scene happen again. But if later in the program you're dealing with anxiety whenever you speak to your boss, for instance, or excessive anger when your spouse makes a mess after you just cleaned up, these real-life tests will occur naturally. You don't need to manufacture them. If you don't "pass," it is not a failure but rather the discovery of other aspects that need tapping.

IF THE SUD WON'T GO DOWN TO 0

On some issues, the SUD simply won't go down to 0. For instance, if you are a competitive athlete or a performing artist, having a bit of anxiety before an event may help bring out your best. Or having some discomfort in the presence of a seemingly nice person who in the past has subjected you to abusive behavior may be a reminder to stay on guard. Or you may actually feel comfortable with a bit of distress around a given issue. Sometimes an area of intense distress has been around for so long that getting it down to a 2 or 3 is such a relief that you may be comfortable leaving it there for a while. What tapping *can do* in any of these situations is decrease your stress response so you can meet the challenges with your undivided emotional attention and full creativity. For most issues, bringing your SUD close to or down to 0 is attainable and desirable, even if it requires multiple rounds of tapping.

Emma's Test

"Even as I recalled the TV studio scene as vividly as I could, I felt no tension in my body or mind, so the SUD is 0. I will know for sure the next time I need to perform or speak in front of a group of people because that usually feels like something close to a panic attack. If I stay calm, I'll know that neutralizing these memories from my childhood really carried over! But even if I do feel anxious, it's reassuring to know I can use the tapping to turn it around."

Your Turn

Test your results by making the memory as vivid as possible, fully stepping into the scene with your imagination. Give your experience an SUD rating. If it is 0, you are done. Reflect on any guiding models associated with that memory. Are they changing along with your response to the memory? If the SUD has not stayed at 0 after you've tested it, notice what came up for you and tap on it as another aspect of the memory that needs your attention. Then test again. If you can't get it down, the following chapter will provide more advanced tools.

SHORTCUTS TO THE BASIC TAPPING PROTOCOL

Since each round of tapping takes only a minute or less, you may wonder why we would even introduce shortcuts. After all, how much shorter than a minute do we need? But to fully resolve an issue may require many rounds of tapping as you go through the steps and focus on multiple aspects.

To this point, we've been encouraging you to follow all the steps in the Basic Tapping Protocol. This grounds you in the procedures and provides the context if shortcuts are to be introduced. But if you are working on complex issues where many trips through the Protocol will be needed, streamlining the process has obvious advantages. Most advanced tapping practitioners are able to fluidly jump around within the Protocol, skipping a step here, dwelling on an issue there. This comes with experience and is part of the art of energy psychology, but here are five concrete shortcuts you can already begin to use depending on the situation:

1. Skipping the Acceptance Statement

The Acceptance Statement reminds you that whatever difficulties may be caused by the outmoded guiding model you are trying to change, you were doing the best you knew how given your circumstances and internal resources when you developed the model. Affirming this validates your ability to take the next steps. We usually use the Acceptance Statement at the start of each tapping cycle because it requires only a few seconds and serves good purposes, but particularly when we are on a roll in pursuing an issue, we might go through multiple rounds of tapping before returning to another Acceptance Statement.

2. Shortening the Tapping Sequence

Tapping on the acupoints specified for a "round" of tapping is the primary ingredient of the Basic Tapping Protocol. This sequence is already a shortcut. Of the hundreds of acupoints on the body, the Basic Tapping Protocol uses only 12. Research shows that this is usually enough for the tapping to be effective. The minimum number of points needed, or the precise points that will be the most optimal, are still questions for further research. We usually use all dozen points, but sometimes as a session progresses, we will switch to using only a few acupoints as we focus on a particular issue or aspect, quickly moving through the points multiple times while stating Reminder Phrases. The four points that are useful for this situation happen to be part of the Daily Energy Routine discussed in the Appendix. They are the points:

1. Under the eyes

2. At the collarbone

3. Over the Heart Chakra

4. On the sides of the chest (about four to six inches below the armpits)

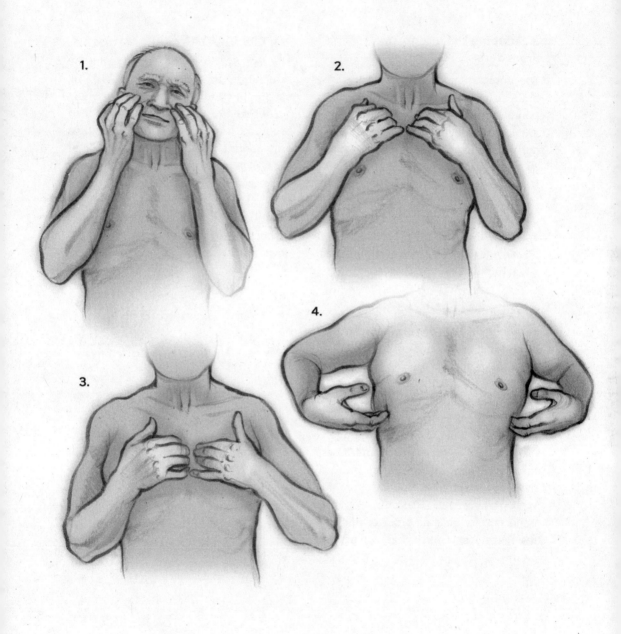

Figure 2.5. You can move through these quickly multiple times as you focus on a particular issue, sensation, or other aspect.

3. Skipping the Integration Procedure

The Integration Procedure allows the brain to take a breather from the emotional focus in order to process it. We find it very valuable, almost always use it during the first tapping cycle, and rarely go through three cycles without using it. However, sometimes you have gained momentum on a particular issue and don't want to interrupt it. As long as you are doing the Integration Procedure periodically, go with your own intuition about when to skip it.

4. Skipping the SUD Rating

Frequently assessing how you are responding to the tapping and the wording you are using provides instant feedback that frequently leads to shifts in your focus. Again, however, it is not necessary to use it every time. In fact, some people find that shifting into the analytical mindset required to do the assessment interferes with the more intuitive flow they enter when doing the tapping. While taking the SUD rating remains important for gauging progress and finding next steps, come to your own balance on this.

5. Using the Eye Sweep

The Eye Sweep is the last step in the Integration Procedure. It can also be used alone and may be a useful shortcut when the SUD intensity has been brought down to a 2 or less. It requires only about six seconds, and because of the way you are consciously sending any remaining disturbed energies out your eyes as they go in an upward motion, we have found that the Eye Sweep alone is a shortcut that can often get the SUD down quickly.

The Basic 12-Step Tapping Protocol on a Page

Phase 1 Preparation Phase:

- Choose your initial focus.

- Rate your discomfort about it.

- Create a Reminder Phrase to keep it psychologically active.

- Formulate an Acceptance Statement about the issue and the feelings it triggers.

Phase 2 The Tapping Cycle:

- Anchor your Acceptance Statement.

- Complete the first round of tapping (while saying your Reminder Phrase).

- Practice the Integration Procedure.

- Complete the second round of tapping (again with your Reminder Phrase).

- Take a new SUD rating.

Phase 3 Adjusting the Protocol:

- Modify your Acceptance Statement.

- Address the aspects of the situation by going beyond your Reminder Phrase.

Phase 4 Testing Your Results

ON TO CHAPTER 3

If your memory still has an emotional charge, bring it to Chapter 3. If it no longer has a charge, we will ask you to select a new issue as you learn the detective work for resolving challenging issues.

CHAPTER 3

The Detective Work

Breaking an issue into smaller parts and tapping on them individually is the biggest key to EFT success.[1]

—Gary Craig

Founder of EFT

IF YOU'VE BEEN APPLYING the Basic Tapping Protocol but your issue isn't getting resolved, you probably don't know all the reasons. This chapter shows you how to conduct the detective work that can help you resolve or at least make significant headway on most issues. The approach presented in the previous chapter is simple, quick, and easy to apply once you've internalized the steps, and it will usually lead to the results you are hoping for. If it doesn't, however, the more complex journey this chapter will take you through probably will.

You can focus either on whatever is unresolved from the previous chapter or any other issue you choose. By the end of this chapter, you will understand some of the most powerful tools energy psychology has to offer. You can proceed through the chapter in any of three ways:

- If your SUD rating on the memory you worked with in the previous chapter hasn't decreased to your satisfaction, this chapter will show you the next steps.

- You may have a particular issue in mind that you would like to work with using this book. If so, you can apply the Basic Tapping Protocol to it by going through the previous chapter, but instead of a memory, focus on the issue you have chosen.

- You can skip this chapter for now and move on to Part II, returning any time you feel stuck as you advance through the remainder of the book.

CHOOSE YOUR FOCUS

Begin by deciding whether you will continue with your memory from the previous chapter, select a new area of focus, or jump to Part II.

Our test driver for this chapter, Leah, is a New York talent agent in her mid-40s. She had received individual coaching from a tapping practitioner to build her confidence for working with celebrities, so she was familiar with the approach.

Leah's Focus

Leah hadn't been able to get the SUD on her troubling memory down to 0 by the end of Chapter 2, so she continued with it. The memory was from when she was seven and at school. She felt too embarrassed to ask to use the bathroom during class, and after trying to "let a little bit out," the inevitable happened. She was mortified, writing in her journal: "My memory of the sensation of wet pants and socks continues to give me shivers (quick tensing of muscles in my upper arms and shoulders). With this sensation were the thoughts that I'm disgusting, undesirable, and that I disappoint others. The level of distress around this started at 10 but was down to 3 by the end of Chapter 2."

Your Turn

Choose the area you wish to focus upon that may require some detective work. If you are going to a new topic, you can choose any type of issue you wish: another troubling memory; something that triggers an unwanted emotional response, such as anger, jealousy, or fear; a place you are stuck in your life; a difficult relationship . . . anything that matters to you. Describe your focus for this chapter in your journal with as much detail as you wish and give an SUD rating to the amount of discomfort or distress that thinking about the issue causes in your mind and/or body right now.

If you are focusing on a new issue, the first step is to apply the entire Basic Tapping Protocol from the previous chapter to that issue before you continue with this chapter. But you don't need to reread Chapter 2 to apply the Basic Tapping Protocol. A list of the steps is on p. 79, and if you need more detail, you can scan the chapter for the "Your Turn" headings, which give instructions for each step. It should be a familiar process by now, and it should continue to get easier as you internalize the steps as you proceed through the book.

REASONS THE BASIC TAPPING PROTOCOL MAY NOT HAVE BEEN ENOUGH

The Basic Tapping Protocol is the place to begin with any concern where you apply tapping, but for longstanding multilayered issues, some detective work is often also needed. In law enforcement, detective work is oriented toward finding and interpreting clues to solve crimes. In energy psychology, detective work is oriented toward finding and resolving whatever is in the way of successfully reaching the goal of your tapping. This process involves recognizing and eliminating psychological blocks to your progress. Several types of obstacles tend to occur, and we will guide you in how to overcome each. The topics we will cover include:

1. Disharmony in your body's energies

2. Unrecognized internal objections to reaching your goal

3. Additional reasons not to change

4. Cognitive distortions and self-limiting beliefs

5. Digging into the roots of the problem

6. Resolving conflicts that are preventing progress

And finally, as the obstacles have been overcome

7. Installing a new guiding model

We will discuss these one at a time and provide instructions for applying the principles governing each issue to the goal you have chosen. It is not necessary, however, to work through every step in this comprehensive guide, though you might find each to be interesting. Also, if after *any* of the steps, your SUD on your initial problem has gone down to 0, you can jump to the seventh step (p. 117) to reinforce the progress and return to the others when your work with a different topic warrants it.

1. DISHARMONY IN YOUR BODY'S ENERGIES

Wholesome physical practices impact your mental health. Exercise that raises your heart rate every day, sufficient sleep, and a healthy diet have a positive influence on your ability to think, learn, and adapt. Tapping protocols will generally be helpful whether or not you are taking good physical care of yourself, but attending to the basics of physical health is going to serve you in many ways. While we encourage you to develop healthy physical habits, that isn't the purpose of this book. However, there is one area in which your physical state can significantly interfere with the beneficial potentials of acupoint tapping—disharmony in your body's energies.

This disharmony may involve hyperarousal, blockages, or depletion. You might experience *hyperarousal* as agitation or anxiety. *Blockages* are often registered as pain or confusion. *Depleted* energies can be experienced as mental exhaustion or depression. While depleted energies may be corrected by a good night's sleep, feeling run-down isn't always due to a lack of rest. It may arise because of imbalances in your energy system.

Energy techniques can help with any of these physical manifestations of energy imbalances. Rather than masking symptoms, as many medications do, energy techniques address physical problems by correcting them at their *energetic* foundations. Similarly, when disharmonies in your body's energies are preventing tapping from having the intended psychological effects, applying an energy intervention does not bury the emotional problem. Rather, it clears your mind so you can deal with the problem more effectively. And it restores your brain's electromagnetic activity to a state in which tapping on emotional issues will be effective again. Just tapping on the 12 acupuncture points without any words or focus on a problem is a quick way of balancing your energies. The breathing technique you learned in Chapter 1 is another.

Decades ago, we developed a sequence of exercises that we call the "Daily Energy Routine" (DER). Requiring only about five to seven minutes, it is designed to establish positive "energy habits" in your body that strengthen your immune system and help you navigate through common everyday stresses. In fact, some energy psychology practitioners have all their clients do the DER prior to each tapping session. If you're interested in learning more about this practice and its benefits, you can go to der.energytapping.com. More information can also be found in the Appendix.

Leah's Energy Routine

Leah experimented with the best times to use the DER. She found that doing it before her workout at the gym was a great warm-up that made the workout go more smoothly. The most valuable time she found, however, was to take a few minutes to do the DER before meeting with a client. She then went into these meetings with her mind clear, her mood positive, and her confidence strong.

Your Turn

Any time that tapping isn't having the desired effect, a powerful correction is to shift your energies. You can use any of the energy-balancing exercises in the Appendix. For instance, if your SUD seems stuck, you can place one hand on your forehead, the other on the back of your head, and take five deep breaths, in through your nose and out through your mouth. Then go through another tapping cycle. See if your SUD goes down. You can use this, the DER, or any other energy-balancing technique in the Appendix at any point that you feel a bit scattered or discouraged as you work through this book.

2. UNRECOGNIZED INTERNAL OBJECTIONS TO REACHING YOUR GOAL

While the Basic Tapping Protocol alone can rapidly reduce or even eliminate fear, anxiety, or anger, many concerns require additional steps, some involving how to deal with objections you may not know you have about resolving your issue. In guiding you in this additional work, we are committed to keeping our suggestions consistent with the best available concepts and practices from the mental health field. With that in mind, we'll take a little detour to look at cognitive behavioral therapy (CBT), which is considered, in many clinical settings to be the "treatment of choice" for a wide range of psychological conditions.[2] In Chapter 2, we identified CBT as the *third wave* of psychotherapy, with the somatic component of energy psychology making it a *fourth wave* approach.

Cognitive Behavioral Therapy and Energy Psychology: Similarities and Differences

CBT is centered on the fact that our thoughts influence our feelings and shape our behavior. The therapy is oriented toward changing the messages in our self-talk. This can help you overcome many difficulties such as anxiety and depression and bring greater success and happiness into your life. CBT and acupoint tapping protocols share important features. Both devote substantial attention to beliefs and feelings; both have procedures for overcoming the emotional damage caused by trauma or other adverse events; and when first introduced, each received a notably cold reception from the clinical community.

David Burns, a psychiatrist in the Stanford School of Medicine and one of the most highly regarded practitioners, teachers, and proponents of CBT, notes that when it first appeared, "most psychiatrists and psychologists considered CBT a form of quackery."[3] CBT has countered these perceptions with literally thousands of clinical trials demonstrating its effectiveness. While CBT is still widely seen as the gold standard for treating a broad range of psychological conditions, more than 170 peer-reviewed clinical trials published in English-language journals (and more than 90 additional studies in non-English language journals, originating primarily in hospitals, clinics, and universities) have now shown tapping protocols to be effective, durable, and unusually fast.[4] In relation to CBT, 10 studies to date have compared CBT with protocols that include tapping on acupoints.[5] In all 10 studies, the tapping protocols produced clinical outcomes that were at least equivalent. Several of the studies demonstrated advantages of tapping over CBT in speed and the stability of improvements.

You will see in this and subsequent chapters the power of adding acupoint tapping to the fundamental CBT concept of changing your self-talk. This involves both the inner talk you are aware of and the subliminal talk that doesn't reach your awareness. Both forms of self-talk are intricately linked with the internal guiding models that shape your life.

Even without tapping, however, when CBT is effective, it can be very effective. Dr. Burns' book *Feeling Good*,[6] which teaches people how to apply CBT to anxiety, depression, and other mental health challenges, has sold more than five million copies. Studies independent of Burns' research have shown that some two-thirds of the people who have read *Feeling Good* while on a wait list for psychotherapy made such substantial emotional gains based on using the book alone that "they no longer required treatment."[7]

Puzzling about the one-third who didn't experience such benefits, Dr. Burns formulated procedures that directly address the person's motivation. In one sense, motivation for overcoming psychological and behavioral difficulties is not a problem. Everyone wants to feel better and to be successful in whatever matters to them. All therapists understand this. But all therapists also understand that *conscious* resistance to doing what is necessary for change and *unconscious* resistance to attaining what one desires are two core dynamics in many of the problems that lead people to seek help. Such resistance counters our intentions. One of the main components Dr. Burns added to CBT for working with motivation and resistance involves accepting oneself and one's resistance. Both the updated approach to CBT and standard energy psychology protocols address resistance directly, but again, tapping adds another dimension.

Overcoming Resistance by Accepting What Is

Accepting yourself and the difficulties you face decreases, somewhat paradoxically, your resistance to overcoming those difficulties. This shift of emphasis early in CBT treatments markedly increased speed and improved treatment outcomes.[8] Dr. Burns' approach acknowledges, understands, and accepts where you are as well as your resistance to change. This is akin to Carl Rogers' cardinal insight, emphasized in Chapter 2, that accepting what you want to change in yourself is often a requirement for willfully and successfully changing it.[9]

The Basic Tapping Protocol addresses motivation and resistance in a number of ways. An essential component of the Protocol is the Acceptance Statement— for example, *"Even though [name the emotional response, automatic thought, or problematic behavior you want to change], I accept myself just as I am."* Rather than mobilizing your energies against yourself, you are building an association between what you want to change and self-acceptance. Then you use energy techniques to implant this pairing into your nervous system. Issues of motivation and resistance may further be resolved as you explore and tap on *aspects* of the concern related to motivation or resistance.

Psychological Reversals

If the Basic Tapping Protocol has stopped reducing your SUD, another area to explore (beyond accepting the problem and bringing better harmony and balance to your body's energies with procedures like the Daily Energy Routine) is whether additional focus needs to be brought to internal resistance about resolving the issue. The term *Psychological Reversal* is used in energy psychology to describe this territory.

A Psychological Reversal is at play when unconscious resistance is interfering with a desired outcome. It is as if a part of you seems to want the opposite of what you consciously desire, or you do the reverse of what you intend. All forms of therapy have to deal with the dynamics of Psychological Reversals because the decision to change a pattern of thought, behavior, or emotion frequently comes into conflict with the part of the person that initially established that pattern.

Psychological Reversals are usually fought out beneath conscious awareness and often with no resolution. Something is holding you back, but you don't know what it is. For instance, you might want never to "fly off the handle" with your partner, but you find that the more determined you feel, the more reactive your behavior. This is typical of a Psychological Reversal—the harder you try, the more powerful the resistance.

Psychological Reversals may be quite tangential to your life's purpose ("If I learn to sew, I'll be expected to mend the kids' clothes") or central ("If I tell my partner what I need, I won't be loved"). Recognizing a buried Psychological Reversal can be an important step toward resolving the issue you are addressing. But some Psychological Reversals may already be in your awareness, as when the inner conflict is about a secondary gain, such as needing to keep a symptom in order to continue disability insurance or release from certain responsibilities: "If I'm no longer so depressed that I can hardly function, I'll be expected to go back to work." We do not mean to imply in any way that most people hold on to disabilities to retain secondary gains, only that it is a possible dynamic to explore when interventions that should be effective aren't working. Other themes for Psychological Reversals might consciously or unconsciously include, "If I truly learn how to relax and not push myself so hard, I won't achieve as much"; "If I do well on my interview and get that important job, I'll have to move away from my family"; or "If I learn how to cook, I'll get asked to prepare dinner" (David's cover).

Psychological Reversals often appear in clinical practice. A colleague was using a tapping protocol with a woman who was seeking help to get over her fear of flying. The client's SUD went down from a 10 to a 5 but seemed stuck until she was asked how her life would be different if she got over her flying phobia. She divulged that then she would "have to go on those dreadful business trips with my husband." Using the tapping to reduce the charge on that concern didn't cause her to suddenly enjoy the business trips, but it did make it possible for her to deal with the situation instead of hiding behind her phobia. The focus of the next session of her therapy shifted to being more assertive with her husband as well as the formative experiences that made this difficult. Once she had achieved reasonable progress on this, the remaining charge on her fear of flying quickly responded to the tapping.

Identifying Psychological Reversals That May Be Involved with Your Issue

The seven most common types of Psychological Reversals addressed in energy psychology training programs have to do with the following:

- **Desirability:** a conflict about *wanting* to resolve the issue.

- **Plausibility:** a belief that it is not *possible* to overcome the problem.

- **Safety:** a feeling that it is not *safe* to overcome it.

- **Worthiness:** a conviction that you don't *deserve* to overcome it.

- **Sacrifice:** not wanting to *give up* something that would be necessary for overcoming it.

- **Courage and Determination:** not being willing to *do what is necessary* to overcome it.

- **Identity:** a sense that overcoming the problem is not compatible with who you are.

Following is a set of questions you can ask yourself in order to identify Psychological Reversals that might be impeding your progress with the Basic Tapping Protocol:

- **Desirability:** Do I really *want* to fully resolve this problem [or achieve this goal]?

- **Plausibility:** Do I believe it is *possible* to fully resolve this problem [or achieve this goal]?

- **Safety:** Do I feel it is *safe* to fully resolve this problem [or achieve this goal]?

- **Worthiness:** Do I *deserve* to fully resolve this problem [or achieve this goal]?

- **Sacrifice:** What would I have to *give up* if I were to fully resolve this problem [or achieve this goal]?

- **Courage and Determination:** Am I *willing* to do what's necessary to fully resolve this problem [or achieve this goal]?

- **Identity:** Would I still *feel like me* if I fully resolve this problem [or achieve this goal]?

Leah's Psychological Reversals

(Remember that Leah was addressing a disturbing memory of wetting her pants at school.)

- **Do I really want to fully resolve this problem?** *Yes, please.*

- **Do I believe it is possible to fully resolve this problem?** *Probably not. The beliefs that I'm not okay, that I'm disgusting and undesirable, and that I disappoint others are deeply rooted in my past.*

- **Is it safe to fully resolve this problem?** *Yes.*

- **Do I deserve to fully resolve this problem?** *Hmm. Sixty percent yes.*

- **What would I have to give up if I were to fully resolve this problem?** *I'd have to give up the nagging belief that something is wrong with me and that I'm undeserving of healing this.*

- **Am I willing to do what's necessary to fully resolve this problem?** *Yes. But the incident was so long ago that it sort of sucks to have to be going through it now.*

- **Would I still feel like me if I fully resolve this problem?** *Yes, I would still feel like me, just cleaner inside.*

Your Turn

Describe in your journal answers to any of these questions that bring up an internal conflict about resolving your issue. Just naming a Psychological Reversal is a step toward overcoming it. Adding brief energy techniques to what you have identified can usually take you far enough so you can proceed with the Basic Tapping Protocol without the Psychological Reversal interfering with progress. A deceptively simple yet effective formula was already introduced in Chapter 2 ("Even though . . . ," p. 56), and you will be using it throughout the book. The following section shows you how to apply this formula to Psychological Reversals.

Addressing Psychological Reversals with the First Part of Your Acceptance Statement

In our experiences, and in those of tapping practitioners we've spoken with, resolving a Psychological Reversal at the energetic level can usually dispense with the need for a complicated and often lengthy analysis of a problem. It still might not feel completely safe to overcome your fear of heights, or you still might not fully believe that you deserve financial success, but the technique does enough energetically so that tapping on the problem or goal that had been stalled becomes effective again. In Chapter 2 you learned how to adjust your Acceptance Statement as you went from one tapping cycle to another, mostly by inserting modifiers like "still" and "some of": *"Even though I still have some of this problem . . ."*

The original Acceptance Statement can be completely changed at any point in the tapping process to focus on a specific facet of the issue needing attention, including any Psychological Reversals that are keeping your SUD from decreasing. The basic structure of the statement is the same, but the content of the first part of the statement will now focus on the Psychological Reversal. For instance, pertaining to the questions posed above, if you identified a reversal based on any of these questions, the wording might become:

"Even though I don't really want to fully resolve this problem [or achieve this goal] . . ."

"Even though I don't believe it is possible to fully resolve this problem [or achieve this goal] . . ."

"Even though it's not safe for me to fully resolve this problem [or achieve this goal] . . ."

"Even though I don't deserve to fully resolve this problem [or achieve this goal] . . ."

"Even though I don't want to give up [the time, the effort, someone's friendship, etc.] in order to fully resolve this problem [or achieve this goal] . . ."

"Even though I don't have the courage or determination to do what's necessary to fully resolve this problem [or achieve this goal] . . ."

"Even though it wouldn't still feel like me if I were to fully resolve this problem [or achieve this goal] . . ."

Leah's "Even Though" Statements

Tying into the Psychological Reversals she had identified above, Leah wrote,

"Even though I don't believe it is possible to be 100 percent free of these feelings of humiliation and disgust . . ."

"Even though part of me believes I deserve to suffer and hold on to these feelings . . ."

"Even though I don't deserve to heal or be forgiven . . ."

"Even though working through this is really hard, and there are days I don't want to do it . . ."

Your Turn

Craft a phrase that captures the essence of each of the Psychological Reversals you identified, beginning the phrase with "Even though . . . ," and record it in your journal.

Addressing Psychological Reversals with the Second Part of Your Statement

The second part of your revised statement can still be any version of *"I accept myself just as I am"* or it can be completely changed to focus on *choice* and *opportunity*. An Acceptance Statement may at any point be changed into a "Choices Statement." For instance:

*"Even though I don't want to deal with my son's defiance, **I choose right now to tune in to my love for him.**"*

*"Even though it's not possible for me to lose this weight, **I choose to love and accept myself just as I am.**"*

*"Even though it's not safe for me to get over my fear of heights, **I choose to realize that I won't take unnecessary risks even if I do overcome the fear.**"*

*"Even though I don't deserve to be happy when others are suffering, **I choose to know that keeping my spirits up is one of my most precious responsibilities to myself and to those who matter to me.**"*

*"Even though I don't want to risk my friendship with Jake, **I choose to know that it will never be quite right again if I don't tell him how he hurt me.**"*

*"Even though it doesn't feel like me if I accept my boss' stupid decisions without arguing, **I choose my battles with discernment**."*

Notice that while the tone of the wording still supports your acceptance of what you are trying to change, it also maps a more empowering way to think about the situation. This creates a pathway for a *negative thought* to become a positive choice, a link at a deep level between an acknowledgment of a problem and a constructive way of dealing with it. This approach, known as the "Choices Method," can work with any emotional challenge or personal goal, not just Psychological Reversals:

*"Even though I'm so driven by my work that my life is way out of balance, **I choose to recognize that my worth as a person is not about my accomplishments**."*

*"Even though I feel trapped in this abusive relationship, **I choose to know that I deserve to have a loving, supportive partner**."*

*"Even though I feel deprived for not having that extra helping, **I choose to know that my body is fully nourished**."*

*"Even though I don't feel like getting on that crowded plane, **I choose to have a restful and enjoyable flight**."*

Of course, some creativity is required to come up with an empowering *choice* that meaningfully addresses the *"Even though"* portion of the statement. Here is some guidance for formulating that wording.

Origins of the Choices Method

The Choices Method was developed by the psychologist and EFT pioneer Patricia Carrington.[10] It can be tailored to any situation—from feeling sad that your daughter would rather hang out with her friends than join you for a movie to challenges that feel bleak and hopeless. A depressed man in his first psychotherapy session was helped to craft this statement: *"Even though my life is hopeless, I choose to find unexpected help in this therapy."*

The Choices Method can also be applied when a person is grappling with an appalling or disastrous situation or experience. A young man lost two of his closest friends when a drunk driver crashed into the car he was driving. He was the only survivor. He developed this Choices Statement: *"Even though I feel overwhelming guilt that I'm still alive, I choose to know that Sid and Raul would want me to fully live life they were deprived of."*

Writing to her colleagues the day after 9/11 on how to assist people dealing with the psychological aftermath of the attack, Dr. Carrington suggested using phrases such as:

"Even though I am stunned and bewildered, I choose to be a still point amid the chaos."

"Even though I am stunned and bewildered, I choose to learn something absolutely essential for my own life from this event."

"Even though I am stunned and bewildered, I choose to have this dreadful event open my heart."

Finding a phrase that recognizes an empowering choice or opportunity obviously requires some ingenuity, but it is easier than it might seem. For starters, Dr. Carrington has an all-purpose default phrase that you can use under any circumstances:

"I choose to be calm and confident."

This can follow a wide range of "Even though" situations:

"Even though I'm nervous about taking the test, **I choose to be calm and confident.**"

"Even though I'm furious with my husband, **I choose to be calm and confident.**"

"Even though I don't know how to help my daughter with her heartbreak, **I choose to be calm and confident.**"

"Even though I'm feeling judged, **I choose to be calm and confident.**"

"Even though I'm scared about tonight's performance, **I choose to be calm and confident.**"

"Even though everything hangs on this interview, **I choose to be calm and confident.**"

In addition to "I choose to be calm and confident" as a default statement, Dr. Carrington suggests a variety of other phrases that can also get you started, such as:

"Even though . . . , **I choose to find a creative way to . . .**"

"Even though . . . , **I choose to find it fun to . . .**"

"Even though . . . , **I choose to think up new ideas for . . .**"

"Even though . . . , **I choose to let it be easy to . . .**"

"Even though . . . , **I choose to surprise myself by . . .**"

Here's a Choices Statement from a friend who tended to become belligerent during disagreements: "Even though I'm afraid of losing the argument, I choose to surprise myself by finding easy and enjoyable ways to get my point across." Pairing the power of well-crafted self-suggestions with energy methods is a winning combination. Dr. Carrington also recommends inserting words that give your statement more appeal and thus greater potency, such as comfortable, satisfying, delightful, ingenious, safe, or unexpected.

Leah's Choices Statements

Using the Choices Method with her Psychological Reversals, Leah combined the earlier phrases (first part of each sentence) with the following Choices Statements (second part of each sentence):

"*Even though I don't believe it is possible to be 100 percent free of this memory of humiliation and feelings of disgust,* **I choose to be curious and open to shifting my beliefs.**"

"*Even though part of me believes I deserve to suffer and hold on to these feelings,* **I choose to recognize that this self-punishment serves no one.**"

"*Even though I don't deserve to heal or be forgiven,* **I choose to remember that I was just a little girl.**"

"*Even though working through this is really hard, and there are days I don't want to do it,* **I choose to commit to tapping on whatever comes up for me.**"

Your Turn

Complete each of your Psychological Reversal statements with a Choices Statement. Use the Choices Method to formulate an opportunity or empowering way of thinking about the situation. For each statement, say it out loud, again rubbing your chest sore spots with the first phrase and holding your hands over your Heart Chakra with the second. While it might be tempting to rush through if you have a list of statements, take your time. Be deliberate as you focus on each statement. Go through this process two or three times with each Psychological Reversal. Then take another SUD rating on the distress in your mind and/or body caused by your original issue.

Reflections

At any point in doing this detective work, new insights that don't quite fit the book's structure may occur to you. Welcome them. They may shift your direction as you move forward. For instance, Leah wrote in her journal,

I rubbed and tapped on each of the Psychological Reversal statements and retested my SUD. I was disappointed to find that after all those steps, it was still at a 3. I realized, however, that I'm always uncomfortable with the sensation of wetness between my legs and that it had to do with disgust related to some of my earliest sexual experiences. This went much deeper than just what happened in the classroom when I was seven. I realized that dampness between my legs brings up feelings of self-judgment and disgust. I came up with a new, more general Choices Statement: *"Even though I'm disgusted by the sensation of wetness between my legs, I choose to know this is natural and healthy."* This brought up all the feelings of the earlier sexual experiences, and after saying this while rubbing my chest sore spots and holding my Heart Chakra, I tapped through all 12 points while stating phrases such as *"Wetness between my legs," "This is natural," "I'm a healthy woman."*

That is how detective work often unfolds while creating Choices Statements. With the discovery of how her bodily sensation was connected to another issue, Leah creatively applied the Basic Tapping Protocol to clear disproportionate emotions from her memories. Next, she continued to address her discomfort with any dampness between her legs but no longer limited it to what occurred in the classroom. This ultimately had a powerful effect on her enjoyment of her sexuality, an outcome she wasn't looking for and never expected, yet it was welcomed with delight.

3. ADDITIONAL REASONS NOT TO CHANGE

All complex systems resist change. That is how they remain intact. Resistance is both inevitable and inherently self-protective. This also applies to any well-established psychological structures, including your internal guiding models. Psychological Reversals are a type of resistance to changing a guiding model, so you may have already identified reasons not to change, but this section may uncover others that are also worth addressing.

In discussing resistance, Dr. Burns suggests to his colleagues that therapists too often ignore the *resilience* in their clients that *produces* resistance. He asks,

> What if the negative thinking patterns, feelings, and behaviors that keep them stuck have powerful unconscious advantages serving vital, even life-preserving purposes? . . . What if their resistance to change reveals something positive, beautiful, and even healthy about them?[11]

Dr. Burns goes on to suggest that before trying to bring about change, first "explore the many *good* reasons a client might have for not changing."[12]

He has found that putting unconscious resistance to change front and center can transform it into the kind of self-understanding that allows change to occur unimpeded. Rather than fight your resistance, the basic guideline is to meet it with curiosity and to find the positive intention hidden within the resistance.

In working with resistance, Dr. Burns addresses *unacknowledged objections to reaching a goal* so they don't impede future progress.[13] For instance, he might reframe guilt and shame as evidence that you have a well-developed moral compass (despite the fact that far more effective ways exist for maintaining a moral compass). Feelings of inadequacy may be recognized as growing out of humility and high standards. Anger might show a willingness to step up with passion for a good purpose. Hopelessness may be keeping you from having expectations that are likely to be disappointing, even as it is also keeping you from actively improving your situation. You will see how tapping can be applied to these insights as we examine why you *shouldn't* change.

Creating a List of Your Reasons Not to Change

If your SUD is not going down after rebalancing your body's energies and addressing any Psychological Reversals you have identified, the next area to explore is whether you have strong and valid reasons *not* to change. This doesn't necessarily mean that in the final analysis you won't still pursue the change you are envisioning but rather you have given the reasons not to change enough consideration that they don't turn up as unconscious resistance and sabotage your efforts.

A simple but useful format for tapping on these reasons not to make the desired change is *"If I . . . , then . . ."* Here are some examples:

> *"**If I** keep revisiting these dark thoughts, **then** I will be ready no matter what bad things happen."*

> *"**If I** am super-strict in disciplining my son, **then** he won't turn out to be a juvenile delinquent like my brother did."*

> *"**If I** keep this extra weight, **then** men won't bother me."*

> *"**If I** remain angry at my husband, **then** I will be making it clear to him that he is never to betray me again."*

> *"**If I** hide my accomplishments, **then** my sister won't feel jealous and take it out on me."*

> *"**If I** stay anxious and fearful, **then** I'll be safer because I'll be more vigilant."*

> *"**If I** let myself feel and show my happiness, **then** people will see me as shallow and uncaring about the suffering of others."*

> *"**If I** continue to judge myself harshly, **then** I will keep improving."*

> *"**If I** remain depressed, **then** people will have to recognize all the bad things in my life."*

Leah's Reasons Not to Change

No longer focusing on the classroom humiliation, Leah shifted her attention to her discomfort and sense of disgust about dampness between her legs. She made the following list of reasons not to change:

"If I maintain the belief that wetness between my legs is disgusting . . ."

". . . then I will never have to say yes to sex."

". . . then I will stay on a righteous path."

". . . then I will be more pure, clean, holy, and acceptable to God."

Your Turn

Make a list of your objections to overcoming your problem or reaching your goal. Use the *"If I . . . , then . . ."* format. If you are having difficulty finding any objections to overcoming your problem, we suggest you look deeper. Many problems persist in part because of the conscious or unconscious reasons for maintaining them, whether rational or not.

Working with Your Reasons Not to Change

Once you have recognized your reasons not to change, two steps will help you move forward.

1. Embrace these reasons rather than remain unconsciously entangled in them.

2. Use tapping to reduce the charge on both sides of your *"If I . . . , then . . ."* statements.

If you accept that these reasons exist, you can make a more informed decision about whether to proceed with your efforts to make that change. Then *if* you still choose to make the change after addressing each of your objections in this manner, you will have made your subsequent actions more likely to bring about the change you desire.

Leah Addressing Her Reasons Not to Change

Leah built a chart to track her progress with the tapping. The SUD number represents the subjective strength of the reason not to change.

SUD BEFORE TAPPING	IF I	THEN	SUD AFTER TAPPING
8	. . . maintain the belief that wetness between my legs is disgusting	. . . I will never have to say yes to sex.	0
6	. . . maintain the belief that wetness between my legs is disgusting	. . . I will stay on a righteous path.	3
6	. . . maintain the belief that wetness between my legs is disgusting	. . . I will be more pure, clean, holy, and acceptable to God.	3

Leah did extensive journaling after tapping on each issue:

After tapping on the first reason, *"I will never have to say yes to sex,"* a memory emerged that I've stuffed away for years. I was at a party, and a boy I didn't particularly like trapped me in a dark room. He started touching me in intimate places, and it felt good, so I let him continue. Someone walked in and turned on the lights, abruptly putting an end to it, but my guilt afterward was enormous.

I tapped on that guilt. It responded quickly. I found it easy to forgive myself for being young and confused, and it was down to 0 after just a few rounds. I then returned to tapping on *"If I maintain the belief that wetness between my legs is disgusting, I will never have to say yes to sex."* What came was not only an acceptance that the belief served me in some ways but also an affirmation that it is okay to say no to sex, and that I never *have to* say yes. I don't need to feel disgust in order to say no.

I felt a sense of freedom in recognizing that I can choose to be sexually intimate or not. My discomfort around the statement shifted to a 0 when I acknowledged the impact of early religious messaging I received about sex and sinfulness. The pastor at the church I attended growing up emphasized that sin is so vile, so abhorrent, and so disgusting that it literally makes God sick. Hearing that message made a significant and lasting impression on me. I believed that I was doomed to spend eternity in hell.

The underlying beliefs that I am not pure, clean, holy, or righteous and that I disgust God had been deeply ingrained over time. Even though my current spiritual framework has evolved, the early programming that I received tends to creep up when I scratch the surface of a current emotional pattern. My adult self knows that consensual sex is a choice that I'm free to make. The old programming should not even apply to my present life, but it still seems to be running in the background. My discomfort after tapping is still there, but it is down to 3.

Your Turn

The purpose here is to increase your acceptance that each reason not to change has some validity. Even if you choose to override it, you are recognizing it. Review your reasons *not to change* and give each an SUD rating on how strongly you feel it. Start with the reason not to change that feels strongest. Using the *"If I . . . , then . . ."* wording, go through a round with the 12 acupoints, tapping on the *"If I . . ."* phrase at one point and the *"then . . ."* phrase on the next. Keep rotating between the phrases as you tap. Insert additional phrases as new wordings come to you. This can be reasonably free-form, or you can stay with the initial phrases. When you feel like you have done a substantial piece of work, take another SUD rating on the grip that this reason not to change has on you. If it still has a charge, notice aspects that still need to be addressed and tap on them.

Once you have the SUD down as far as you can, go to any additional reasons not to change that seem primary at this point. Complete this process for each of them. Do the Integration Procedure from time to time. When you have done as much as you can or choose to do at this point, give another SUD rating to your original issue.

As you saw with Leah, working with your reasons not to change can take you on a journey that will have positive consequences on issues that are different from your initial focus. As you also saw with Leah, the steps to this point may not have completely resolved all the issues related to your original concern. If not, a cognitive distortion may be keeping the problem from being resolved.

4. COGNITIVE DISTORTIONS AND SELF-LIMITING BELIEFS

Caitlin had a long list of reasons not to confront her son, Colm, about mistakes she believed he was making in raising his daughter, Mona. Among her reasons for staying silent were that *if* Caitlin spoke up, *then* it would make Colm feel angry and betrayed that she wasn't supporting him when he was trying to be a good father. The more she tapped on statements such as *"If I tell Colm the truth, then he will feel betrayed by me,"* the more advisable it looked to stay silent. But this is not what the situation required. While feeling relief with the thought that she wouldn't have to engage in

an unpleasant interaction with her son, she also wanted to help him be a better parent.

What broke the logjam for her was recognizing that her guiding model about herself as Colm's mother was this: "My main job at this point in Colm's life is to make him happy." She had been able to set reasonable boundaries while he was growing up, but now that he was an adult, doing anything that would really upset him was unthinkable to her. He already had enough challenges without a doting grandmother adding to his burdens. Because of the harm being done to her granddaughter, however, she realized that her aversion to hurting Colm had made her ineffective as the family elder in relation to her grandchild.

To address the dilemma, she came up with this Choices Statement: *"Even though I believe it's my job to make Colm happy,* ***I choose to recognize that this keeps me from being effective or even truthful about Mona."*** As she worked with this insight, she was able to recognize the faulty thinking about her role as Colm's mother, which is known in CBT as "countering distorted thoughts."

How CBT Counters Distorted Thoughts and Beliefs

CBT recognizes that many of the problems that bring people into psychotherapy trace to faulty ways of thinking, and the approach is designed to refute these.[14] Among the types of cognitive distortions that are frequently addressed in CBT (as well as in energy psychology) are summarized in the following table.

Cognitive Distortions Table

COGNITIVE DISTORTION	DYNAMIC	EXAMPLES
All-or-nothing thinking	No shades of gray	"I'm a bad person." "The situation is hopeless."
Overgeneralization	A few experiences become a rule or expectation	"Relationships are dangerous." "Therapy doesn't work."
Negative orientation	Filtering out the positive and focusing on the negative	"I've failed as a parent." "Life is nothing but sorrow."
Unrealistic expectations	Failure to recognize the difficulties in a situation	"I'll have it done by tomorrow." "Marriage will be easy."
Irrational conclusions	Judgments based on emotions or insufficient facts	"No one will ever understand me." "The election was stolen."
Catastrophizing	Dwelling on the worst possible outcomes	"The plane will go down." "Then the parachute won't open."
Blaming	A focus on finding fault with yourself or others	"It's my fault that she died." "He caused me to fail."
Magnification	Exaggerating the importance of insignificant events	"My talk was a disaster—three people left early."
Minimization	Discounting evidence of danger or of success	"He wouldn't dare hurt me again." "I was just lucky."

Distortions are often at the core of anxiety disorders, depression, marital and job difficulties, parenting failures, and a range of other major life problems. CBT practitioners have developed a talk therapy approach called "cognitive restructuring" to help people recognize and change faulty thought patterns. The goal is to interrupt destructive or self-defeating ways of thinking while they are occurring and replace them with thoughts that will be more constructive and life-affirming.

Cognitive restructuring uses logical analysis to counter irrational thoughts. It involves questioning basic assumptions and beliefs, gathering evidence about whether they are accurate, doing cost-benefit assessments about the consequences of holding to particular ways of thinking, and instilling alternatives to self-defeating thought patterns. Active techniques used in cognitive restructuring include keeping a log of negative thoughts, gathering information by asking others about their perceptions, formulating positive alternatives to negative thinking, and using those positive alternatives until they become habitual. It is laborious, but for many people it is effective.

How Tapping Protocols Counter Distorted Thoughts and Beliefs

Bringing the Basic Tapping Protocol to cognitive restructuring yields an elegant approach that is both less laborious and more powerful. For instance, a Choices Statement can be fashioned to directly address a cognitive distortion:

> *"Even though I believe I'll always be hurt when I get close to someone, I choose to recognize that I'm getting much better at assessing people."*

Not only does the second part provide a logical challenge to the prediction in the first part, the simultaneous acupoint stimulation sends signals to the nervous system that—in ways not yet fully understood—results in weakening the influence of the negative statement and strengthening the impact of the positive statement.

Acupoint tapping on the cognitive distortion usually has a stronger influence on overcoming the negative belief than logic alone. You can tap while stating an old belief, such as *"Part of me believes I'll always be hurt when I get close to someone."* This further reduces the emotional power of the belief. If events that shaped the belief can be identified, tapping on them along with the above steps can often eliminate the belief's power with less effort than a purely cognitive approach.

Positive Reframing

A way to tie it all together is called "reframing," the basic procedure used in CBT for formulating a statement that presents a new outlook on the issue.[15] Effective reframing changes your interpretation of your own story. Tapping on it embeds it into new neural pathways. For instance, people who have had difficult or even traumatic childhoods often think of themselves as being "damaged goods." But they have also survived, and they have learned a great deal about life that was never required for those who grew up in more comfortable circumstances. Tapping on a reframe such as *"I'm a survivor, and I know more than most people about how to succeed through tough challenges"* will be both accurate and empowering.

The timing of a reframe is important if it is to have the desired effect. Reframes will often occur naturally as the tapping progresses, and the tapping substantially enhances the way the reframe will be incorporated. In addition to spontaneous reframes, you may want to actively formulate them. Generally, you wouldn't introduce a reframe that hadn't occurred spontaneously until the SUD rating of the emotional strength of the core belief is down to a 3 or less. Otherwise the mind will have difficulty accepting it as a possibility. We'll return to reframes—which in relation to guiding models can lead to complete "makeovers"—later in the chapter in the section called "Installing a New Guiding Model."

Core Beliefs and Guiding Models

Most of your guiding models have been with you for a long time, instruct you in myriads of ways, and serve you well. But when a guiding model is formed around a cognitive distortion or a core belief that has become outdated, problems inevitably follow. This is why both CBT and energy psychology give so much attention to cognitive distortions. As already emphasized, the Basic Tapping Protocol organically shifts core beliefs. But particularly when a problem won't readily resolve, examining your core beliefs can be a necessary step.

In their book *The Energy of Belief*, tapping therapists Mary Sise, LCSW, and Sheila Sidney Bender, PhD, show how deeply embedded core beliefs may be passed through generations. They describe Jackson, a father of three small children, and how his difficulties with his children traced back to a core belief his own father instilled in him:

Jackson's father was a Vietnam veteran and, as is the history for so many vets, his father witnessed many friends being killed in ambushes and horrific battles. After returning from the war, his father married, and he and his wife had six children, including Jackson. Jackson's father could never again handle noise and chaos at home as it unconsciously reminded him of the war. Whenever Jackson and his siblings were excited and playful, their father would respond with agitation and violence. Inevitably, someone always got hit, at times vigorously. Jackson's mom was always trying to keep the children quiet and the house clean so her husband didn't get upset. No one understood the concept of emotional triggers and how commotion and chaos provoked agitation and anger in Jackson's father because he was being unconsciously reminded of his horrific experiences in the war. Jackson and his siblings grew up believing that there was something wrong with being excited and playful and that something bad would happen if they were having fun.

Jackson is now married with three small children, and he experiences his own intense agitation when they are noisy or having fun. He reflected, "It feels like something is wrong, and I have to silence them." For Jackson, noise became a trigger to his own childhood experiences. Whenever he starts to relax and have fun, he fears something bad will happen to him as it had when he was a young boy.[16]

When a parent's dysfunctional core beliefs impact a child, the child may develop beliefs that mimic the parent's (as happened with Jackson). On the other hand, a child may react against a parent's misguided core belief in ways that become strengths, as when a depressed, pessimistic parent raises a child who develops a markedly positive and hopeful outlook on life. Of course this can also be taken too far, such as if the child becomes adept at denial and develops a Pollyannaish outlook. Reflecting on the core beliefs of your parents or other people who were influential during your childhood can shed new light on deep beliefs you have been taking for granted.

Examining Cognitive Distortions and Limiting Beliefs

Core beliefs that are based on cognitive distortions do not come with the label "Caution: faulty belief, do not trust me." They are called *beliefs* because we believe them. But when they have caused enough damage in your life that you have, in a program like this one, chosen to focus on a difficulty they have created, they are ready to be exposed, challenged, and transformed.

To identify a distortion or faulty belief, do another SUD assessment of your original issue. Notice what is keeping the rating at a higher level than you desire. If it is a sensation or an emotion, tap on it—either naming the emotion or sensation or focusing on it kinesthetically—until you have neutralized it as much as you can. Then take another rating.

If a thought or belief is keeping the SUD at a higher level, revisit the above examples of cognitive distortions to see if any apply. If you are able to identify a cognitive distortion in your mental model, you have taken a large step toward correcting it.

Leah's Limiting Beliefs

Leah identified three beliefs based on cognitive distortions that were getting in the way of resolving her issue. The first involved *all-or-nothing thinking*: "I am a bad person and unworthy of forgiveness," which she rated at a 4 in believability. The second involved a *negative orientation*: "I am vile and disgusting to God," which she rated at a 6. The third involved *catastrophizing*: "I am sinful by nature and doomed to spend eternity in hell," which she rated at a 2.

Your Turn

Describe in your journal any faulty beliefs or cognitive distortions you have identified. Choose one and give it an SUD rating of how believable it feels to you. Ten means the distortion you have identified feels like a completely believable, indisputable fact. It doesn't feel like a distortion. Zero, on the other hand, means you don't believe this cognitive distortion at all, even if it is still hanging around somewhere in your psyche.

Crafting Counterarguments

Next you will be crafting a statement that counters the cognitive distortion or unrealistic belief and putting it into the by-now familiar format of *"Even though a part of me believes [state the belief or distortion as if it were true]"* followed by *"I choose to [a statement that challenges the belief]."* For instance:

"Even though part of me believes that my worth as a person is measured by my achievements, I choose to discover how that is only a small part of the story."

"Even though part of me believes that men will always hurt me, I choose to recognize how much stronger I've become."

"Even though part of me believes I will always be poor and struggling, I choose to be alert for opportunities that will help me thrive."

The following table is keyed to the most common forms of cognitive distortion.

Cognitive Distortions and Sample Corrections Table

COGNITIVE DISTORTION	"EVEN THOUGH PART OF ME BELIEVES . . .	I CHOOSE TO . . .
All-or-nothing thinking	I'm a bad person,	see the kindness in my intentions."
Overgeneralization	all relationships are dangerous,	recognize that my failures are teaching me how to create a joyful partnership."
Negative orientation	I've failed as a parent,	remember all the ways I've provided Noah with what he needs."
Unrealistic expectations	marriage will be easy,	expect challenges and to be ready for them."
Irrational conclusions	I'm absolutely going to fail,	discover abilities I don't know I have for rising to the occasion."
Catastrophizing	the plane will go down,	focus on the four billion passengers who have safe flights every year."
Blaming	he caused me to fail,	learn from my mistakes and not repeat them."
Magnification	my talk was a disaster since three people left early,	register the praise I received from the majority who did enjoy it."
Minimization	he won't hurt me again,	remain vigilant based on past patterns."

These counterarguments don't need to offset the cognitive distortion with overwhelming logic, just so long as the rebuttal feels valid. And if you can't come up with a strong counter, you can always use this default: *"Even though part of me believes [state the belief], I choose to know this belief isn't serving me."*

Your statement can also use humor instead of one of the more customary wordings, as in this example from our colleagues Ann Adams and Karin Davidson:

> *"Even though I learned by first grade that relationships don't work, it's vitally important that I keep believing the relationship advice of a six-year-old because everyone knows that six-year-olds are experts on adult relationships."*[17]

> *"Even though part of me believes that I am vile and disgusting to God, **I choose to pause and experience awe as I notice the perfection of nature and realize that I am part of it!**"*

> *"Even though part of me believes I am sinful by nature and am doomed to spend eternity in hell, **I choose to notice how it feels to soak in the energy of love, which I believe is the true essence of God.**"*

Leah's Counters to Her Limiting Beliefs

Based on her limiting beliefs listed earlier, Leah formulated the following Choices Statements:

> *"Even though part of me believes I am a bad person and unworthy of forgiveness, **I choose to forgive myself for blindly accepting the beliefs and programming of my childhood.**"*

Your Turn

Give an SUD rating to the power each cognitive distortion you have identified has over you. Taking them one at a time, create a Choices Statement in the form of *"Even though part of me believes . . . , I choose to . . ."* and record it in your journal. As you read each statement, rub your chest sore spots as you say the first phrase and hold your hands over your Heart Chakra with the second. Repeat three times for each cognitive distortion. The next procedure will go further in defusing these distortions.

Leah's Tapping on Her Cognitive Distortions and Limiting Beliefs

Leah made a chart that summarized this whole process:

COGNITIVE DISTORTION	"EVEN THOUGH PART OF ME BELIEVES . . .	I CHOOSE TO . . .	SUD BEFORE TAPPING	SUD AFTER TAPPING
All-or-nothing thinking	I am a bad person and unworthy of forgiveness,	forgive myself for blindly accepting the beliefs and programming of my childhood."	4	0
Negative orientation	I disgust God and am a disgusting person,	pause and experience awe as I notice the perfection of nature, and realize that I am part of it!"	6	2
Catastrophizing	I am sinful by nature and am doomed to spend eternity in hell,	notice how it feels to soak in the energy of love, which I believe is the true essence of God."	2	0

Your Turn: Eliminating Cognitive Distortions

For each cognitive distortion:

- Go through another tapping cycle: 1) Choices Statement, 2) the 12 acupoints stating the cognitive distortion ("*Part of me believes . . .*") at each point, 3) the Integration Procedure, and 4) another trip through the 12 points.

- Give another SUD rating on how believable the cognitive distortion feels now.

- You may wonder if giving words to the distortion you want to change serves to reinforce it. But as we've seen, the opposite occurs. Tapping sends signals to your brain that reduce the neurological grip the belief has on you.

- Stay alert for sensations or emotions that are keeping your SUD rating from going down and take a detour to tap on any you notice. Then return to the faulty belief or cognitive distortion.

- Repeat the process until the SUD rating begins to decrease for your cognitive distortion.

- As the SUD begins to decrease, alternate between saying the cognitive distortion and the counterargument (the *"I choose . . ."* statement), so at one tapping point you are saying one and on the next point you are saying the other.

After three rounds of tapping with these alternating statements, give another SUD rating to your original issue. If a negatively charged memory emerges of an event that was a factor in shaping the cognitive distortion or limiting belief, just note it. It will be addressed in the following sections.

Recap of the Chapter to This Point

We know this is a demanding chapter. But please remember that it is not necessary to go through every technique. We are attempting to cover all the areas where detective work might be needed to make progress on a tough issue. This guides you in going for a deep and permanent change on a longstanding issue. We think each topic is worth considering, but you can pick and choose. Also remember that if you feel overwhelmed at any point, you might shift to energy techniques (the Daily Energy Routine or the Appendix) or even set the book aside for a day or two and let your unconscious mind do some of the work. You will often find that when you return to the program, some blocks will have dissolved or fresh insights will have appeared. In any case, let's take stock of where we are in the process:

1. You have focused on an unresolved experience or other concern that matters to you.

2. You have taken steps to:
   a) Balance your energies
   b) Overcome Psychological Reversals
   c) Address other internal objections to changing the situation

d) Replace cognitive distortions and faulty beliefs with Choices Statements

3. If your original issue feels totally resolved (SUD of 0), wonderful! Proceed to "Installing a New Guiding Model" on page 117. If your issue is not yet resolved to your satisfaction, continue here to dig deeper.

5. DIGGING INTO THE ROOTS OF THE PROBLEM

If the SUD of your original issue is still above 0 or above a low number you find acceptable, you may need to go deeper into formative experiences that set you up for the current problem. Difficult childhood experiences are often at the root of self-limiting core beliefs and guiding models. Such experiences may also set into motion self-defeating patterns of behavior that occur with little thought. Some of these may have emerged and been addressed in the earlier sections, as you saw with Leah. But some may need special focus. For instance, unless unprocessed material from the past has been resolved, a person who has been abused may reflexively abuse others, as you saw with Jackson, or may become habitually fearful and withdrawn.

While reflecting on how your past may be interfering with your progress can be revealing, a more systematic approach is called the "Affect Bridge."[18] As applied in energy psychology, you focus on a *feeling* or *sensation* that comes to mind when you take the SUD rating and you "ride it back" in time to an earlier experience. You might ask yourself to go back to:

... *one of the first times I felt scared of someone.*

... *one of the first times I was rejected.*

... *one of the first times I exploded with anger.*

... *one of the first times I had this feeling of pressure over my heart.*

... *one of the first times I couldn't catch my breath.*

You may be surprised by how quickly a parallel experience from your past comes to you and how clearly it relates to the current situation, particularly when the "bridge" is a feeling or a sensation. Some people using the technique have sensed themselves moving backward in time over an actual bridge. Others have experienced gliding back on a stream into their past. Many just see or sense an image that links to the memory.

If you identify a memory that played a pivotal role in the concern that is on the table, treat it as a separate issue for the Basic Tapping Protocol. Give it its own SUD rating, Reminder Phrase, Acceptance and Choices Statements, and proceed with the rest of the Protocol.

Leah's Affect Bridge

When Leah did another SUD rating on the statement *"Part of me believes that I am vile and disgusting to God,"* the intensity had gone back up again, from 3 to 5. This type of fluctuation is not unusual with a longstanding complex issue involving one's identity. When reflecting on a sermon she heard in childhood, she described feeling "a sense of hopelessness wash over me." She used this feeling of hopelessness for her Affect Bridge, riding it back in time. She continued in her journal:

This feeling was accompanied by sensations including a heaviness in my chest, tightness in my throat, pressure behind my eyes as tears were forming, and a pit in my stomach. Fear of spending eternity in hell had been ingrained prior to that experience, but this was the first time I recall feeling hopeless about the possibility of going to heaven. I had also been taught that God loved me and wanted to spend eternity with me in heaven (John 3:16—"For God so loved the world . . ."). Yet in that moment, I knew that no matter what I did or how hard I tried, I would never get to heaven. I was a "lukewarm sinner," and I disgusted God.

I tapped on the memory of the preacher saying, "You're lukewarm!" and "God will spew you out of his mouth!" and feelings of panic and a deep sense of shame spread through me. SUD level jumped to a 9. Because I noticed feeling flooded and overwhelmed, I shifted my focus to staying grounded and embodied. I paused and did an energy routine and then returned to tapping. I kept my eyes open and tapped on the phrase *"Even though the preacher said, 'You are lukewarm and God will spew you out of his mouth,' in this moment, you are safe."* It felt more comforting to speak to myself in third person, as if I was talking to the part of me that believed I was disgusting to God. After several rounds of tapping, the SUD level went back to a 2, but it still had some charge.

Another cognitive distortion and related memories involving the sense of hopelessness and despair bubbled up. The distortion "It's all my fault, and I could have stopped it from happening" came into focus. It was linked to multiple memories and events (SUD rating of 6). I added the Choices Statement, *"I choose to acknowledge that I responded the best way I knew how at the time."*

I tapped through the sense of hopelessness that was connected to the thought "It's all my fault," to the sinking pit in my stomach, and to the feelings of guilt and shame. Each time I returned to the Choices Statement (shortened to *"I did the best I could at the time"*), I had a tearful emotional release. The thought "It's all my fault; I could have stopped it from happening" went down to an SUD of 3.

Of all our test drivers, Leah's journey through this chapter was one of the most complex. She began with a humiliating incident that occurred in third grade and wound up working with core issues involving her identity, safety, sexuality, and relationship with God. She was meticulous in addressing and writing down every aspect that emerged. Your detective work may not stray so far from your original issue, but if it does, Leah's account provides an informative model.

Your Turn: Affect Bridge

Here are the steps for your Affect Bridge:

- Take another SUD reading on the current state of the issue that has been your focus in this chapter.

- Identify a feeling, sensation, or thought that plays into the SUD number.

- "Ride" it back in time to one of the first times you had this feeling or sensation.

- Apply the Basic Tapping Protocol to this memory (as you did in the previous chapter).

- Once you get this and any other memories that may call for your attention as low as you can get them, give another SUD rating to your original issue in this chapter.

Remember, a round of tapping takes only about minute, so the *actual steps* for these first five ways of lowering a resistant SUD rating can, once you've had some practice with the methods, often be completed in less time than it took to read the instructions.

Second Recap of Chapter 3: The Five Areas of Detective Work to This Point

To quickly review:

1. Go through the steps in the Daily Energy Routine (p. 84) and rerate the SUD.

2. Identify any Psychological Reversals using the Choices Method with each (p. 92), and rerate the SUD.

3. Identify any other areas of resistance to resolving the issue, put them into the "If I . . . , then . . ." format (p. 96), tap on each, and rerate the SUD.

4. Identify any cognitive distortions or self-limiting beliefs (p. 100), tap on each as described, and rerate the SUD.

5. Use the Affect Bridge (p. 109) to revisit any unresolved experiences from your past that are playing into the current issue, apply the Basic Tapping Protocol to address them, and rerate the SUD.

6. RESOLVING CONFLICTS THAT ARE PREVENTING PROGRESS

Dr. Burns has noted that "although we may be suffering and desperately want to change, there may be powerful conflicting forces that keep us stuck."[19] If your SUD is still higher than 0 after taking all these steps, an *internal conflict* not settled by the techniques used to this point may require further attention before the issue is fully resolved. Internal conflicts are a normal and natural part of life. Just as a guiding model has many parts, your psyche holds many guiding models. These are always in a dynamic interplay, working with one another, forming compromises, and sometimes fighting one another. The part of you that is afraid of getting rejected may be conflicting with the part of you that longs to be in a deeply committed relationship. The part of you that wants to relax and be nurtured may be screaming at the part of you that is driven to take on challenging assignments and give them your all.

Most of these inner negotiations take place outside your awareness. Despite the inevitable conflicts, the psyche is usually able to maintain reasonable equilibrium. Sometimes, however, the inner conflicts upset that equilibrium to the point that your state of mind, your ability to effectively pursue what matters to you, and your overall sense of well-being are disrupted. Most forms of psychotherapy have ways of dealing with such conflicting parts. For instance:

- Carl Jung (1875–1961), the legendary Swiss psychiatrist, introduced "active imagination" around 1915 as a technique in which the contents of the unconscious mind were translated into images and personified as separate entities that would create narratives and communicate with one another.

- Around that time, the Romanian American psychiatrist Jacob Moreno (1889–1974) introduced "psychodrama," a technique in which people would use dramatization techniques to role-play inner parts or unresolved experiences.

- The German-born psychiatrist Fritz Perls (1893–1970), the founder of Gestalt therapy, adapted psychodramatic methods in his "two-chair technique," also called "parts work," where one part is given a voice and posture in a dialogue with another part. (For Perls, it was often between what he called the "top dog" and the "underdog.")

- The Canadian-born psychiatrist Eric Berne (1910–1970), the founder of Transactional Analysis, focused on three internal "parts" or "ego states": the parent, the child, and the adult.

- The American-born family therapist Richard Schwartz views and works with the inner parts as a "family" in his highly popular Internal Family Systems model.

- CBT also uses dialogue. In fact, David Burns has called its "Externalization of Voices" technique—in which a dialogue is enacted between a person's negative thoughts and positive thoughts—perhaps the "most powerful of all the CBT techniques."[20]

Each of these approaches provides a creative way of addressing the same issue: we all have fragmentary parts that need to be brought into communication and harmony if we are to function at our best. For instance, your *inner child* might be saying, "I want to play"; your *inner parent* might be saying, "You've got to work"; and your inner adult might be negotiating between the two of them. Giving voice, posture, and interaction among these internal parts is a potent way of bringing them into greater cooperation. Energy psychology, you may not be too surprised to hear, adds acupoint tapping to this type of internal dialogue. Maggie Adkins, a highly regarded EFT practitioner and teacher in Australia, explains that the purpose of inner dialogues that use tapping is to "make friends—to create a new and better relationship—with whatever part of us is presenting an issue."[21] In addition to dialogues between these parts, she distinguishes several other categories for such dialogues:

- Dialogues with your inner child

- Dialogues with a physical sensation or body part

- Dialogues between yourself and your entire body

As you carry out the dialogue, you tap. Tap on an acupoint while one part is speaking. Then go to the next point in the 12-point sequence when the other part is speaking. Move to subsequent points as the exchanges go back and forth. Some people will actually switch chairs, or at least postures and facial expressions, as they role-play each part.

This can be a wonderfully creative process, but it varies so much from one person and one situation to another that we don't have a set of guidelines about how to carry out the dialogue. A few basics, however, are for each part to state what it needs, to listen respectfully to what the other part needs, and to agree to do what it is able and willing to do to accommodate the needs of the other part.

You can imagine how Jackson's (p. 103) inner dialogue might have unfolded after the Affect Bridge brought him back to an incident when he was 10:

10-year-old Jackson: *We were having so much fun, and then he came home and yelled at us. This time, I was the one who got slapped. I feel the stinging on my face. I don't know what I did wrong. I only know that I'm a bad boy.* [While tapping.]

Jackson's adult voice: *That must be very confusing. And very painful.* [While tapping.]

10-year-old Jackson: [With tears welling up.] *It is! It really is. I try to be good. I try to be quiet. I try not to make a mess. But sometimes I forget.* [While tapping.]

Adult: *Yes, I know how hard you try. And your tears tell me how unfair it feels. I can see that you really want to do what your daddy expects.* [While tapping.]

10-year-old Jackson: *I really do. But I mess up all the time. I'm very bad!* [While tapping.]

Adult: *I know you believe that. But I want to tell you something, Jackson. Your daddy isn't like most dads. Did you know that?* [While tapping.]

10-year-old Jackson: *I don't know what you mean. He's the only daddy I have.* [While tapping.]

Adult: *Yes, how would you know? But most dads like to see their kids play. Most dads like to see their kids having fun.* [While tapping.]

10-year-old Jackson: *Not my daddy. He has rules. And if we break the rules, we are bad.* [While tapping.]

Adult: *What I want you to understand is that it is the rules that are bad, not you.* [While tapping.]

10-year-old Jackson: *I don't know what you mean.* [While tapping.]

Adult: *You know how your face hurt when he slapped you?* [While tapping.]

10-year-old Jackson: *Yes, it hurt a lot. It still hurts.* [While tapping.]

Adult: *Your daddy was damaged a long time ago so that when things get loud or the room gets cluttered, it hurts him. Kind of how your face hurts. It's a different kind of hurt, but it is real.* [While tapping.]

10-year-old Jackson: *I don't understand.* [While tapping.]

Adult: *Your face still hurts even though you're not getting hit. If I didn't know he hit you, I wouldn't know your face hurts. It's kind of like that. You can't see his pain, and you don't know what caused it. But he has a lot of pain inside. And when you are loud, it makes his pain worse. And that's why he gets angry.* [While tapping.]

10-year-old Jackson: *Because I was bad.* [While tapping.]

Adult: *What I'm trying to show you is that you're not bad. Your daddy has something wrong with him. Something is broken inside of him.* [While tapping.]

10-year-old Jackson: *Why can't he fix it?* [While tapping.]

Adult: *He can't.* [While tapping.]

10-year-old Jackson: *Can I fix it for him?* [While tapping.]

Adult: *No, you can't fix it either.* [While tapping.]

10-year-old Jackson: *Then what should I do?* [While tapping.]

Adult: *That's tricky. You're in a difficult situation. If you make noise or make a mess, he will punish you. So you need to keep trying to follow his rules when he is around.* [While tapping.]

10-year-old Jackson: *I already know that!* [While tapping.]

Adult: *But here's the thing. When he punishes you, it's not because you're a bad boy. Yes, you need to follow his rules the best you can. But you also need to be able to play and be loud when he's not around.* [While tapping.]

10-year-old Jackson: *But I'm always scared of getting loud or having fun, whether he's around or not.* [While tapping.]

Adult: *I know. I can see what happens to you when you are grown up. You have learned so completely that it's not safe to be loud or messy, so noise and clutter bothers you the way it bothers your daddy.* [While tapping.]

10-year-old Jackson: *How do you know that?* [While tapping.]

Adult: *I'm from your future, coming back to visit you. I want you to know that you are a good boy. I want you to know that you are in a difficult and unnatural situation. I see it, and I am so sorry about it!* [While tapping.]

10-year-old Jackson: *Thank you.* [While tapping.]

Adult: *But I'm about to say something that will surprise you. Right now you are 10. But I am the you of your future. I am no longer in the situation from when I was 10.* [While tapping.]

10-year-old Jackson: *This is weird!* [While tapping.]

Adult: *Yes. And here's the tricky part. Right now you are here in the future with me. And even though you are still 10 after all these years, I'm an adult now. And I can help you realize that your daddy's rules aren't the world's rules. The part of you that believes you are bad and that believes that noise and clutter are dangerous can start to heal.* [While tapping.]

10-year-old Jackson: *I do feel safe here talking to you. Can I really stop being so afraid?* [While tapping.]

Adult: *That's what I have in mind for both of us. You see, I'm all grown up now. I have children of my own, as you will. And I get mad at them for the same reasons your daddy got mad at you. If you can feel safe with me, we can both heal from the time that it was so dangerous for you as a little boy to be natural.* [While tapping.]

Leah's Inner Dialogue

Leah also carried out a lengthy inner dialogue, though for our example here, we will stay with Jackson's. After Leah's dialogue, she revisited and tapped on the cognitive distortion that had been at a 2: *"I disgust God and am a disgusting person."* It had gone down to a 0, as had the original memory from third grade.

Your Turn

Your inner dialogue may take any of many forms. For instance, instead of time-traveling for a dialogue with your "inner child," as you saw with Jackson, you might create a dialogue that gives voice to

a physical sensation such as a heaviness in your heart, a body part like your heart or lungs, or your entire body. By generating signals that maintain balance in your body's energy system, the tapping propels the dialogue into a healing space.

Whether with a sensation, a body part, your entire body, or two sides of your personality, create a dialogue that addresses an internal conflict that may be preventing progress on resolving your issue. If you went back to an earlier memory during the Affect Bridge, your dialogue could be with yourself at the age you were during the memory. What did you need? How were you hurt? Describe these in vivid detail. Speak from your heart. It doesn't need to be as dramatic as Jackson's dialogue, only true to your experience. What still needs to be healed? Listen well.

From your "adult ego state," what guidance can you give this child? Play with the ability to time-travel or personify parts that this format allows. Express your love, caring, and encouragement. Continually tap through the dialogue, proceeding until the two parts have reached as much mutual understanding and cooperation as possible. At the end, give another SUD rating to your original issue.

Will This Ever End?

As long as we are on this Earth we are forever facing new challenges, from bonding as an infant to the adjustments that are necessary in old age. To meet them effectively, we keep revising and updating our guiding models, consciously or not. While it is useful to process thoughts and emotions that are in the way of your health, happiness, and effectiveness, we caution you to avoid becoming obsessive about trying to get everything "cleaned up." Go easy on yourself, as would a loving and effective therapist. Dawson Church put the situation into perspective like this:

> One of the questions people frequently ask is, "Do I ever get to the end of my emotional processing?" It's like the question asked of a notorious French courtesan, "Does your sexual appetite wane as you age?" She replied, "How would I know? I'm only 85."[22]

7. INSTALLING A NEW GUIDING MODEL

We have looked at six different types of detective work for identifying and overcoming obstacles to reaching your original goal.

Somewhere along the way, your rating of the amount of internal distress when bringing your original issue to mind may have gone down to 0. But even if it is still at 3 or lower, you can do a reframe of the guiding model that has been interfering with the changes you wish to institute. And you can use tapping to "install" that revised guiding model into your nervous system.

If your SUD is still in the midrange (4 to 6), you might repeat some of the techniques in this chapter or search for other aspects of the issue to bring it down to 3 or less. If your SUD is still at a 7 or higher after going through all these procedures, there is still another effective option. We all have issues that could benefit from outside guidance, and you've come upon a challenge that you may at some point want to tackle with the help of a seasoned tapping practitioner or another source of professional support. In addition, even if you haven't made a major breakthrough, you've been developing skills that you will be able to apply to other concerns.

If your SUD is at 3 or lower, the reframing is already occurring in your psyche, and you can speed it along with a final procedure that actively translates the changes in your psyche into changes in your life. The first step is to imagine how your life will be when this issue is no longer in your way. Next, turn this vision into a statement. If the issue was an exaggerated distrust of others, the statement might be *"I'm learning to see the good in people and in their intentions."* If the issue was a fear of crowds, the statement might be *"I'm starting to enjoy being where people gather in large groups."* If the issue was that you never find the time to savor your family, the statement might be *"I like it when I feel my tenderness, and that is happening more and more with my family."*

Creating an Affirmation

You may recognize that these phrases are *affirmations*—statements you desire to be true even while the reality of that truth is still in progress. Affirmations are useful for installing a new guiding model. For an effective affirmation:

- Put it in first person, present tense.

- Make it short, simple, and direct.

- Affirm *wants* rather than *don't-wants*.

- Affirm *wants* rather than *shoulds*.

- Affirm a goal you believe is realistically possible to attain.

- Affirm a goal that is also a "stretch," so it is large enough to be exciting.

Your affirmation needs balance between being a possibility you believe you could achieve and a possibility that would stretch you to another level. Stretching stimulates excitement and motivation. The goal of raising your annual income from $50,000 to $51,000 is not likely to get your juices flowing. The prospect of moving up to $80,000 or $100,000 may do it, and this principle holds whether the goal has to do with more money, less weight, better relationships, more vibrant health, or greater achievement.

On the other hand, affirmations *don't* work very well if they:

- Reflect what you think you *should* want rather than what you really want

- Call for too large a step or for changes that are far beyond what you believe is possible

- Are worded in a way that doesn't engage your enthusiasm

- Are repeated mindlessly

Here are some examples of well-worded affirmations:

"I see the opportunity in every challenge my son presents."

"I'm at ease around new people and look forward to meeting them."

"I stay in a grounded, heart-centered space in the face of my husband's criticisms."

"I am completing my book with ease, joy, and brilliance."

"I enjoy my exercise program and feel drawn to it every day."

"I am attracted to healthy foods and eating habits."

"I find ways to bring more and more play into my day."

"I am making a full recovery quickly, easily, and joyfully."

"I am wealthy" (or for easier believability, *"I am becoming wealthy"*) . . . or healthy, happy in my marriage, etc.

"I appreciate every moment" (or *"I am learning to appreciate every moment"*).

Leah's Affirmation

"I consistently approach myself with compassion and forgiveness."

Your Turn

Imagine that you have succeeded in making the change you have been envisioning. Create an affirmation, patterned after the above examples, that briefly describes what has occurred for that change to have been made and write it in your journal. Tap it in by stating it as you tap each of the 12 energy points.

While many self-help programs that use affirmations stop with having stated the affirmations, the following steps—neutralizing Tail-Enders, making your affirmations concrete, and stimulating energy points—will add power to them.

Identifying Tail-Enders

A Tail-Ender is a specific form of Psychological Reversal. Psychological Reversals can form around *any* internal objection to reaching your goal. This might involve the goal's ultimate desirability, the sacrifices you might need to make to reach the goal, the plausibility of reaching the goal, whether it would be safe to attain the goal, and issues involving your self-worth or identity. A Tail-Ender is a Psychological Reversal that is based on an internal belief that the goal is *not possible* or *not desirable*. Gary Craig called this type of Psychological Reversal a Tail-Ender because it is invisibly (unconsciously) tacked onto the end of an affirmation. For instance, the affirmation *"I maintain balance and harmony between my career and my personal life . . ."* might have as a Tail-Ender:

"but of course my work responsibilities always come first."

If the affirmation is *"I eat and exercise so I will maintain my ideal weight,"* possible Tail-Enders might be, *"but if I am at my ideal weight . . .*

. . . men will hit on me and expect sex."

. . . I will weigh less than Mom, and she will be jealous and angry."

. . . I will feel emotionally vulnerable."

. . . I will have to give up the comfort and pleasure of eating what I want."

. . . I won't know if a man loves me for myself or for my body."

Leah's Tail-Enders

Leah's affirmation seemed straightforward enough: *"I consistently approach myself with compassion and forgiveness."* But the invisible phrases her psyche placed at the end of it were *"unless it has to do with pleasure"* and *"unless I disappoint someone."*

Your Turn

To identify any Tail-Enders that your psyche has invisibly added to your affirmation, see what happens as you try to complete these statements in your journal:

- The thing about me that makes it impossible for me to reach this goal is . . .

- If there were an emotional reason for me not reaching this goal, it would be . . .

- To reach this goal, I would have to . . .

- What I really want, rather than just this goal, is . . .

- Thinking about this goal reminds me of . . .

- I would be more willing to reach this goal if first . . .

If any of the above statements brings up a Tail-Ender, note it in your journal.

Neutralizing Tail-Enders

The Basic Tapping Protocol can be used to neutralize Tail-Enders. Follow these basic steps:

1. Shorten the Tail-Ender to about a dozen words or less so it can serve as your Reminder Phrase.

2. Give a 0-to-10 SUD rating on how large of an obstacle the Tail-Ender seems to be.

3. Craft an Acceptance or Choices Statement, such as *"Even though I will feel emotionally vulnerable if I lose weight, I love and deeply accept myself"* or *". . . , I choose to continue to build better boundaries."*

4. Go through another cycle, repeating the Tail-Ender at each of the 12 acupoints, doing the Integration Procedure, and again running through the tapping points.

5. Give another SUD rating to how strong an obstacle the Tail-Ender seems to be.

6. Continue to work with aspects and any of the techniques in this chapter to neutralize each Tail-Ender as much as you can.

How Leah Defeated Her Tail-Ender

"My first Tail-Ender elicited only a 3, so going through the tapping sequence quickly got it down to a 0, and I tapped on *'Embracing pleasure.'* I am enjoying this new take on pleasure, particularly appreciating the greater sense of freedom around my sexuality! My second Tail-Ender about disappointing someone started at a 7, and I had to visit a time in my childhood to get it down to a 2. From there, it was relatively easy to get it down to a 0 by tapping on *'I choose to know I do my best and my best is plenty good.'*"

Your Turn

Go through the six-step process for neutralizing any Tail-Enders that have tacked themselves onto your affirmation. Once you have removed or neutralized the Tail-Enders, you can tap directly on your affirmation. You don't need to give it an SUD rating or do the Integration Procedure at this point. Just tap while you state the affirmation at each acupoint.

If any unpleasant emotions, sensations, or objections arise as you tap, shift your focus to these. As they lose their power, return to the affirmation. Do at least three rounds of tapping on your affirmation before moving to the next step. If you wish, describe the experience in your journal.

Making Your Affirmation Concrete

So far, your affirmation has probably been a relatively general statement. Now you will be making it concrete by envisioning a situation related to the original problem where it would be challenging to implement your affirmation. The process was described earlier as "testing your results," but now you will be taking it a step further, not just testing whether the SUD is down to 0 but giving a rating of how believable it is to you that you can respond in the new way.

After Rosa's SUD about her anger toward her daughter was reduced to 0 (Chapter 2), she was asked to imagine a situation in which it would be difficult to "keep your cool." Rosa only had to look to the previous school night when she had told Carmen to be home by 9 pm. Carmen was belligerently defiant, bringing herself inches from Rosa's face, screaming. She would not back off.

The therapist asked Rosa to see herself responding in exactly the way she would like to play out this scenario. Rosa saw herself calmly telling Carmen to back off and, when Carmen wouldn't, calmly naming a consequence that mattered to Carmen. In this case, Carmen was earning points for doing chores, and she could use the points to obtain things such as makeup and clothing. Rosa saw herself matter-of-factly telling Carmen that she could continue the conversation respectfully or she could lose 20 points. Rosa rated the *believability* of her being able to pull this off as relatively strong.

For this technique, the rating is not an SUD (Subjective Units of Distress) but an SUB (Subjective Units of Believability). With an SUD, you want to bring the number down to 0 or near 0. With an SUB, you want to bring it up toward 10. Rosa's SUB rating was a 6, showing a fair degree of confidence, and she was able to bring it up to an 8 with another tapping cycle.

Leah's Challenging Scene

To make her affirmation concrete, Leah imagined displeasing someone. In her scene, she showed up for an appointment with a client without having been able to give the portfolio she had produced adequate time. The client's disappointment was obvious. Her belief that she could meet this situation with self-love, self-compassion, self-forgiveness, and skill was at 5 (the SUB), which, as you will see, she increased with the following technique.

Your Turn

You have already crafted an affirmation statement that describes a desirable change, and you have neutralized the Tail-Enders. Now you will test it. Imagine a scene in which, like Rosa's and Leah's, it would be challenging to have the emotional and behavioral responses you desire. Visualize the scene like a movie. In this movie, your response to the challenge is one you consider to be ideal. Give the scene an SUB rating of 0 (no believability) to 10 (complete believability).

Embedding Your Affirmation into Your Nervous System

Once you have (1) properly worded an affirmation for a goal you consider worthy and realistic, (2) neutralized the Tail-Enders, and (3) paired it with vivid imagery of having the desired response in a challenging situation, the last step, applying the Basic Tapping Protocol, will make it as reliable an approach as we've ever seen for shifting neural pathways to support a goal.

Only two adjustments to the Protocol are needed to do this. Along with saying your affirmation at each tapping point, you also visualize your success in the challenging situation. And you word the first part of your Acceptance or Choices Statement like this:

> "Even though I only believe [state your affirmation] at [your SUB rating], I love and accept myself just the way I am."

For Rosa, after a few tapping cycles, stating her affirmation and visualizing herself remaining calm in the face of Carmen's provocations, Rosa was up to an SUB of 9. If the SUB is up to 8 or higher, that's usually a promising sign that you will be successful in translating the affirmation into your life. Often it can't get to a 10 in believability until you've experienced the new response in an actual situation.

Leah's Empowering Vision

Leah's revised statement was "Even though I am only 50 percent confident I will approach myself with compassion and forgiveness, I love and accept myself as I am." She again brought to mind the scene with her client as she tapped while envisioning herself explaining to her client, with total self-acceptance, that the portfolio didn't meet her standards either, admitting that she ran out of time, and saying with utter confidence that the next time they meet, the portfolio will be at least as good as the samples that got the client to hire her in the first place. This process was done in her imagination, eyes closed, while tapping and envisioning herself staying in a space of self-love, self-compassion, and self-forgiveness. The believability went up to an 8.

Your Turn

Tap on your affirmation, combined with the vision of successfully carrying it out in a challenging situation:

1. Start with taking an SUB rating on the likelihood that you will respond to the challenging situation as you hope.

2. Tap on the 12 acupoints while visualizing, articulating, or feeling yourself carrying out your desired response.

3. Do the Integration Procedure.

4. Tap on the points again.

5. Take another SUB rating.

6. Identify aspects or Tail-Enders while you are doing the rating.

7. Tap them down.

8. Continue the process until the SUB is 8 or higher.

Sometimes as you go through these steps, you will see reasons to modify your affirmation statement. Do that as necessary. Reflect in your journal on the entire process of installing a new guiding model.

ENLISTING YOUR DREAM LIFE

Even as you consciously take the steps in this chapter to make improvements in a specific area of your life, a subconscious part of you is actively working on your personal development. Your dreams provide a glimpse into these unconscious inner workings and allow you to engage with them. The psychologist Steven Ungerleider noted that "inventors, scientists, and writers have credited major accomplishments to ideas that came to them in their dreams."[23]

Robert Hoss, PhD, a dream researcher and the director of the Society for the Study of Dreams, has, with his wife, psychotherapist Lynne Hoss, pioneered the application of acupoint tapping in working with dreams.[24] Their powerful model, which they call "Dream to Freedom," can be applied if (1) you have a dream while you are working with any topic in this book, or (2) you feel stuck and want to *incubate* a dream to call on the wisdom of your unconscious mind for help in that area. A primer for how to use their technique in these ways can be found at dreams.energytapping.com.

IN CLOSING

Formulating the words that accompany your tapping is the *art* of applying an energy psychology approach, but it also follows the principles laid out in this and the previous chapter. As a session progresses, it generally follows this pattern: the opening phases identify, acknowledge, and accept the problem or issue; the focus then moves on to recognizing the obstacles to change and to tapping down the emotional components of those obstacles; and it ends with Choices Statements that emphasize and install the desired outcome.

While this chapter is more complex than any other in the entire book, it teaches many of the most important skills and procedures energy psychology has to offer. The key principle is that if you stop making progress on an issue that matters to you, you can take well-defined steps of detective work to discover what needs to be resolved next and use the procedures taught in this chapter to resolve it. You can return to this chapter at any point in the book that you need a boost.

An article that David wrote, "Words to Tap By," while not essential, may be a useful adjunct to the procedures in this chapter and can be found at tapping-words.energytapping.com. Another article, which was a distillation of more than 800 interviews and survey returns from practitioners and clients, provides a glimpse into the perceptions of a wide range of individuals who use energy psychology, and it synthesizes guidelines for using the approach (800surveys.energytapping.com).

Chapter 3 Recap

Here are the basic steps:

1. Balance your energies.

2. Identify, accept, and neutralize any Psychological Reversals.

3. Identify, accept, and diffuse any other reasons not to change.

4. Identify and transform cognitive distortions and self-limiting beliefs, replacing them with positive inner talk.

5. Find the roots of the problem in your past and resolve lingering issues.

6. Resolve other conflicts that are preventing progress.

7. Consciously install the new guiding model.

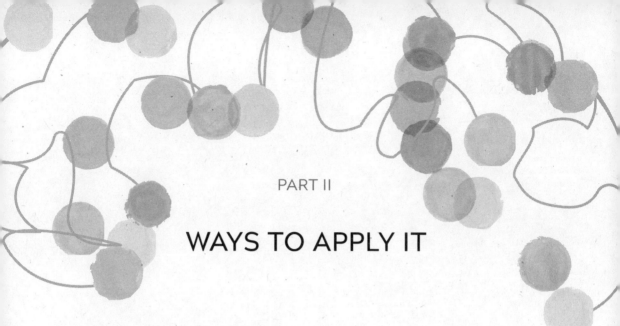

PART II

WAYS TO APPLY IT

THE MOST FREQUENT REASONS people seek help from a therapist are the topics of the first six chapters in Part II. They include:

Chapter 4: Worry, Anxiety, and PTSD

Chapter 5: Sadness and Depression

Chapter 6: Habits and Addictions

Chapter 7: Peak Performance

Chapter 8: Relationships

Chapter 9: When Disaster Strikes

Everyone deals at some point with worry, sadness, self-defeating habits, relationship difficulties, and the desire to perform at their best. Chapters 4 through 8 guide you in applying the Basic Tapping Protocol in each of these areas. Chapter 9 focuses on the uses of energy psychology in communities following a disaster. Finally, Chapter 10 broadens the scope to the social implications of energy psychology.

Chapters 4 through 8 all begin with a "Quick Fix" box and then take you much deeper into the issues involved with the topic. Chapters 4, 5, and 6 also address their topics by offering:

- Case examples demonstrating how PTSD, depression, and addictions have been treated effectively using an acupoint tapping approach

- An overview of the best practices in the mental health field for working with these conditions

- A discussion of how psychotherapists or people in psychotherapy can tailor a tapping approach to build on those best practices

Each chapter in this section assumes a basic understanding of the material in Chapters 2 and 3. With that, you can move through these chapters in any order, as their themes call to you.

You may find yourself going on a profound and multifaceted journey with any one of these chapters as they are each ambitious and substantial. So please pace yourself with compassion and patience.

CHAPTER 4

Worry, Anxiety, and PTSD

Tapping is so successful in stopping phobias, anxiety, PTSD,
and other problems [because] not only does tapping halt the
stress response . . . it retrains the limbic system.[1]

—Nick Ortner
Founder, The Tapping Solution

YOUR NERVOUS SYSTEM CAN be hijacked by adverse experiences, causing it to work against you.[2] To start with a heartrending example, a dozen years after the 1994 genocide in Rwanda, 50 children at the El Shaddai Orphanage in Kigali, still suffered with severe symptoms of PTSD, including anxiety, depression, flashbacks, nightmares, and insomnia. Many of these children, now adolescents, had witnessed their parents being slaughtered. Three of our close colleagues brought Thought Field Therapy to the orphanage. The outcomes of the treatment were measured using an established PTSD symptom checklist completed by the orphans' caregivers before and following the single-session treatments.

The improvements vastly exceeded those of any previous peer-reviewed study of a PTSD treatment in terms of speed, degree of effectiveness, and percentage of subjects who were helped.[3] After a single tapping session (using translators), 47 of the 50 orphans were no longer in the PTSD range on the standardized assessment. Remarkably, benefits were sustained on a one-year follow-up on the same measure with no additional treatments. One of the investigators, the psychologist Caroline Sakai, described the experience of a 15-year-old girl who was three years old at the time of the 1994 genocide:

She'd been hiding with her family and other villagers inside the local church. The church was stormed by men with machetes, who started a massacre. The girl's father told her and other children to run and to not look back for any reason. She obeyed and was running as fast as she could, but then she heard her father "screaming like a crazy man." She remembered what her father had said, but his screams were so compelling that she did turn back and, in horror, watched as a group of men with machetes murdered him.

A day didn't pass in the ensuing 12 years without her experiencing flashbacks to that scene. Her sleep was plagued by nightmares tracing to the memory. In her treatment session, I asked her to bring the flashbacks to mind and to imitate me as I tapped on a selected set of acupuncture points while she told the story of the flashbacks. After a few minutes, her heart-wrenching sobbing and depressed affect suddenly transformed into smiles. When I asked her what happened, she reported having accessed fond memories. For the first time, she could remember her father and family playing together. She said that until then, she had no childhood memories from before the genocide.

We might have stopped there, but I instead directed her back to what happened in the church. The interpreter shot me a look, as if to ask, "Why are you bringing it back up again when she was doing fine?" But I was going for a complete treatment. The girl started crying again. She told of seeing other people being killed. She reflected that she was alive because of her father's quick thinking, distracting the men's attention while telling the children to run.

The girl cried again when she reexperienced the horrors she witnessed while hiding outside with another young child. The two of them were the only survivors from their entire village. Again, the tapping allowed her to have the memory without reliving the terror of the experience.

After about 15 or 20 minutes addressing one scene after another, the girl smiled and began to talk about her family. Her mother didn't allow the children to eat sweet fruits because they weren't good for their teeth. But her father would sneak them home in his pockets and when her mother wasn't looking, he'd give them to the children. She was laughing wholeheartedly as she relayed this, and the translator and I were laughing with her.

Over the following days, she described how, for the first time, she had no flashbacks or nightmares and could sleep well. She looked cheerful and told me how elated she was about having happy memories of her family. Her test scores had gone from well above the PTSD cutoff to well below it after this single treatment session and remained there on the follow-up assessment a year later.[4]

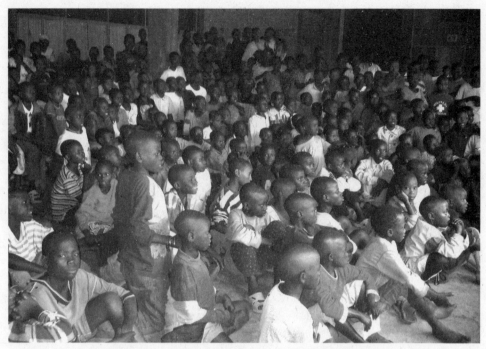

Figure 4.1. Orphaned Rwandan children and adolescents who were taught
a basic tapping protocol by Dr. Caroline Sakai and her team.

The powerful impact of a single tapping session on 47 of the 50 adolescents surprised everyone, including the investigators. They were careful not to imply in speaking with us that just one session is sufficient for treating PTSD. Some people, for instance, may be neurologically poised for a major breakthrough. Still, the number of sessions that have been required for successful treatment with acupoint tapping protocols has been relatively low in comparison with other methods.[5] Even a single tapping session lowered subjective stress and anxiety from an average SUD of 7.7 to 2.5 in a large-scale study involving 1,722 individuals treated by 287 practitioners.[6]

THE SHARED THREAD AMONG WORRY, ANXIETY, AND PTSD

Worry, anxiety, and PTSD fall along a continuum from mild to extreme distress. They are all connected by fear. William James, who served as chair of Harvard University's Department of Psychology from 1875 to 1907, noted that the great challenge for psychological education is "to make our nervous system our ally instead of our enemy."[7] That is the theme of this chapter.

Fear appears early on the evolutionary chain. Mice, our distant mammalian relatives, have highly specific brain circuits for fear, and evolution has maintained this arrangement in the human brain.[8] These circuits trigger automatic life-saving strategies—fight, flight, or freeze—in the face of real and present danger. They are preprogrammed responses to a sense of *immediate* threat. Anxiety, on the other hand, is the body and mind *anticipating* that something dreadful *will* happen. Anxiety can persist over time and isn't always related to an obvious danger.

Recent brain research has, however, revealed a surprising finding about the relationship between fear and anxiety. Although each is a distinctly different emotional state, both use the same neural circuits.[9] PTSD is considered an anxiety disorder because, as with other anxiety disorders, the symptoms arise despite no immediate threat. But PTSD takes anxiety into another dimension, involving serious (though reversible) damage to the nervous system. Both anxiety and PTSD include physiological as well as subjective components. The physiological elements may include heart palpitations, hyperventilation, sweating, trembling, stomach tightness, or nausea. The subjective elements may include feelings of dread, nervousness, panic, impending danger, or doom. Difficulties with sleep and concentration are also common with each.

Worry, which is yet another mental state, tends to first engage the problem-solving regions of your brain. Anxiety may build on worry, but it involves additional physiological and subjective components. With the complexity of modern life, in which our primary stressors are social or psychological, our worries and anxieties become connected to situations or imagined situations that have nothing to do with physical danger. Yet the same fight-flight-freeze chemistry is activated, and the costs to health and inner peace of such distress when it is persistent are well-documented.[10]

In addition to fight-flight-freeze, another response to childhood trauma can lead to *people-pleasing* tendencies. This can be a problem in all subsequent relationships. It is a reason, for instance, that some people stay with an abusive partner.

A tapping approach can help curb excessive worry, counter unwarranted fear and anxiety, overcome "please and appease" tendencies, and heal the extreme manifestations of trauma, such as PTSD or other changes to the nervous system caused by overwhelming distress. We'll begin with worry.

EVERYDAY WORRIES

Everyone experiences worry, and we all have plenty to worry about: health, finances, parenting, loved ones, work, attractiveness, status, upcoming performances, aging. At a more global level, we are compelled to witness rising sea levels, rampant wildfires, and devastating storms. We all wonder if any of these are going to impact us or our family. Is the economy going to collapse? Is crime, terrorism, or nuclear or biological warfare in our future? Are our freedoms and way of life in jeopardy?

Worry directs your attention. It can do this for better or for worse. It helps you anticipate what might go wrong and prepares you to be ready if it does. It helps you focus your problem-solving abilities to prevent what can be prevented. But the worry that can lead to creative strategies that empower you to meet or prevent problems can also become an unrelenting state that swells into anxiety and obsessive fear. It can serve as a psychological straitjacket that narrows your vistas and hampers your most creative responses to the challenges you face.

While anxiety permeates your body, worry starts largely in your mind. A Chinese proverb sums up the way worry can move into anxiety with a vivid metaphor: "That the birds of worry and care fly over your head, this you cannot change; but that they build nests in your hair, this you can prevent."

OVERCOMING EXCESSIVE WORRY

Worry can progress from the way your mind focuses on what needs your attention to ruminating about all the things that *could* go wrong or obsessing about things you can't control. Crossing into these territories squanders your creative energy and drains your life force. Websites that advise people on how to defeat worry or obsessive fear suggest that you train your brain to stop the fear response (one site we found counsels "Just Say No to Fear"), but their instructions on how to do this are thin. However, add tapping to commonsense measures, and you have an effective approach.

Tapping can make strategies such as "accept what you cannot change" and "train your brain to turn off irrational fears" become effective by sending deactivating signals to the brain areas involved with anxiety and fear while sending activating signals to the areas involved with fear management. While it is not well understood how the body knows to get the activating and deactivating signals to the right places, both clinical experience and several imaging studies suggest that it does.[11]

GETTING STARTED

Before we move into ways to apply the Basic Tapping Protocol to worry, we've created the kind of "tapping script" referred to in the Introduction. The one-size-fits-all "Quick Fix" box on the next page gives you an idea of how tapping can be applied to excessive worry. While it doesn't personalize the approach as the chapter's subsequent instructions do, it is likely to yield some benefit and, in any case, will prime you for the following, more complete approach.

Quick Fix: Worry

You can apply this "Quick Fix" tapping script to a worry you feel is out of proportion. Bring your worry to mind and give it a 0-to-10 SUD rating. Say out loud the first statement below as you tap on the Top-of-the-Head Point. Then say the next statement while tapping on the next point. Go through each statement, cycling through the 12 tapping points as you move from one statement to the next. Skip any phrases that don't fit for you.[12]

"Even though I feel worried about [name worry],

I love myself and completely accept that I have this worry.

Even though this worry is draining me and feels intense,

I choose to know that I can release it.

Even though I don't know how to let go of this worry,

I'm open to moving forward.

I feel this worry in my [name the body part].

I know it's draining me.

I'm tapping to reduce this feeling.

And I choose to start to let it go and find greater peace.

Although it sometimes seems safer to worry than to let go,

I'm willing to consider feeling safe without this worry.

I don't need to carry this heavy feeling anymore.

I choose to release this worry and feel lighter.

I breathe in relaxation and breathe out the worry.

Even though I felt overwhelmed by this worry,

I choose to let it start to fade and to move forward with confidence.

I choose to focus on what I can control.

I choose to do what I can to release this worry.

I choose to let the universe guide me toward the right path.

I will find sources of support to help me through this.

I am calm and confident as I allow this worry to fade."

After going through this sequence two or three times, you will probably find that the texture of the worry is already softening. Gauge this with another SUD rating on your worry. Even if the worry still feels excessive, you will have prepared yourself to overcome it by next applying the Basic Tapping Protocol, as shown in this chapter.

WORRY IS A PHYSIOLOGICAL AND PSYCHOLOGICAL STATE

While anxiety engages your brain's fear centers more intensely, a simple worry still affects your body. Your *physiological* response to a worry reveals how your primitive brain or early programming assesses a situation. Quelling that response with energy techniques allows you to engage your advanced problem-solving faculties, unfettered by evolutionary instincts that were more useful in the environment of your distant ancestors or early difficulties from your own life that have not been fully processed.

Excessive worry as a *psychological* state often traces to a guiding model with a pessimistic orientation. For instance, you may overestimate the possibility that things will turn out badly, jump immediately to worst-case scenarios, or treat every anxious thought as fact. This may be a product of your early experiences, but it is also a tendency we have all inherited. Our ancestors needed to anticipate famines, predators, invaders, and other existential threats. Being alert for a hungry lion nearby had greater survival value than finding the sweetest fruits, so they stayed attuned to the many physical dangers lurking in the wild.

As a distant descendent of these survivors, you are still hardwired to give more weight and attention to problems than pleasures. This pessimistic orientation of the human psyche is sometimes called our "negativity bias."[13] The neuropsychologist Rick Hanson famously summarized this arrangement: "Your brain is like Velcro for negative experiences and like Teflon for positive ones."[14] But the responses that are essential in the face of physical danger are often counterproductive when triggered by the psychological stressors of today.

APPLYING THE BASIC TAPPING PROTOCOL TO AN EXCESSIVE WORRY

We are about to walk you through the Basic Tapping Protocol tailored for addressing a worry that you feel may be excessive. Declawing such a worry doesn't mean going into denial about the issues involved. Rather, it means reducing the worry's emotional hold on you. We will briefly describe each of the 12 steps of the Protocol presented in Chapter 2, list the page numbers that describe that step in greater detail, and offer commentary on applying that step to worry. While 12 steps may feel intimidating, you will probably be able to work your way through them in 20 to 30 minutes (unless they unearth deeper issues you decide to address here).

1. THE PREPARATION PHASE

Many worries usefully operate in a "constructive zone," bringing a focus to problems that require your attention. Some, however, become part of the problem you are worrying about or add new dimensions to it. When the worry distorts the facts of a situation, the situation becomes more difficult to handle. For instance, you are worried about how to tell your adult daughter that you don't want to join her family for Thanksgiving. You can't bring yourself to break the news, and you get sick the day before the planned gathering.

Preparation Phase, Step 1: Choose Your Focus (p. 50)

Identify an excessive worry or one that drains your spirit. Some people have dozens of worries. If that's the case for you, choose just one for now. You can apply the same approach to others later if you wish. If nothing comes to mind, imagine something bad that could occur. You don't need to terrify yourself with the worst things you can conjure. Just bring into your awareness something you could lose or a circumstance that could change for the worse.

As with Chapters 2 and 3, our test drivers provided us with their journal entries as they moved through this chapter. We will include reports from two of them. Robert is a happily married bank executive and father of two sons who were born after his first son died of a brain tumor at age three. Robert had no previous experience with tapping. Ava is a 49-year-old therapist, experienced in tapping, who provides clinical services at a mental health clinic and is also an administrator there.

Ava's Worry

"I'm worried about a promotion that would give me additional responsibilities without the authority to make decisions or affect change. My supervisor tends to micromanage, withholds information about plans and initiatives, and shifts course without warning. When I do make decisions, I'm worried that I'll be criticized, blamed, reprimanded, and otherwise unsupported. I'm worried that I'll end up being the scapegoat for anything that goes awry and get 'thrown under the bus.'"

Your Turn

In your journal, briefly describe the worry you have selected. It doesn't need to be as traumatizing as Robert's or as central to your daily life experiences as Ava's, but do select something that matters to you. If your worry is more like a background thought, you can work with it by using phrases such as "Part of me worries that . . ."

Robert's Worry

"I worry every day that one of our other sons will come down with a terrible illness."

Preparation Phase, Step 2: Rate Your Discomfort about It (p. 53)

Focus on your worry and give it a 0-to-10 SUD rating. You are rating the discomfort you feel in your mind and/or body as you tune in to the worry. Your emphasis here is on the way the worry is draining your spirit. Write the number in your journal next to your description of your worry.

Your Turn

Notice the thoughts and sensations that come to you as you bring your worry to mind. Give a 0-to-10 SUD rating on the intensity of your worry based on these sensations and your sense of distress.

Robert's Initial SUD

The sensations Robert identified included an intense pressure in his chest, moving up through his throat and settling behind his eyes as if trying to force tears through them. His fear of losing his sons was enormous. His SUD was a 10.

Ava's Initial SUD

When tuning in to her worry, Ava kept seeing her supervisor in her mind and thinking about his unfairness. She also noticed an uncomfortable sensation on the right side under her rib cage. She rated her worry as an 8.

Preparation Phase, Step 3: Create a Reminder Phrase (p. 55)

Your Reminder Phrase keeps your worry psychologically active while you do the tapping. It doesn't need to completely describe the situation, just enough so you know what it means.

Robert's Reminder Phrase

"Cancer could strike again."

Ava's Reminder Phrase

"I'll be thrown under the bus."

Your Turn

Write down a few words that will keep your worry activated as you tap.

Preparation Phase, Step 4: Formulate Your Acceptance Statement (p. 55)

Your Acceptance Statement is simply a description of your issue followed by accepting yourself and/or accepting yourself for having this issue.

Robert's Acceptance Statement

"Even though I have this overwhelming terror that Mason or Oliver might get cancer, I accept my fears."

Ava's Acceptance Statement

"Even though I'm worried that I'll be blamed for everything that goes wrong at work if I take this promotion, I deeply and completely accept myself."

Your Turn

Building on your Reminder Phrase, write your Acceptance Statement in your journal.

2. THE TAPPING CYCLE

The core of an energy psychology session involves anchoring your Acceptance Statement, tapping while repeating your Reminder Phrase, practicing the Integration Procedure, tapping again, and taking a new SUD rating. We take you through each step here.

The Tapping Cycle, Step 1: Anchor Your Acceptance Statement (p. 57)

Find your chest sore spots and massage them as you say the first part of your Acceptance Statement. Place your hands over your Heart Chakra at the center of your chest as you say the second part. Repeat twice. Do this now.

The Tapping Cycle, Steps 2-4: Tap, Integrate, Tap (pp. 60-63)

Now do a tapping round while saying your Reminder Phrase at each acupoint (Step 2). Follow this with the Integration Procedure (Step 3) and another round of tapping paired with your Reminder Phrase (Step 4). Remember to state your Reminder Phrase with enough emphasis and feeling that it doesn't become rote.

These three steps should take less than three minutes. We want to reemphasize that you are not embedding the worry deeper into your psyche, though this is how it might seem at first. Rather, the tapping sends deactivating signals to fear and threat centers of your brain triggered by the worry.

The Tapping Cycle, Step 5: Take a New SUD Rating (p. 63)

Following the first round of tapping, the Integration Procedure, and another round of tapping (as above), give your worry another SUD rating. Repeat this process until your SUD won't go down any further.

Robert's New SUD Rating

Robert was of course working with an extremely intense and difficult issue. It did go down to an 8 after he noticed "I no longer have that choking feeling," but it stayed at an 8 after two more rounds of tapping.

Ava's New SUD Rating

Ava wrote in her journal:

After three rounds of tapping on "the uncomfortable sensations under my ribs," the sensation was gone (SUD down to 0), but I noticed tightness in my throat, which I rated at an 8. As I felt into this sensation, I associated it with an inability to speak up or be heard. I tapped on it while thinking of not being heard. After two rounds of tapping, I began to yawn. The tightness in my throat had decreased and my worry about additional responsibilities without authority was at a 4.

Your Turn

Thinking of your original worry, give it a 0-to-10 SUD rating on how much discomfort it evokes in your mind and/or body right now. Note the number in your journal. Repeat the "Tapping Cycle" Steps 2–5, staying with the same Reminder Phrase. If your SUD number is unchanged after two times through Steps 2–5, go on to the next section, "Adjusting the Protocol." If your SUD has gone down, continue to repeat Steps 2–5 until it doesn't go down any farther. At that point, or at any time the number has increased (which usually means another aspect of the worry has emerged), also move to the following section.

3. ADJUSTING THE PROTOCOL

Once you have gone through an initial cycle of the Protocol, you can make adjustments so the wording stays attuned to who you are and how you are progressing.

Adjusting the Protocol, Step 1: Turning Your Acceptance Statement into a Choices Statement (p. 64)

Review your initial Acceptance Statement. You will slightly modify the first part by simply acknowledging that some of the charge might still be there even after the tapping. The reason for this is, again, that the unconscious mind is very literal, so making these minor adjustments keeps you better attuned to what has unfolded. For instance, *"Even though part of me worries that this will be a setback . . ."* becomes *"Even though part of me **still** has **some** worry that this will be a setback . . ."*

You can stay with this slightly revised Acceptance Statement, using it before subsequent rounds of tapping. A time comes, however, as the SUD diminishes, that it is useful to transform the Acceptance Statement into a Choices Statement (p. 92). The reason we don't usually introduce the Choices Statement until the SUD has gone down substantially is that the Choices Statement may introduce a solution before you are ready to embrace that solution. But once you are ready, the second part of your statement (following the *"Even though"* part) might become something like:

"I choose to be calm and confident."

"I choose to learn something absolutely essential for my own life from this situation."

"I choose to have this worry open my heart."

"I choose to have this difficult challenge make me stronger."

"I choose to discover new resources in myself."

"I choose to embrace the fact that I can't control what I can't control."

The format for the Choices Statement is already familiar to you: *"Even though I'm worried that [describe your worry], I choose to [describe the choice]."* If a believable Choices Statement to counter the first phrase isn't occurring to you, continue to use the Acceptance Statement.

Robert's Choices Statement

"Even though I still have much of this overwhelming terror that Mason or Oliver might get cancer, I choose to have fond memories of Bobby's legacy."

And:

"I choose to live in appreciation about my two healthy sons rather than fear of something extremely unlikely."

Adjusting the Protocol, Step 2: Address the Aspects of the Situation by Going Beyond Your Reminder Phrase (p. 66)

Tracking the physical and psychological aspects of your worry is an inner journey that may go in various directions. For many people and many worries, the steps you have taken to this point will reduce the intensity and persistence of the worry considerably. You may, however, still find some aspects that, if attended to, can take it down further. Bringing in aspects may also raise additional issues, which you can address one by one with the Basic Tapping Protocol. Part of the power of acupoint tapping is how quickly you can resolve an issue and move on to the next.

You may notice as you examine the aspects of your worry that one aspect may seem to oppose another. For instance, one aspect may be feelings related to a difficult experience, such as being sad and hurt. Another aspect might be a part of you attempting to protect yourself from reliving those negative feelings by, for instance, avoiding situations that might evoke the feelings. Just work with whatever comes into your awareness and stay with the flow if, after tapping one aspect down (e.g., *I allow myself to feel my feelings*"), another emerges (e.g., the sadness and hurt the first aspect was protecting you from experiencing). Likewise, after clearing one worry, another worry may be waiting in the wings. A great strength of tapping is that you can bring an accepting awareness to each aspect that arises in the present moment and resolve each of them. We will describe both Robert's and Ava's experiences as they focused on aspects that arose.

Additional Aspects of Robert's Worry

For Robert, the unresolved aspect of his worry—the experience of Bobby's painful illness and death—was huge. Memories of that time flooded him when he explored why his SUD rating seemed stuck at an 8. What began with a protocol that is effective for reducing most worries evolved into helping to heal the most tragic event of his life.

Robert and his wife had spoken with a grief counselor in the months following Bobby's death, and they also participated in an eight-week support group for parents who had lost a child. They found these to be helpful, but oceans of grief remained. Robert managed to suppress much of this as time passed and he resumed his daily activities and responsibilities. It was in the persistent worry that one of their other sons would become ill, however, that his grief refused to remain submerged.

This stubborn reminder that illness had struck like lightning and could strike again had cast a dark cloud over Robert's life. It hampered his ability to fully enjoy what was by almost any standard highly fortunate circumstances: a good marriage, two delightful and healthy sons, a job he enjoyed, and a comfortable lifestyle. In a follow-up visit with their grief counselor a year after Bobby's passing, Robert described his unrelenting sadness. He happened to mention the opportunity to be a test driver for the book you are now reading. While the grief counselor wasn't trained in energy psychology, she was familiar with the method and encouraged Robert to apply it to his memories of the period from Bobby's diagnosis through his death. Robert did this in a systematic manner, going through the steps of the Basic Tapping Protocol.

Dozens of memories were readily available to him. He tapped on the moment he realized Bobby's symptoms were of concern; the office visit where the doctor announced that Bobby's headaches were due to a brain tumor; the first time he tried to explain to Bobby the medical situation; several instances where Bobby's pain from the pressure caused by the tumor was hard to console; the despair and helplessness he felt when strategizing with his wife about how to manage Bobby's illness; moments of recognizing Bobby's deterioration; Bobby's death; and seeing Bobby in the casket. He addressed these one or two at a time, usually in sessions of about 15 to 20 minutes each. Some memories required more than one session. He did all the steps in the Basic Tapping Protocol, including tapping on aspects that would emerge as he took subsequent SUD ratings.

Each of Robert's memories started with a high SUD rating—an extreme sense of distress in his body and mind when he recalled the experience. The tapping didn't make the memories less horrible, but it allowed Robert to remember the experience without reliving its agony. He reached a point where the "generalization effect" discussed earlier (p. 72) was set into motion so that other memories he had initially identified didn't need more attention.

While it was painful to revisit these memories in vivid detail, the relief was so palpable that he was motivated to return to the process to tackle the next memory. He attended to every memory he had initially listed or that came up during the tapping in the space of about a week, with one or two sessions nearly every day.

After this arduous process, he again rated the worry about his remaining sons becoming sick and gave it a new SUD. It had gone down from an 8 to a 4. He then went through Chapter 3, which is designed to take you further if the Basic Tapping Protocol isn't producing the full outcome you desire. His energies took a hit whenever he went into this worry, so doing a simple energy technique was immediately soothing.

Robert also easily identified a Psychological Reversal: "If I stop worrying, it will happen." At a deep level, he believed that it wasn't safe to stop worrying. This responded to the techniques for working with Psychological Reversals and cognitive distortions. The single most powerful procedure was the inner dialogue. Robert realized he wanted to say some things to Bobby, and he imagined Bobby was right there as he told him, while tearfully tapping, how much he loved him, how much he missed him, and finally how it was time for him to move on from the overwhelming grief he had been carrying since Bobby's death.

After taking these steps, Robert's SUD on his worry was down to 2, which he felt was okay, almost as a tribute to how deeply he loved his first child and a recognition that some things are out of his control. While taking the SUD down to 0 is ideal, taking it down to 1 or 2 may, again, be perfect in many situations, such as Robert's, or if a tenacious old model is being gradually dismantled, or when an athlete or performer finds that a little bit of anxiety helps them do their best. The steps Robert needed to take to deal with his worry had required him to squarely face and then process an indescribably painful emotional wound, taking a giant leap toward healing it.

We selected his story because we wanted to illustrate the web of issues that can be tangled around a single worry and to show that tapping can effectively address each issue tied to a worry rooted in an even devastating experience. Many worries, however, will become less intrusive after working with the bodily sensations they evoke. Most worries will be reshaped into a more grounded guiding model after practicing the basic steps outlined above. While not as traumatic as Robert's, Ava's worry also led her to some challenging moments.

Additional Aspects of Ava's Worry

Ava began with the modified Acceptance Statement and Reminder Phrase, *"Thrown under the bus."* As she was tapping, she had thought, "You didn't do it right. That's not how we do it here." The following is from her journal:

I continued tapping, following my inner voice. I realized the voice sounded like my supervisor, which also sounded like my mother. I thought back to an earlier time that I had that feeling or heard someone say, "You didn't do it right," and landed on an event from middle childhood (about eight) when I was chastised for not cleaning my room well enough. I felt proud of how well I had cleaned my room and called her to see. Instead of delivering praise, my mom ran her finger across the top of the doorjamb, revealing dust, and stated, "Looks like you missed a spot." I felt crushed, embarrassed, and angry. I tapped on the statement: *"Even though my mom found dust on the doorjamb, and it feels like I've been kicked in the gut, I choose to recognize that this was about my mom, not me."* But the SUD was still a 9.

Aspects:

- *Seeing my mom at the doorjamb, holding up her finger to reveal dust.*

- *Hearing my mom say, "Looks like you missed a spot."*

- *It feels like a kick in the gut.*

- *Being ashamed for not cleaning well enough.*

- *Thinking, "I did a bad job."*

- *Deciding that no matter how hard I work, it won't be good enough.*

Reminder Phrase: *"You missed a spot."*

I became tearful as I tapped on the phrase, *"You missed a spot."* I continued tapping and added the integration (eyes, humming, counting). After three rounds, my SUD was down to 7.

I continued tapping through aspects as I cried, recalling that when I was a child, I was afraid to cry for fear of being punished. I rocked back and forth while holding energy relaxation points. I envisioned my current self holding my younger self, stating "That was really unkind" while she cried. Once she seemed more regulated, I pointed out some of the things she had done well (organized the books on the bookshelf, arranged things neatly in the closet, cleaned under the bed, vacuumed, etc.). She didn't respond, but she allowed me to approach and comfort her while she cried.

My SUD remained at 7 on the statement, *"You missed a spot."*

I noticed what felt like a knot in my diaphragm and

observed it for a few moments to feel into its qualities. The knot felt dense and dark and tightly wound, like the inner core of a baseball. I tapped on the sensation, color, and density of the energy in my diaphragm. The knot loosened slightly and then moved up into my chest and throat. I belched several times and continued tapping. The sensation of the knot SUD reduced to a 5. I rechecked *"You missed a spot,"* and the SUD had gone down from 7 to 3.

Returning to the original memory, I heard my mom say, "You missed a spot," and her voice seemed more playful, as if she was making a joke. (Since my room was so clean, she had to really search for anything out of place or dirty, and there was no way I could have reached the top of the doorjamb.)

I closed my eyes and placed my adult self back into the scene at the point my mom left the room. Instead of my eight-year-old self being upset, she asked for a boost so she could reach the top of the doorjamb to dust it. After she wiped the dust, I stayed and invited her to read together. I stayed while my child self showed me her books and talked about things she liked to do. We agreed to go swimming together.

My SUD level on *"You missed a spot"* reduced to zero.

I revisited my Choices Statement: *"Even though I still have some fear that I'll be blamed for everything that goes wrong at work if I accept this promotion, I choose to embrace that even though that might happen, I can move forward with joy and confidence."*

The SUD had reduced to 0. I realized "That's her stuff to work through" when I imagined my supervisor blaming me for things going wrong.

Your Turn

Many worries will respond to the Basic Tapping Protocol without the elaborate steps illustrated by Robert's and Ava's experiences. As you continue to work with your worry, notice what opportunities come to mind for focusing on its aspects or exploring your past.

4. TESTING YOUR RESULTS (p. 74)

This last step in the Basic Tapping Protocol, "Testing Your Results," is taken when all the other work on the issue has been completed. In it, you will imagine a situation that tests whether the new SUD rating is stable. Note that the imagined situation is *not* that what you are worried about has occurred. It is a situation that triggers your worry that it *might* occur. If, as your life goes on, the situation does occur, you will be more psychologically prepared to meet it if you have separated the worry from unhelpful physiological and emotional responses and made its guidance as constructive as possible. For Robert, it would have made no sense to test his results while the SUD was still at an 8. But once it was down to a 2, which he felt was appropriate given the history, he was ready to imagine a situation that would test the stability of his gains.

Robert's Challenge

Robert conjured the image of a good friend having just learned that his daughter had been diagnosed with diabetes. Robert was able to imagine himself consoling and counseling the friend without being plunged into terror for his own sons. This was a relief, and a bit of a surprise, demonstrating that the progress he made on his terrifying worry was substantial and stable.

Ava's Challenge

"I played out an imagined scene of myself in the new supervisory role. My boss came into my office and started to confront me about a decision I had made. I listened and provided feedback but did not feel myself becoming activated or defensive. My SUD remained at 0."

Your Turn

Imagine a situation that would challenge your progress. Play out the scenario vividly in your mind. If your improvements prove to be stable, you have done as much as you can to keep this particular worry in a constructive zone. If the SUD shoots back up, notice the sensations or thoughts that led to the higher rating. You may wish to tap on them or repeat some of the earlier steps. If it is a major area of discontent that isn't responding to the techniques in this chapter, and you are intent on resolving it now, Chapter 3 offers powerful guidance.

OVERCOMING ANXIETY

Moving now from worry into anxiety, anxiety has reached epidemic proportions worldwide, affecting more than 40 million people in the US alone, including many children and young adults. While some forms of anxiety, such as obsessive-compulsive disorder (OCD) are very difficult to treat, treatments are available. Yet only about a third of those living with acute anxiety in the US are receiving treatment, and the consequences of not receiving adequate help for chronic anxiety can be substantial. Left untreated, anxiety is considered a "gateway" disorder that often leads to physical illness, depression, or drug and alcohol abuse.[15] Even mild anxiety can have serious long-term effects. A study of 68,222 adults found that simply having low-level chronic anxiety resulted in a 20 percent greater risk of dying during the eight-year course of the investigation, along with other physical and emotional problems.[16]

Research on Tapping for Overcoming Anxiety

Clinical studies show that acupoint tapping protocols are highly effective for treating anxiety. A 2016 statistical analysis assessed the 14 peer-reviewed clinical trials that had been conducted by the time of the study.[17] Published in the prestigious *Journal of Nervous and Mental Disease*, a total of 658 people receiving treatment showed that acupoint tapping had a strong impact on reducing the disorder. Here are some examples of the individual studies cited in that analysis:

- The anxiety level of women about to receive surgery declined by 74 percent after a single tapping session.

- Anxiety among war veterans dropped by 42 percent after six EFT sessions.

- People with a fear of public speaking reached statistically significant improvements after a 45-minute tapping session.

- High school students with test anxiety about their university entrance exams had a 37 percent drop in their anxiety levels after a brief tapping program.

These changes weren't just subjective. Cortisol is a stress hormone produced by your body. While it is essential for managing stress, too much cortisol can cause anxiety and activate the fight-or-flight response without any external cause.[18] A single tapping session has been shown to significantly reduce cortisol levels[19] and facilitate positive changes in gene expression.[20] The impact of tapping on hormones, gene expression, and other physiological states[21] are underlying dynamics in its effectiveness with psychological disorders.

Case Report: Treatment for an Anxiety Disorder

Emily was in her 20s when she scheduled a session with David for anxieties that had been getting in the way of her life for many years. They were particularly strong when she had to be around other people or even if she had to consider being in a social situation. She was terrified she would say something or do something and get made fun of. Going to work as a salesclerk in a department store was a daily torment. She would say as little as possible while still being polite to shoppers. She also vigilantly avoided friendships and never accepted the dating invitations that would occasionally come from an interested customer. Asked when she believed these feelings began, she described an incident shortly after starting college. She was having lunch with several new friends and mentioned how attracted she was to a campus football hero. One of the girls said, "Hell will freeze over before he'd go out with you!" The other girls chimed in with derisive laughter. Emily never returned to college.

While touched by the poignancy of this story, David sensed that Emily's fear of judgment went back much further. While being guided in the Affect Bridge (p. 109), Emily recalled a forgotten incident from kindergarten when she was on the playground. It was a windy day. Emily was chasing a girl who had made off with a doll she had been playing with. The wind caught Emily's skirt so that everyone could see her undergarments.

But that day, Emily had forgotten to wear any. As kindergartners are prone to do, this was all the kids talked about for the rest of the day.

Emily was beyond humiliated, and the tapping had to address the many aspects of this incident, such as the moment she noticed others were looking at her and realizing what they were seeing, the flush of embarrassment in her chest and face, the voices of other children making fun of her, her anger at herself for having forgotten to put on her panties, the feeling of wanting to disappear. Once every aspect she could identify had been neutralized, with its SUD down to 0, the incident from college was also brought down to 0. This was all in the first session.

In the next session, they focused on situations that triggered her anxiety. Her dread of going to work was prominent, as well as specific incidents that occurred during work, such as when she had to assist a loud, tight-knit group of women who had entered the store that week. Her tapping focused on not only distant and recent memories but also the related physical sensations, which in Emily's case included feeling her heart racing, sweating, and stomach discomfort. Finally, with the memories, triggers, and physical sensations relatively neutralized, the third session addressed her guiding model that being around people was a sure path to being ridiculed. She could then tap while imagining future situations where she was around other people with no anxiety.

At the fourth and final session addressing her anxiety, Emily reported that she had accepted a dinner invitation from one of her customers and had a wonderful evening. A couple of years later, Emily arranged another session about her problems with a new boyfriend. The session began with her reflecting how, after our brief work together, she stopped avoiding social situations and with that, the old guiding model that kept her terrified of doing something embarrassing had faded into a distant memory.

Applying Tapping to Anxiety

Many of the steps for addressing a worry also apply to working with anxiety, so we won't be taking you through another process as we did for worry, but we will discuss some additional areas to concentrate on if you are using the book for addressing anxiety. These points are condensed but convey the essential principles.

- We cannot overemphasize the importance of attending to your body when working with anxiety. Keep yourself well-nourished and hydrated. Use energy medicine techniques such as the Daily Energy Routine (der.energytapping.com) to calm yourself when needed and to establish a baseline of calm through regular use.

- When anxiety does arise, scan for sensations that accompany it. Tune in to and tap on them periodically using the Basic Tapping Protocol.

- Identify, examine, and tap on early experiences that were formative in the onset of your anxiety. Use the Affect Bridge (p. 109) to find incidents that may not be immediately apparent.

- Describe in your journal the guiding model perpetuating your anxiety and keep tracking it. Notice how it shifts as you process unresolved emotions from earlier experiences. Challenge any cognitive distortions or self-defeating beliefs, as you learned to do in Chapter 3.

- Identify triggers that provoke your anxiety and use tapping to neutralize them individually.

- Be meticulous in the "Testing Your Results" phase (p. 74), imagining situations that would have made you anxious before the tapping work.

- If your SUD goes up with the "Test Your Results" procedure, receive that as useful information. An obvious next step would be to tap on the scenario you are imagining. Another would be to look for additional aspects that are keeping the SUD from going down. If you're not sure and want to take this to a deeper level, proceed through the detective work presented in Chapter 3.

As always, outside resources are available if you have gone as far as you can with self-help tools and want a more complete resolution of excessive worry, anxiety, or related concerns. Licensed mental health professionals who are trained in tapping as well as life coaches specializing in the method can be found in almost every major city.[22] Remote video sessions are also proving to be an effective way of receiving guided tapping sessions.

PANIC ATTACKS

A panic attack involves extreme anxiety condensed into several minutes that seem interminable. The physical components may include rapid breathing or shortness of breath; chest or stomach pain; sweating; trembling; and/or a rapid, fluttering, or pounding of the heart. The mind may be experiencing intense fear, anxiety, or a vivid sense of impending doom or death. You can't talk yourself out of a panic attack, but you can take simple physical and energy-informed steps that can stop one. Here is a poignant example.

Tapping During a Panic Attack

A friend of ours, a college history professor who had been learning EFT, shared this account with us of how he turned to tapping during a panic attack. It is from his journal reflections, edited for readability:

My wife was out of town, and I found myself ruminating one night on all the terrible things that could happen, from the deaths of loved ones to losing everything in a fire to being buried alive in an earthquake to a painful illness to actual torture. I get into these horrifying spaces often, and it's not by choice. I know too much about history to deny that these kinds of things can and do happen. When I go into these spaces, terrible images just seem to intrude into my mind. I don't know why. Maybe I have some twisted, deep logic that imagining these scenarios is helping prepare me should one of them come my way or is even in some mysterious way preventing them from happening. I know that isn't how it works, but I keep falling into these dark holes.

This time, however, the horrifying daydreams developed into something more than my usual terror tour of what can go wrong. I started to tumble into a physical reaction I couldn't control: heart pounding, shallow breath, trembling, wanting to run but not knowing where or how. I thought to myself, "I'm having a panic attack!"

I'd never had a panic attack before, but as anyone who has had one knows, the overwhelming sense of panic is horrible. And no end is in sight, making it immeasurably worse. The leap into my observer self, by naming what was happening as a panic attack, might have given me enough distance from being totally immersed in the anxiety to realize that it was only temporary. But suddenly, just as this thought was starting to give some comfort, another thought intruded: "Every dreadful thing you're fearing is a possibility. You are seeing things as they *really* are. Your usual denial won't get you out of this one. The 'panic attack' you are having right now is forever!"

I felt trapped, and the panic wasn't subsiding. While I wasn't thinking very clearly, naming it a panic attack immediately brought up that tapping can help with anxiety. So I began tapping on the EFT points. My first words were, "Even though I'm having a panic attack, I accept what is happening." I didn't know if this would help, but I noticed after the first time I said this phrase, I took a long inhale. By the third time, I was calm enough to examine what was going on; I was out of the *panic attack*. My breathing and heart rate were heading back to normal—but my mind was still filled with anxiety.

I was absorbed in the blunt truth that we human beings are totally vulnerable. Our lives and the lives of those we love can be snuffed out in an instant. In any case, pain and suffering are likely to be part of our future. These are realities we usually cope with by trying to tuck them as far away in the recesses of our minds as we can so that we are able to get on with our lives. But I was caught in vivid imagery of how these terrible things might play out, so they were front and center, and there was no "off" switch.

After exploring every angle I could think of for getting out of this waking nightmare, I reluctantly realized that the *only* effective way out is to surrender. Loss and death are going to come with or without my consent. Tapping on accepting this instead of being *obsessed with wishing I could change what can't be changed* calmed me further. There is nothing in my repertoire for stopping death, acts of nature, or social collapse. I tapped on *"It's not on my shoulders to prevent what I can't prevent."* With that, I was able to go to sleep last night.

Today I feel calm as I reflect on last night's experience from a centered space. I can savor that my life is good and let that fortify me. I can deal with whatever happens rather than torturing myself about what might happen.

Four Steps for Stopping a Panic Attack

As you just saw with our friend, acknowledging that a panic attack is occurring is the first step in taking immediate control of the situation. No one needs to have this experience. It's not like a good cry that leaves you feeling cleansed and refreshed. Rather, panic leaves you scared, shakes your confidence, and has you worrying that it could happen again and wanting to avoid the types of situations in which it occurred.

If you've ever had a panic attack, which is often traumatizing, tap on the memory of your first or worst attack, as you did for a difficult memory in Chapter 2. This is to disperse the emotional residue of your past experiences. Then practice these four simple steps to internalize them, so they will be there when you need them.

1. Recognize what is happening and **remind yourself that despite how it feels, it will pass** and cause no physical harm. If panic attacks are a recurring issue for you, rehearse these words so they will be available to you if you need them: *"I am having a panic attack and can bring calm back to my body right now."* You should, however, also educate yourself on how to recognize the difference between a heart attack and a panic attack, because this may be vital information in that moment.[23] People having a panic attack often believe they are having a heart attack because both share some common symptoms, such as chest pains and altered breathing.

2. Next, **anchor yourself to the here and now**. Look at your feet. Look at your hands. Hold the base of the ring finger of one hand with the thumb and index finger of your other hand. Besides grounding you in the present moment, this also activates points on your ring finger that ease the fight-or-flight response. You will probably find your breathing start to regulate.

3. Continue to focus on regulating your breathing as you **place one open hand over your forehead and the other on the back of your head** just above your neck. One of our colleagues, the psychologist Tara Cousineau, calls this the "brain hug." It activates points that calm the body and reduce distress.

4. As you feel the panic subsiding, continue the same breathing as you place one hand on your chest and, with the four fingers of your other hand, tap on the ridge below the fourth and fifth fingers on the back of the hand that is on your chest (see Figure 2.4 on p. 62). These are points you already know from the Basic Tapping Protocol. They turn off the fight-or-flight response. If you find it helpful, imagine yourself in a comfortable place. During a calm time, you may want to cultivate an image of a "safe place" you can revisit when needed.

If you are in the midst of a panic attack and you use this process, you will probably have steered yourself into a much calmer space. The physical residue of a panic attack may, however, include tightness that remains in your body. A technique called "progressive muscle relaxation" can release this tightness (as might a brisk walk, a run, a swim, a bath, or anything else that relaxes you). Progressive muscle relaxation involves going through each muscle group in your body (e.g., your hands, arms, feet, legs, abdomen, chest, groin, neck, face), tightening all the muscles in that area for six seconds while holding your breath. Then say or think "Relax" as you release the muscles while slowly letting your breath out your mouth. Then move on to the next muscle group.

Once the physical stresses of the experience have been soothed, you may want to bring your attention to any troubling thoughts related to the panic attack or triggers that may have preceded it and set it off. You can address these using the Basic Tapping Protocol.

OVERCOMING POST-TRAUMATIC DISTRESS

If you are experiencing moderate to severe psychological symptoms of trauma, abuse, or physical injury, you may experience a host of symptoms such as flashbacks, nightmares, sleep difficulties, problems concentrating, extreme startle reactions, self-destructive choices (e.g., substance abuse or taking unnecessary risks), angry outbursts, overwhelming guilt, shame, sadness, helplessness, or denial of the traumatic event. You may avoid places, activities, or people that remind you of the traumatic situation.

We must emphasize that no book can responsibly promise to facilitate the level of healing that is achievable for you. While it is possible to overcome PTSD on a self-help basis, we strongly encourage you to seek treatment from a qualified practitioner and to use this chapter in conjunction with that person.

This section is written for mental health professionals interested in using tapping with clients dealing with serious trauma-based disorders and for those clients. We are not imparting secrets that should be withheld from people who have been traumatized. This discussion may in fact be of great interest to people receiving treatment for these types of conditions as well as for their family and friends.

While the earlier guidelines in this chapter for addressing worry, excessive fear, anxiety, and panic may all apply, there is no substitute for being with a caring, knowledgeable, skilled guide if deep emotional wounds are opened as part of the healing process. Our goal is to identify recognized "best practices," particularly from the clinical literature on PTSD,[24] and present ways to incorporate them into a therapist-assisted acupoint tapping approach.

What Is PTSD?

PTSD is considered an "anxiety disorder," with its symptoms and disruption to life at the extreme end of anxiety conditions, which also include phobias, generalized anxiety disorder, panic attacks, and obsessive-compulsive disorders. Among the most common causes of PTSD are witnessing or being directly involved in violence; being the victim of sexual or physical abuse, either as an adult or in childhood; and being involved in either serious accidents or natural disasters such as tornadoes, hurricanes, floods, tsunamis, and wildfires. Traumatic distress occurs when you have been in a dangerous situation you can't control and your coping mechanisms are overwhelmed.

The Body Keeps the Score. *The Body Keeps the Score*,[25] Bessel van der Kolk's book and earlier paper of this title, heralded a shift in the mental health field's understanding of trauma and how it needs to be treated. The book stayed in the number one slot on the *New York Times* paperback nonfiction list for 27 of the remarkable 232 weeks it was on that list. We were honored to present on energy approaches for treating trauma at his prestigious International Trauma Conference in 2015 (the 26th annual gathering—he still hosts the conference each year and has invited us back). We consider Dr. van der Kolk a cherished friend and colleague. He has identified three pivotal ways that PTSD changes the brain:

1. The amygdala, the primitive part of the brain involved in identifying threat, *amplifies any signs of danger*;

2. The thalamus, which is involved in orchestrating sensory information, *loses its ability to filter irrelevant information*, leading to overwhelm and confusion even in ordinary situations;

3. The neurological system involved in generating your sense of self, which runs through midline structures of the brain, becomes blunted, resulting in *dampened responses to pleasure, excitement, sensation, and connection.*

Abram Kardiner, MD, one of the foremost pioneers in the understanding and treatment of PTSD, underlined the physiological *nucleus* of PTSD.[26] The brain's threat centers relive experiences from the past or interpret ordinary experiences as fraught with danger. Effective psychotherapy can shift this neurological pattern, reversing each of the three brain changes identified by Dr. van der Kolk.

PTSD and the Nervous System. Your nervous system responds to threats with the familiar fight-flight-freeze response. The prototype for this strategy is found in the earliest multi-celled creatures, and it remains a central defense mechanism in all mammals. The fight-or-flight reactions are initiated in the amygdala. Heart rate and respiration increase as fuel in the form of glucose is pumped throughout the body to prepare for fighting or fleeing. Freezing is an even more primitive response. It is used in the animal kingdom when "playing dead" or trying to be unnoticed are the only available defense strategies. A child may experience this when, for instance, trapped and being molested by an adult. The freeze response is governed by the vagus nerve, the longest nerve in your body, which extends from your brain stem to your belly and through many organs.

Like the amygdala, and often in collaboration with it, the vagus nerve appraises safety or danger, friend or foe, before you are conscious of these assessments.[27] If danger has been identified, primitive fight-flight-freeze responses are set into motion. When safety has been reestablished, the vagus nerve calls off these responses and, according to the psychologist Stephen Porges' provocative polyvagal theory, activates its "social engagement system," a more advanced evolutionary development.[28] Since PTSD keeps the person in a threat response even when danger is not present, therapies that can stimulate the vagus nerve's social engagement system are an antidote to PTSD.

The psychologist Robert Schwarz has described how acupoint tapping treatments can keep the vagus nerve's social engagement system as its default, rather than the more primitive threat response.[29] When a person with PTSD thinks about a core traumatic event, or anything emotionally connected to that event, the vagus nerve causes the body to automatically react as if the person is not safe. It's extremely difficult to talk oneself out of this response. Acupoint tapping appears to send deactivating signals to the vagus nerve while the vagus nerve initiates an alarm. The alarm

is interrupted, and the experience changes profoundly. Now the body stays calm as the person thinks of the event, and the social engagement system can be set in motion.

This presumably works in conjunction with the deactivating signals that acupoint tapping sends to the amygdala. As these shifts become established with tapping, people who have suffered with PTSD can rebuild their lives more creatively, without the weight of continually reliving the worst traumas of their lives. Nonetheless, PTSD is notoriously difficult to treat effectively. CBT and its variations are still considered the standards of care for treating PTSD in many conventional treatment settings,[30] yet two-thirds of service members and veterans completing a course of cognitive-oriented therapy in the peer-reviewed studies published in the *35 years* between 1980 and 2015 still met PTSD diagnostic criteria *after* treatment![31] High dropout rates have also been a problem in CBT treatments of PTSD.[32] Acupoint tapping protocols, on the other hand, are showing themselves to be highly effective.

The Research on Using Tapping with PTSD

The first high-quality controlled study of energy psychology for veterans with PTSD had a low dropout rate and found that 86 percent of the 49 veterans treated no longer tested in the PTSD range after six one-hour tapping sessions (see Figure 4.2).[33] The study has been replicated,[34] and subsequent research has produced strong evidence supporting these findings.[35]

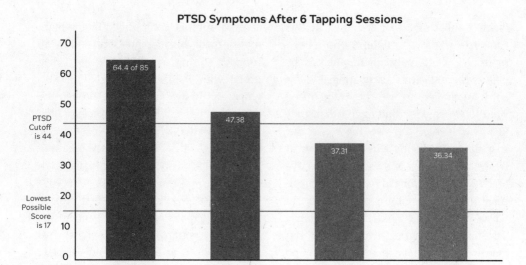

Figure 4.2. The researchers used the military version of the standardized "PTSD Checklist" (PCL-M) before and after the tapping treatments.

An analysis of data from seven independent studies examined outcomes for a total of 247 patients receiving tapping treatments for PTSD. The study found high "effect sizes," a statistical measure of impact, which indicates strong improvements.[36] One of these investigations examined the use of tapping for treating PTSD in a public health facility in Scotland.[37] The patients were allowed to receive up to eight treatment sessions. Voluntary termination of treatment occurred, however, after an average of 3.8 sessions, with large improvements reported on post-treatment measures.

In a study of group treatment of 218 veterans and their spouses, 83 percent of the veterans and 29 percent of the spouses initially tested positive for PTSD (for spouses, a dynamic known as "vicarious PTSD" often takes hold).[38] After a week-long residential retreat that included four days of EFT and other energy psychology techniques, symptoms had dropped dramatically. On a six-week follow-up, only 28 percent of the veterans (down from 83 percent) and 4 percent of the spouses (down from 29 percent) tested in the PTSD range.

In an analysis comparing 36 studies of a variety of treatments for helping children who had been traumatized in human-made or natural disasters, only one of the studies used an energy psychology approach.[39] Others used more conventional treatments such as CBT and Narrative Exposure Therapy. The tapping therapy had the highest effect size of all 36 studies. Since only one tapping application was included in this comparison study, it might not have been representative. A subsequent analysis by different investigators, comparing 17 different interventions for treating traumatized youth, supported this finding.[40] In that study, EFT was one of the two most effective therapies in reducing PTSD symptoms at treatment endpoint and the most effective of the 17 interventions in retaining improvement in PTSD symptoms on follow-up. In terms of potential bias, in neither study were the investigators advocates of a tapping approach. In fact, their reports gave no attention to the tapping therapies beyond listing their high effect sizes.

A 10-minute video showing excerpts using an acupoint tapping approach in the rapid treatment of four combat veterans who had PTSD can be viewed at vetcases.com.[41]

Tapping in the Treatment of PTSD

After learning of the early study showing an 86 percent success rate with 49 veterans after six tapping sessions,[42] David contacted the study's principal investigator and asked whether he could interview some of the therapists involved. One of them, Ingrid Dinter, described to him her work with Keith, an infantry soldier who'd served in the Mekong Delta during the Vietnam War. He'd reported in his initial session that he'd seen "many casualties on both sides." More than three decades later, he was still tormented with nightmares and repeated flashbacks. "Sometimes I think I see Viet Cong soldiers behind bushes and trees," he explained. His

severe insomnia, complicated by the nightmares, made him fatigued and unable to function during the day. He'd been diagnosed with PTSD but reported that his group and individual therapy through the US Department of Veterans Affairs hadn't helped with his symptoms.

During Keith's six sessions with Ingrid, he tapped on acupoints while focusing on traumatic war memories and other psychological stressors. In their first session, he reported that since the war's conclusion, he'd rarely gotten more than one to two hours of sleep at a stretch and averaged about two nightmares each night. By the end of the six sessions, he was getting seven to eight hours of uninterrupted sleep and was having no nightmares. He related that other symptoms, such as intrusive memories, startle reactions, and overwhelming guilt had abated as well. A six-month follow-up interview and further testing showed that the improvements held. In brief, the core of his treatment involved tapping on traumatic memories and on triggers in his current life that elicited PTSD symptoms.

Using Tapping to Achieve the Goals of the Best Practices for Treating PTSD. The brochure from one of Dr. van der Kolk's professional trainings promises therapists that after going through the program, they will have "the knowledge you need to provide your clients":

- A way to find words that describe the deep and painful effects of trauma

- Tools to regulate their emotions, even when they are unexpectedly triggered

- The ability to trust other human beings after the shameful and horrific details of their trauma

- The opportunity to be fully alive in the present, not stuck in the past

While this book can't replicate a thorough professional training program such as Dr. van der Kolk's, the Basic Tapping Protocol can address and, perhaps to a surprising degree, take clients far in accomplishing each of these objectives. Consider the tools you have already acquired in Chapters 2 and 3 (each bulleted point corresponds with one of the objectives listed in Dr. van der Kolk's training programs):

- You learned to move between current experiences and earlier distress or trauma while reducing the emotional pain of each, a process by which you, step by step (from one SUD reading to the next), are able to *"find words that describe the deep and painful effects of trauma."*

- You were provided with potent tools for sending deactivating signals to emotional centers of your brain, which quickly *"regulate your emotions, even when they are unexpectedly triggered."*

- You can put earlier destructive experiences into context by neutralizing the emotional harm they created, opening the way to *"trust other human beings"* despite

the horrific treacheries that may have been involved in your trauma.

- You can clear the emotional aftermath of traumatic or other distressing experiences, making it possible for you *"to be fully alive in the present, not stuck in the past."*

Considerations for Using Tapping with PTSD

Although it is beyond our scope here to offer a complete instructional manual for professionals applying acupoint tapping to PTSD and other trauma-based challenges, here is what we can offer. The following subsections are organized according to issues that frequently emerge even when the best therapeutic practices are applied with trauma, and they show where to bring in tapping. The issues we address here include:

1. Establishing trust

2. Preventing retraumatization, flashbacks, and nightmares

3. Hopelessness

4. Dissociation

5. Guilt and shame

6. Anger and forgiveness

7. Freezing

8. Depression

9. Post-traumatic growth

For each of these topics, we will discuss some of the core dynamics and then show how to apply the Basic Tapping Protocol by formulating Acceptance and/or Choices Statements that address the salient issues. Stating these phrases out loud while using the "Sore Spots/Heart Chakra" technique and tapping will be a good start in each area. Then apply, where necessary, the Basic Tapping Protocol (Chapter 2) and work with aspects, inner conflicts, Psychological Reversals, and cognitive distortions (Chapter 3) as the treatment unfolds. Of course, not every issue will arise for every person, the order in which they arise will vary, and several issues may be on the front burner at once. Still, an effective trauma therapist is prepared to recognize and address these issues if and when they present themselves.

1. Establishing Trust. Most people who have been traumatized carry deep wounds in the most tender areas of their psyche. Unless their traumatic experiences have been processed and largely healed, being asked to describe in detail what occurred before a substantial amount of rapport and trust have been established may be received as a sign that the person asking is not attuned to the traumatized person's inner life. Traumatized brains are often dedicated, however unsuccessfully, to *not* reliving the trauma.

After preliminaries, you might introduce tapping to address an issue that isn't directly related to the traumatic event, such as to ease a mild area of worry or distress, to bring some relief to a physical symptom, or simply reduce discomfort about entering therapy. Experiencing the effectiveness of acupoint tapping is one of the quickest ways to establish trust in the therapy and the therapist. Once this occurs, you and the person can begin to approach the traumatic history more directly.

EFT practitioners have developed what they call the "Gentle Approaches," such as the "Tearless Trauma" technique and "sneaking up on the problem."[43] Skillful reframing (p. 102) can also quickly build bridges. For instance, a way to begin exploring traumatic events with a combat veteran might begin with the following Acceptance Statement, which provides a framework as the therapy proceeds:

"Even though I've been through more than you could ever understand, I accept myself and recognize that my experiences would have been beyond any normal person's coping abilities."[44]

As the "Sore Spots/Heart Chakra" technique and the tapping reduce the distrust, anger, or resentment, revising the second part makes it an empowering Choices Statement:

"Even though I've been through more than you could ever understand, I choose to be surprisingly at peace with that and find out what you've got to offer."

When do you transition from an Acceptance Statement to a Choices Statement? Not before the person is ready. The Choices Statement may be the therapist's agenda before it is the client's agenda, so it requires sensitive attunement on the therapist's part to not lead where the person isn't ready to go. With each of the following issues, you would begin with the "Sore Spot/Heart Chakra" technique (rubbing chest sore spots with the first phrase and placing the client's hands over the Heart Chakra with the second). Then proceed, as necessary, to the Basic Tapping Protocol, followed by detective work.

2. Preventing Retraumatization, Flashbacks, and Nightmares. Among the most delicate issues in treating people who have been traumatized is not having the therapy cause them to vividly *relive* the trauma. They are reliving it enough spontaneously, and each time they do, the dysfunctional brain patterns that are part of PTSD are deepened, which reinforces helplessness and hopelessness. The therapist must keep it safe for the person to revisit the past without reactivating the full emotional trauma of the original experience. This is where the clinical concept of a "window of tolerance" applies, where the emotion needs to be active enough to process but not so intense as to overwhelm.

The moment a client seems to be going into substantial fear, pain, or anger about the precipitating event, the focus of the tapping can shift to the emotion or physical sensations the person is experiencing in that moment. Through such prompt symptom reduction, you are training the limbic system to stay calm even when provoked by difficult memories or fantasies. As emotions and physical sensations are soothed, the tapping might then proceed to the critical issue of safety, beginning with an *"I accept myself"* statement that moves into an empowering Choices Statement such as:

> *"Even though I thought I was going to die, I choose to recognize that it was a long time ago, and I'm safe now."*

Traumatic events can become encapsulated in the brain and reexperienced in endless loops during *waking* (*flashbacks*) or *sleep* (*nightmares*). Intrusive flashbacks come in two forms that deeply entrench the damage caused by the trauma into the emotional brain. In the milder form, the person is aware of who they are and where they are. They may experience the terror of the original incident, but they are conscious of the here and now. In the more extreme form, the person experiences the emotions as if the event *is* occurring. They may not even remember the original event—much of the brain goes offline during such episodes—but the emotions and bodily reactions are vivid and often overwhelming.

But flashbacks also serve a purpose. By forcefully keeping the unresolved wound in the person's awareness, flashbacks and nightmares can be reminders about where healing is needed. Once trust and safety have been established, it becomes possible to use tapping so the person can recall what happened, even in great detail, without *reliving* the experience. This is a marker on the path to overcoming the ongoing trauma of PTSD. As it occurs, the intrusive memories tend to stop and peaceful sleep returns. Listening carefully to the traumatized person's descriptions of flashbacks and nightmares can set some of the agenda for the tapping. As the tapping lowers the SUD, the initial *"I accept myself"* statement might move into an empowering Choices Statement such as:

> *"Even though this memory has haunted me for years, I choose to know that I'm taking steps to tame it."*

3. Hopelessness. A person who has been navigating PTSD for years—perhaps after various attempts to overcome the symptoms using psychotherapy, medication, or other means—may not expect that very much will come from this latest attempt to find relief. If that is the case, address the resistance relatively early in the treatment. As the tapping lowers the SUD, the "I accept myself" statement might move into an empowering Choices Statement, such as:

> *"Even though it seems I'll never again experience success, happiness, or love, I choose to be open to a level of healing that I don't expect."*

4. Dissociation. In dissociation, thoughts, emotions, memories, surroundings, and identity become compartmentalized, and the normal continuity among them breaks down. The person may feel detached from their body or disconnected from the world. Dissociation often originates as a self-protective technique in which the psyche of an abused or severely neglected child creates an alternative reality to escape from fully experiencing unbearable situations. The type of flashback in which the person has no recognition of where they are or what is occurring involves dissociation. Additional features of dissociation may also emerge, such as *depersonalization* (feeling that the self is detached from the body or is not even real) and *derealization* (feeling that the world is far away or is not even real).

If a person dissociates during a session—losing orientation to time and place—reestablishing contact with the therapist and the environment is the first step. This might involve instructions to focus attention on objects in the room, on the therapist's voice, or on the person's breathing, followed by tapping on phrases such as *"I'm safe now," "I'm here with [therapist's name]," "My body is becoming calm and centered."* As therapy progresses, a key goal that counters dissociation is for the traumatic history to become integrated into a coherent story about the person's life. Techniques for bringing this about include dialogues among internal "parts," as presented in Chapter 3. As the tapping lowers the SUD, the *"I accept myself"* statement might move into an empowering Choices Statement that focuses on conflicts between two internal parts or on the action of one of the parts, such as:

"Even though part of me spaces out when I am reminded of what happened, I choose to use tapping until I can look that memory in the face without flinching."

5. Guilt and Shame. Guilt is rooted in negative self-judgment about something you *did*. Shame is rooted in negative self-judgment about who you *are*, as if something about you is fundamentally flawed. Either or both forms of self-judgment are often dynamics in PTSD. Survivor guilt about having lived after a disaster in which others did not or guilt about not having prevented an accident or other tragedy or about actions committed during warfare can plague a person forever after. Being abused as a child or violated as an adult may lead to shame that you were treated that way because you deserved to be.

Guilt can weigh down the spirit, but its positive function is that past mistakes can be reviewed so they aren't repeated. Shame weighs down the spirit with no constructive psychological purpose we've been able to identify. Addressing guilt or shame is often an important component in treating PTSD. Each responds well to the Basic Tapping Protocol, with particular emphasis on self-acceptance. An Acceptance Statement to get started might be this: *"Even though the accident was my fault, I deeply accept my sadness about what happened."* A Choices Statement might emphasize ways of moving forward: *"Even though the accident was my fault, I choose to learn from what happened, make amends where I can, and move forward as a wiser person."*

6. Anger and Forgiveness. Anger and blame toward one's abuser or another perpetrator of harm and suffering are natural responses. Anger is neurologically based in the "fight" part of the limbic system's "fight-or-flight" response to danger. A function of anger that persists following a traumatic event guards against repetition of the mistreatment by the same party. Angry outbursts can also serve as reminders of the need to release pent-up energies that no longer serve a useful function. To forgive someone who was responsible for cruelty or atrocities may, however, seem unthinkable. It might seem like condoning the behavior or even like colluding with the person to commit future violence.

On the other hand, anger, blame, and hate keep the abused person emotionally and energetically connected with the abuser. Desmond Tutu, a recipient of the Nobel Peace Prize for his role in leading the Truth and Reconciliation Commission in South Africa following decades of oppression, torture, and other horrible mistreatment, put it like this for a BBC television audience: "Holding onto your resentment means you are locked into your victimhood—and you allow your perpetrator to have a hold over your life. When you forgive, you let go, it sets you free."[45] Dealing with accumulated anger and the question of forgiveness is often an important part of the healing process when working with PTSD. Again, the Basic Tapping Protocol can be usefully applied. After the tapping has lowered the SUD, the "I accept myself" statement might move into Choices Statements such as:

"Even though what I was put through is unforgivable, I choose to come to inner peace despite what happened."

"Even though my rage toward him has no bottom, I choose to consider what forgiveness might look like."

7. Freezing. When a person is in a traumatic situation where resistance or escape is not possible, the "freeze" part of the fight-flight-freeze response is activated. Shame about having become immobilized when overpowered by a rapist may need to be addressed as part of healing, as alluded to earlier. But the nervous system may stay locked in the freeze response long after the traumatic event. The vagus nerve, which controls the freeze response, can, if provoked by fear or fearful memories, slow the heart, dilate blood vessels, and deprive the brain of oxygen. When a person goes into freeze during a therapy session, almost any active form of engagement by the therapist may feel intrusive. Recognizing and calmly accepting this allows the freeze response to begin to diminish. Sometimes the person will be so frozen that they won't be able to tap.

Encouraging simple movements is a start toward helping them unfreeze. They will usually be able to move their eyes or move their head slightly. Moving the eyes from side to side can help disengage the branch of the vagus nerve that initiates shutdown and activate the branch involved with social engagement. Using a Choices Statement, even without tapping, might be the next step. Simply having the person repeat after you (or just think it if they can't say it): *"Even though I feel completely isolated, I choose to know that I can communicate yes or no by nodding my head."* When they are ready to rub the chest sore spots, hold their Heart Chakra, and tap to the words, an empowering Choices Statement might be:

"Even though I sometimes become immobilized, I choose to know that this is part of my healing."

8. Depression. PTSD and clinical depression share some common symptoms: episodes of overwhelming sadness, difficulties with sleep (too much or too little), loss of interest in activities that had been pleasurable. While depression and PTSD are different conditions with different neurological underpinnings, about half of the people diagnosed with PTSD also meet the diagnostic criteria for depression. When depression and PTSD co-occur, each needs attention. The following chapter goes into more depth about clinical depression, but for starters, an Acceptance Statement might move into a Choices Statement such as:

"Even though I'm sad and depressed, I choose to know I am taking steps to find my way out of this dark place."

9. Post-Traumatic Growth. Severely traumatized and incapacitated people can and do rebuild their lives back *better*. Nearly half of trauma survivors evidence "post-traumatic growth" after healing from PTSD.[46] The three ways PTSD changes the brain described earlier—amplified signs of danger, inability to filter information, and a blunted sense of self—can all be reversed. Personal strength is restored. An appreciation of life is reestablished. The imagination becomes more constructive. The ability to make plans returns. The compulsion to repeat symbolic versions of the trauma to counter the dampened ability to experience the excitement and sensations of ordinary life cease. Damaged relationships may be repaired, productive work resumed, new creative endeavors discovered, and the enjoyment of life restored! Peter Levine, PhD, the originator of Somatic Experiencing, one of the most widely used approaches for treating trauma, has observed that "while trauma can be hell on earth, trauma resolved is a gift of the gods."[47] To get started:

"Even though [name the trauma] has interfered with my life in so many ways, I choose to recognize how it has also made me wiser and stronger."

Working with Combat Veterans

Because so many who have gone into battle to protect their nation and their loved ones return with PTSD, we want to close this chapter with a focus on the special considerations when treating combat veterans. We asked Ingrid Dinter—who had treated Keith in the earlier account—to share her understanding of the difference when working with those who have served in a nation's military and others living with PTSD. She began by explaining how veterans are trained to protect their country. They take a vow that they are willing to sacrifice their lives to protect their people and their nation's constitution. This leads to a different mindset from someone who has been raped, in an accident, or in any other situation where the trauma was unexpected and their sense of safety obliterated without warning.

As a result, many veterans do not feel victimized in the same way as almost anyone else experiencing PTSD. They instead tend to accept that "I was just doing my job." More common, however, are guilt, shame, and rage due to a wide range of compelling dynamics, from participation in something that seems wrong, tragic outcomes due to a weak chain of command, death of a buddy, immoral personal acts, betrayal by one's government, or a dismissive or even contemptuous way of being met upon coming home. Any of these can trigger guilt, shame, or rage. On the other hand, the bond between the brothers and sisters in arms and the pride in their service is strong and lasts a lifetime. For many, this is an ongoing blessing after enduring the horrors of war.

Although most veterans would far prefer to talk about their war experiences with a fellow veteran than with a therapist, Dinter understands she is not part of that community. Instead, she takes the position of representing the community the veteran vowed to defend. She offers her sincere gratitude, honor, and respect for their service and holds the space of being a member of the community into which they are reintegrating. She finds this approach to be the basis for creating a "sacred bond," for becoming a buddy who has the veteran's back as they mentally return to the war zone for therapeutic purposes. She makes it very clear that she does not judge, condone, or excuse anything that happened. Her job is only to help the veteran release the emotional weight of the memories and triggers. This opens the door to deeper healing and finding new meaning and purpose in their lives.

While Ingrid felt the above guidelines were valid for veterans, she asked us to highlight a few other considerations. More than just "establishing trust" (our first consideration), she emphasized the importance of completely and deeply acknowledging the person's experience and their understanding of it. She seeks further clarification with requests such as, "Tell me more. I wasn't there. Help me understand." She fully respects that whatever the answers, they are the person's experience. This is not to be questioned, challenged, or judged. She models acceptance and proceeds to offer or elicit phrases that accept each aspect of the related events, thoughts, and emotions; and she has the person tap on every one of them. She is open to the possibility that the person's understanding of the experience may change, but she does not try to change it. Instead, by using tapping to reduce the charge on the experience, she knows that the understanding will change organically.

Dinter often has the person tell a story about anything that emerges, a story with a beginning, a middle, and an end. This may be a memory, a flashback, or even a nightmare. When using this technique, called the "Tell the Story" technique in EFT, the person is instructed to begin to tell their story in whatever way they can but to stop and tap as soon as they feel emotion coming up. In the tapping sequences, Dinter replaces statements such as *"I love and accept myself"* with statements that better reflect military values, such as *"I honor and respect myself."* She also emphasized that in her experience—after identifying each event, emotion, and memory separately, and tapping on them individually—the risk of flashbacks and retraumatization can be greatly reduced. The story eventually loses its power to cause the person to relive the trauma.

ON TO CHAPTER 5

This chapter has taken you on a journey from (1) selecting and addressing an area of personal worry; to (2) understanding the additional physiological and psychological dimensions that are involved when a worry has progressed into anxiety; to (3) the steps for taming a panic attack, to (4) applying tapping to the best practices psychotherapists use in working with PTSD. We recognize that for some people, the content of this chapter will be challenging, and we are also aware that the next chapter focuses on another difficult facet of the human experience: sadness and depression. While much can be gained by addressing these issues directly, as acupoint tapping protocols allow, we again remind you to pace yourself, take breaks, and use energy exercises or other forms of emotional self-care or external support as you move through this material.

CHAPTER 5

Sadness and Depression

Talk therapy can provide empathy, support, and practical suggestions
for addressing depression. Acupoint tapping, however, can bring
about rapid shifts in the physiological roots of the condition.[1]

—Robert Schwarz, PsyD
Executive Director, Association for Comprehensive Energy Psychology

THE ANONYMOUS CANADIAN POET who uses the pen name Atticus offers a powerful metaphor, pointing out that being depressed is like being colorblind yet continually being told about the world's wonderful colors.[2] Sadness and depression fall along the same continuum, but depression is more deeply embedded in the body's chemistry. Energy psychology has been effective in treating both. We'll begin with sadness.

APPLYING TAPPING TO HEARTBREAKING SADNESS

Margaret was a 48-year-old waitress who had been living alone since her divorce three years earlier. Her two adult daughters, with her three young grandchildren, had moved to different states to follow their husbands' employment. Margaret got to see each family for a few days about twice a year. These visits were the most gratifying part of her life, but the families were so busy that they didn't come to see her, and she couldn't afford to take time off from work to be with them nearly as much as she would have liked.

Margaret's husband had announced that he was leaving her for another woman two days before her 45th birthday. She never saw it coming. The period around her birthdays became a time of immense sadness, and this sadness seemed to intensify and become longer each year. Margaret had a few close friends whom she had known for decades. One of them was in therapy with a social worker who was learning EFT and needed practice clients. As Margaret's 48th birthday approached and her sadness grew, her friend encouraged her to schedule a session.

After carefully listening to Margaret's description of the divorce and her sadness about it, the therapist asked her to feel into her sadness and imagine it as a color. It was a dark, heavy, smokey blob in her chest and neck. Margaret rated its intensity as a 10. Her breathing was restricted, and her throat was tight. She was guided through the same protocol you have been learning: *"Even though I have this heavy, smokey blob in my chest, I accept myself and my feelings."* This was followed by tapping on the 12 acupoints, using phrases like *"This sadness,"* *"This tightness in my throat,"* and *"This smokey blob in my chest"*; then the Integration Procedure followed by further tapping.

This got the SUD down to 7, but when she went within to rate it, rage at her ex-husband filled her. It was a high 10. Her main takeaway from the divorce had been that she wasn't good enough. She had failed him. It was her fault that he left her. Her daughters had expressed a great deal of anger at their father for leaving, but in her heart of hearts, Margaret felt she was to blame. Suddenly and unexpectedly, three years' worth of buried rage surfaced and overwhelmed her.

The session then focused on helping her to accept the anger. She responded well to a series of statements such as *"Even though I could kill the bastard, I accept myself and my feelings!"* The session then moved into an imaginary dialogue (p. 113) where she expressed her authentic anger to her ex-husband as she tapped. By the end of the first session, her sadness imagery wasn't as dark and heavy, and she rated it as a 5.

That night she had a dream about her father who left the family when Margaret was four. In the dream, Margaret was tried in court and found guilty of being responsible for her father's abandonment of the family. She ruminated about this for the rest of the week until she could address it at her second session. By the end of that session, the tapping had greatly reduced the guilt she had been carrying her whole life for the breakup of her family, and she had made a connection between that and how she had been carrying the blame for the demise of her own marriage. The result was a tremendous release of energy. She was almost euphoric about a giant load having been lifted.

By the time of her birthday, she wanted to celebrate, for the first time since the divorce. She asked the friend who had referred her to the therapist if they could go out for a festive birthday dinner.

HONORING YOUR SADNESS

While you can't avoid bouts of sadness, you can meet them in ways that are constructive and even empowering. You can also use your sadness as a gateway into unresolved experiences from your past, as we saw with Margaret. Sadness seems to have a reorienting purpose within the psyche. During periods of sadness, the communication between the parts of the brain involved with emotion and memory increases.[3] When we are sad, we also tend to be more motivated to take on difficult tasks to improve our lives.

Whatever the benefits of a sad state, however, no one wants to hang out there. Nonetheless, to master your internal states, you need to begin by accepting that you are feeling what you are feeling. While denying or distracting yourself from sad feelings may force them out of your awareness, this temporary reprieve allows them to grow in your subconscious. When this occurs, the repressed feelings will still have an impact—and probably a worse one. Repressing your sadness also prevents you from garnering the benefits of sadness as a way to reorient yourself.

Instead of running from feelings of sadness, you can honor them by letting them be, even encouraging them with reflective activities such as writing in a journal, listening to the blues, watching a poignant movie, expressing your sadness in artistic activities, talking about it with a friend, or allowing yourself to cry. As you contemplate what the sadness seems to be communicating, you can use that information. Themes that may emerge might include memories pushing for a new level of emotional resolution, changes you need to make in your life, changes that have occurred in your life that you need to adapt to, negative thinking that needs to be countered, or emotions calling for attention. Tapping can help you with any of these. To get started, begin with the following "Quick Fix."

Quick Fix: Sadness

Bring to mind a loss or other source of sadness that you would like to further process so you retain its important messages but are no longer carrying the emotional burden. Give an SUD rating to the amount of distress you feel in your mind and/or body when you think about this sadness. Say out loud the first statement below as you tap on the Top-of-the-Head Point. Then say the next statement while tapping on the next point. Go through each statement, cycling through the 12 tapping points as you move from one statement to the next. Skip any phrases that don't fit for you.

"*Even though I am feeling so sad about [name it] right now,*

I completely accept that I am sad.

Even though this feeling is weighing me down and draining my energy,

I give myself permission to acknowledge it and feel it.

Even though I'm not sure how to let go of this sadness,

I choose to see myself without it.

I feel this sadness in my [name where].

As I tap to reduce this sadness, I can begin to relax.

I can let go of this sadness without forgetting the lessons it holds.

My sadness is teaching me [state whatever comes to mind].

I choose to be gentle and patient with myself as I work through my sadness.

Even though part of me might feel guilty or disloyal if I let go of this sadness,

I know that releasing it is best for my well-being.

Even though I've been holding on to this sadness,

I choose to trust my intuition and do what is best for me.

I'm ready to release some of this sadness and open myself to new sources of comfort and joy.

Even though I don't know what the future holds,

I choose to trust that there is a path toward greater peace.

I know I am capable of creating a more positive future for myself.

I choose to let this sadness begin to fade.

I choose to embrace feelings of peace, clarity, and happiness."

After going through this sequence two or three times, you will probably find that the texture of the sadness is already softening. Gauge this with another SUD rating on your sadness. Even if your sadness still feels excessive, you will have prepared yourself to go deeper into overcoming it by next applying the Basic Tapping Protocol, as shown in this chapter.

DISCOVERING WHAT YOUR SADNESS HAS TO TEACH YOU

If you happen to be feeling a little sad, or a lot sad, you may want to use the Basic Tapping Protocol, as adjusted for sadness in this chapter, to mine that sadness for buried gems—insights that can be used to cultivate a happier and more fulfilling life. If sadness and depression aren't relevant to you right now, feel free to move on to another chapter. This one will always be available if you need it.

Getting Started

The process goes along the lines of the Basic Tapping Protocol, but it places greater emphasis on the Choices Statement. Here we introduce you to 38-year-old Noah, one of the program's test drivers who had no previous experience with energy psychology.

Noah's Initial SUD, Reminder Phrase, and Acceptance Statement

Noah was still heartbroken about a divorce from two years earlier. He rated his sadness at a 10. His Reminder Phrase was *"Overwhelming sadness."* The Acceptance Statement he built on it was, *"Even though I'm still heartbroken about the divorce, I deeply and completely accept this overwhelming sadness."*

Your Turn

Describe your sadness in your journal and give it an SUD rating. Create a Reminder Phrase and an Acceptance Statement that, as usual, incorporates the Reminder Phrase. Then proceed as follows:

The Initial Tapping Rounds

Apply the remainder of the Basic Tapping Protocol to your sadness:

1. State your Acceptance Statement out loud three times, rubbing your chest sore spots with the first phrase and placing your hands over your Heart Chakra with the second.

2. Go through the 12 tapping points as you say your Reminder Phrase at each point.

3. Do the Integration Procedure.

4. Tap through the points again, stating your Reminder Phrase at each point.

5. Take a breath and give another SUD rating to the amount of sadness you feel in your body and mind.

6. Repeat this process, beginning with your Acceptance Statement each time, and then the tapping, until your SUD is down to a 4 or less.

If your SUD is above 4 and has stopped going down after two tapping cycles with the same Reminder Phrase, it is time to make a shift. Identify an aspect of the situation requiring attention. Work with it as described on page 66. Then return to your initial sadness. If this still doesn't bring it below 4, proceed through the other detective work discussed in Chapter 3.

Noah's Initial Tapping Rounds

It took some work for Noah to get the SUD on his sadness down to 4. The Basic Tapping Protocol got it from the original 10 down to 8, but it didn't move from there after three more tapping cycles. Looking for aspects, he identified a stinging feeling around his heart. After tapping on *"Stinging in my heart,"* his sadness was down to 6. Then some waves of anger at his ex came up. He didn't feel ready to deal with this, so he set the program aside for a few days. When he returned to it, he could easily access the anger. He tapped on several memories that he was angry about and, one by one, reduced the charge on each. He then returned to his sadness, and after a couple more cycles, it was down to a 3.

Your Turn

Go through the above steps until your SUD is down to 4 or less. Be as persistent as necessary, addressing aspects and psychological reversals as they might emerge. Describe the process in your journal.

A New Reminder Phrase Keyed to a Function of Your Sadness

Five possible functions your sadness may serve include:

1. Makes me more motivated to do things that will improve the quality of my life.

2. Tells me about something needing attention.

3. Reveals cognitive distortions and negative thinking (p. 100).

4. Activates something unfinished from my past that needs another layer of resolution.

5. Calls for me to go into "reset" mode about something that is important to me, such as work, relationships, or use of time.

Once the intensity of your sadness is down to 4 or less, you are ready to formulate a new Reminder Phrase and a Choices Statement that will not only help alleviate your sadness further but also help you glean the benefits of any of these functions that your sadness has been serving. Here are some examples tied to the above list:

1. Need to get motivated: *"Still not exercising."*

2. Need to pay attention: *"My son's aggressive behavior."*

3. Need to correct cognitive distortions: *"I always fail."*

4. Need for resolution: *"The trauma when I was eight."*

5. Need for a reset: *"I'm drained at the end of each day."*

Functions of Noah's Sadness and His New Reminder Phrase

Reflecting on possible functions of the intense sadness he was carrying about his divorce led Noah to recognize that he had put his life into freeze mode. His Reminder Phrase was keyed to his need for a major reset: *"Still overwhelmingly sad about my divorce after all this time."*

Your Turn

Begin by choosing one or more functions from the above list that your sadness might be serving, or a sixth function that is a better fit but is not on the list. Create one or more Reminder Phrases related to that function. You will be using them in the subsequent tapping cycles.

Formulating a Choices Statement

Once your sadness is down to an SUD of 4, the next step is to tie a function of your sadness into a Choices Statement that points toward constructive action. You will be selecting the function you believe is the most important. Here are some examples, keyed to the earlier list:

1. **Need to Get Motivated:** *"Even though I've not yet started exercising, I choose to reaffirm that exercise will be worth the effort and to build a habit of regular exercise."*

2. **Need to Pay Attention:** *"Even though I don't want to think about my son's aggressive behavior, I choose to schedule a meeting with his guidance counselor and develop a plan."*

3. **Need to Correct Cognitive Distortions:** *"Even though I believe I will fail again, I choose to talk over my discouragement with [my best friend]."*

4. **Need for Resolution:** *"Even though I've grieved my mother's death from when I was eight so many times, I choose to recognize that it is intruding into my consciousness every day now, and I will give it the attention it is calling for."*

5. **Need for a Reset:** *"Even though I just take it for granted that I feel drained at the end of each day, I choose to become serious about making shifts before I break down physically or mentally."*

Noah's Choices Statement

Noah created a Choices Statement built on his Reminder Phrase: *"Even though I'm still overwhelmingly sad about my divorce, I choose to make this the time that I begin rebuilding my life."* This got his SUD down from a 3 to a 1. He then shifted the focus of the tapping into taking concrete steps for rebuilding his life.

Your Turn

Formulate your new Choices Statement. At the start of each tapping cycle, say it out loud three times, rubbing your chest sore spots with the first phrase and holding your hands over your Heart Chakra with the second. Then proceed to the tapping routine, using your new Reminder Phrase at each tapping point. Again, if your progress gets stuck, look for aspects or proceed through the detective work in Chapter 3. When your SUD is as low as you can get it, describe in your journal your experience working with your sadness. Next we turn to depression.

THE NATURE OF DEPRESSION

Everyone goes through sad moods, but if your sadness persists over an extended period, you may have fallen into depression. Depression is a more physiologically and energetically entrenched mental state than sadness. To establish a framework for using tapping for depression, we'll briefly touch on the nature of the disorder, its prevalence, symptoms, causes, and conventional treatment approaches.

While the above instructions for addressing sadness may still be helpful, more is usually required to restore a brighter outlook if you are depressed. Sadness can serve positive functions—such as to focus your mental abilities on issues requiring your attention—but when sadness moves into depression, it is a different story energetically, chemically, and cognitively. It may rob you of the energy to be effective in addressing whatever has surfaced. Depression may also put a negative and disempowering spin on problems that call for your creative best.

It is difficult for people who have never experienced an episode of major depression to fully grasp what it is like. Based on her personal experience with the condition, Martha Manning, in an extraordinarily perceptive article in *Psychotherapy Networker*, described how her severe recurrent depression

> sweeps right through and tears you up. It threatens your health, your mind, your soul. It makes you a stranger to the people you always called close. It makes you look kindly on death as a merciful exit from a pain that's elusive in description. Not only do you forget who you were, you're horrified by the person you've become. And there are no promises that this time you'll get out intact or alive.... People couldn't comprehend my suffering, and I was totally inept at explaining it.[4]

Prevalence

Approximately 280 million people around the world suffer from some form of depression.[5] In the US, an estimated 21 million adults (projecting from surveys), or 8.4 percent of the population, had an episode of major depression in 2020.[6] For women, the percentage was 10.5 percent, compared with 6.2 percent for men. Prevalence was highest among people in the 12 to 17 age range (17 percent) and again in the 18 to 25 age range (also 17 percent). You may not know, however, if someone is depressed. In fact, for ongoing low-grade depression, the feelings may have become so familiar that you may not realize it if you are depressed.

Symptoms

The formal definition for an episode of "major depression" is that five or more of the following eight symptoms have persisted for at least two weeks and impact daily functioning:

- A depressed mood that lasts for most of the day, nearly every day, with noticeable signs of hopelessness and sadness (for children and adolescents, this can also be an "irritable mood" or angry outbursts)

- Appetite disturbance or significant unintended weight gain or loss (for children, this can be failure to achieve expected weight gain)

- Diminished interest or loss of pleasure in almost all activities

- Insomnia, sleeplessness, or increased amounts of sleep that affect normal schedules

- Fatigue or low energy

- Feelings of worthlessness or excessive guilt on a daily basis

- Inability to concentrate or make decisions

- Recurrent thoughts of death or suicide or suicide attempts[7]

For *chronic* depression (officially designated as "persistent depressive disorder"), five or more of these symptoms must have persisted for at least two years. Chronic depression may be classified into two categories: "low-grade persistent depression" and the more intense "chronic major depression." On the lesser end of the depressive spectrum, a "minor" depressive episode involves three or four of these symptoms persisting for at least two weeks. "Recurrent brief depression" involves more than six episodes in a year with five or more of the symptoms, each lasting at least five days.

Causes

Like many psychological conditions, depression may result from any combination of factors. People with a family history of depression are more vulnerable to the condition, suggesting a genetic component. Some depression accompanies hormonal shifts, such as post-partum depression, menopause, premenstrual cycles, or the hormone changes of adolescence. Depression may also be triggered by a challenging life circumstance, such as a loss, the death of a loved one, an illness, a trauma, or a major disappointment. Negative thinking and depression may form a "depressive loop" where negative thoughts maintain the depression and the depression fosters more negative thinking.

Genetics. Depression is known to run in families. While at least 10 percent of the general population will suffer from a major depressive episode during their lifetime, the chances increase to 20 to 30 percent when a parent or sibling has major depression. This does not, however, in itself prove that depression is inherited. How children are nurtured, disciplined, rewarded, and punished can all influence depression, and a depressed parent may also inadvertently teach ways of thinking that foster depression. However, studies of twins, which are able to isolate many variables, suggest that at least one-third of the likelihood of being afflicted with a major depressive disorder is due to genetic factors.[8] Which genes are not clear. Those controlling the neurotransmitter serotonin appear to be involved, but dozens of gene combinations have been identified as potentially contributing to the condition.[9]

Early History. The term "adverse childhood experiences" (ACEs) describes a wide range of difficult circumstances, events, or conditions, including neglect, abuse, family dysfunction, exposure to substance abuse, mental health problems, extreme economic adversity, bullying, and family or community violence.[10] The greater the number and severity of ACEs, the greater the likelihood of health and mental health disorders, including depression.[11]

Brain Structures. Depression correlates with reduced activity in the vagus nerve, hippocampus, prefrontal cortex, and thalamus. The *vagus nerve* is involved with emotional regulation and sensitivity to stress. The *hippocampus* is involved with learning and memory, and it connects with other parts of the brain that control emotion, particularly the amygdala. The *prefrontal cortex* plays a central role in high-level thinking and planning. The *thalamus* is the coordinating center for processing what your senses take in. Reduced activity in these brain structures helps explain some of the symptoms of depression, such as difficulties thinking clearly, memory

problems, feelings of hopelessness, and loss of motivation. Nonetheless, the precise ways that changes in brain activity play into depression have not been clearly mapped.[12]

Chemical Messengers. Neurotransmitters are chemicals the central nervous system uses to carry signals between nerve cells throughout the brain and body. Serotonin, dopamine, and norepinephrine are three neurotransmitters involved with depression. *Serotonin* is a mood regulator associated with happiness and feelings of calm. Low levels of serotonin may lead to a depressed mood, loss of pleasure, and a sense of worthlessness. *Dopamine*, known as the "feel good" chemical, associates specific activities or experiences with pleasure. Low levels of dopamine may lead to apathy and a loss of motivation. *Norepinephrine* helps the body process adrenaline and is involved with involuntary responses to dangerous or stressful situations. Low levels may lead to fatigue, difficulties concentrating, less interest in pleasurable activities, and decreased motivation and attentiveness.

Brain Inflammation. Inflammation in the brain has been shown to be a potential factor in the development of depression and may also inhibit the effectiveness of antidepressant medication.[13] Changes in diet or the introduction of anti-inflammatories may be a component in the treatment of depression.

Cognitive Distortions. Negative thought patterns may result from depression or may perpetuate it. For instance, a guiding model in which life's challenges are met with a predetermined sense that you will fail breeds depression. Harsh self-criticism breeds depression. Self-limiting beliefs breed depression. The depression then further undercuts your ability to use your resources to help yourself through whatever life presents.

Energy Disruptions. A central premise in energy psychology is that energy disruptions correspond with both physical and mental problems. For that reason, malfunctions in the brain's chemical signaling can be corrected not only by biological interventions (such as antidepressant medication or vagus nerve stimulation devices) but also by working with the body's energy systems. In addition, the neural pathways that support cognitive distortions and outdated guiding models, as we've seen throughout this book, are highly responsive to energy psychology interventions. Correcting cognitive distortions and outdated guiding models using acupoint tapping protocols can be powerful tools in helping to overcome depression.

TAPPING FOR DEPRESSION

Studies of tapping protocols in the treatment of depression have been encouraging. A statistical analysis of data from the first 12 clinical trials using EFT in treating depression showed strong overall improvements for the 398 participants.[14]

The psychologist Fred Gallo coined the term "energy psychology" with his 1998 book of that title (he was also David's first teacher of the method in 2002).[15] One of Dr. Gallo's patients was Jennifer, a high school junior who had been dating Chris for two years. Chris was three years older than Jennifer. Chris developed a serious respiratory condition that deteriorated rapidly, eventually taking his life. Jennifer grieved deeply and soon became clinically depressed. She felt lost without Chris and was plagued by memories of his suffering. She had been seen by a physician who placed her on antidepressant medication. She was also seeing a therapist who was encouraging her to discuss her grief and to review many of the events that transpired during Chris' illness as well as her positive memories of him prior to his becoming ill. Unfortunately none of this was helping, and Jennifer was becoming increasingly depressed. As she was diagnosed with a major depressive disorder that had so far been unresponsive to treatment, psychiatric hospitalization was being considered. Jennifer was referred to Dr. Gallo by her physician for a second opinion and possible treatment. Here is Dr. Gallo's account:

After meeting with Jennifer and establishing rapport, we discussed the treatment I could offer her. I asked if she would be okay with treatment if it didn't cause her upset. She asked if that were really possible and, after my assurance that it was, she smiled and agreed wholeheartedly with that option.

With tapping, Jennifer wouldn't have to become wrapped up with memories and distressing emotions. I guided her to briefly tune in to the images that were contributing to the depression symptoms of sleeplessness, loss of pleasure, crying, poor appetite, etc. She rated her distress at the time with each as 10 on the 0–10 SUD scale. Her most distressing image, however, was of Chris' suffering—having difficulty breathing while simply lying on the couch. She was taken through a tapping treatment and, within a matter of 10 minutes, that image, while still tragic, no longer produced the agonizing inner turmoil.

Next, the focus was on any residual feelings of depression. By this time, the strength of her depression had decreased significantly, down to 4. At that point, I had her tap while focusing on the depression's sensations and emotion, which she described as being "centered in my heart." As the feeling of depression decreased, we continued with the tapping and mindfully observing the depression sensations. Within a few minutes, Jennifer was not feeling depressed at all. Several times throughout the session, she exclaimed, "This is crazy! It's weird, but it's good!"

When Jennifer came in the following week, she indicated that she had not felt depressed for three days after the initial treatment. While the memory of Chris on the couch was no longer causing her distress, other memories were intruding that were triggering depressed feelings. Although I had advised Jennifer not to get caught up in thoughts about Chris, this was easier said than done. So, during this second session, a number of other memories were "neutralized," and the treatment was oriented toward further relieving depressive feelings.

In all, only a few visits were needed to help Jennifer. Her mood improved tremendously. She found it much easier to concentrate. She slept and ate better, and her interest in life and teenage activities returned. I followed her for a few months to ensure she was doing well, and she reported no additional incidents of depression. She had become involved in social activities with friends and several months later started dating again. The depression did not return.

A PRIMER FOR APPLYING TAPPING FOR OVERCOMING DEPRESSION

More than a century of psychotherapeutic interventions with people living with depression, as well as thousands of scientific studies, have revealed some dynamics that are generally shared across all forms of depression. Understanding these dynamics is vital for an energy approach to align with the best practices that are currently available for treating depression. Rather than try to analyze this vast literature, we followed the guidance of 16 of the world's leading experts in working with depression as presented in a definitive symposium of the mental health field's best practices.[16]

The guidance provided in the remainder of the chapter is oriented toward therapists who treat depression as well as for people wishing to overcome it. We want to emphasize that if you are struggling with depression, we strongly recommend that you use these techniques in conjunction with a qualified mental health professional. People who are depressed often feel desperate and don't really believe they can be helped. Pairing a skilled therapist with self-applied tapping is a powerful and promising combination.

As with the guidance for working with PTSD provided in the previous chapter, the following does not attempt to take you step by step through a therapy program for depression. What we offer is guidance for addressing seven areas that are vital for overcoming the condition. For each, we suggest Reminder Phrases, Acceptance Statements, and Choices Statements you can build upon to get you started in applying the Basic Tapping Protocol to that area. The areas covered include:

1. Finding hope that your efforts can make a difference

2. Simple techniques for generating the energy to overcome depression

3. Negative thoughts and beliefs

4. Formative experiences

5. Positive exposure

6. Social connection

7. Relapse prevention

1. Finding Hope That Your Efforts Can Make a Difference

The lethargy and discouragement that define depression are the first obstacles to overcoming it. Not only do depressed people lack the physical energy to take positive actions but they also often don't believe that anything is going to be effective. For instance, while innumerable studies demonstrate that physical exercise combats depression, finding the motivation to maintain a program of regular exercise for its health benefits is hard enough if you aren't depressed. It is exponentially more difficult if you are.

When people struggling with what is known as "learned helplessness" believe they have no control over what happens to them, they begin to think, feel, and act as if they *are* helpless.[17] Learned helplessness is a core dynamic in depression. When people try everything they can think of and are still depressed, they begin to feel hopeless.

Where to Begin. The preparation phase of the Basic Tapping Protocol you learned in Chapter 2 includes crafting an Acceptance Statement. Because of the pessimism that is almost always a companion to depression, accepting your depression already poses some special challenges. If a depressed mood is overshadowing everything else in your life, where do you even begin? It may feel like a distraction or even a step backward to focus on stressful issues in your life, childhood events that may have set you up for depression, or "negative thinking" that to you just feels realistic. Seeking relief from the depression is your only concern, and any other focus may seem off the mark to you.

While for many issues it is better to be as specific as possible, for depression, the experience of depression itself can be your initial focus. You can give it a name (a Reminder Phrase such as *"My depression," "Darkness," "All is bleak"*) and an SUD rating, specifying the intensity of your depression at the moment you are rating it. The other issues mentioned above may emerge later when you are identifying aspects that need to be addressed for further reducing the depression.

Accepting Your Pessimism. This step is particularly critical when you don't really believe that expending effort to overcome your depression is going to pay off. Consciously accepting rather than fighting that belief signals to your psyche that you are paying attention to the obstacles on the road ahead of you. Of course, you most likely don't *want* to stay depressed. But you may not believe there is a way out. So that is where you begin, with any of the following, in any combination, or anything else that might be a better fit for you:

"Even though nothing has helped my depression . . .

"Even though I know this won't work . . .

"Even though tapping looks stupid . . .

"Even though I don't want to do this . . .

"Even though I don't have the energy to do this . . .

"Even though I don't have time for this . . .

"Even though I'll always be depressed . . .

I deeply and completely accept that these are my feelings."

Again, say the first part out loud as you massage your chest sore spots and the second part out loud with your hands over your Heart Chakra. Do each statement that fits for you three times. You can alter the second part in any way you wish.

2. Simple Techniques for Generating the Energy to Overcome Depression

Focusing on your physical energies is a vital next step. Dr. van der Kolk suggests in the best practices program mentioned earlier that if people are too shut down to benefit from therapy, doing activities where they move their bodies is an important step on the path to effective treatment. Simple energy exercises can quickly begin to enliven your body by getting its energies into a better flow.

But when you are depressed, getting yourself motivated enough even to do the easiest of exercises is challenging. Tapping can help. Once you've embraced the reality of your depression with an Acceptance Statement that resonates for you, keep the first part of your statement but shift the second part (right column above) to make it a Choices Statement, such as

". . . I'm willing to see if some easy techniques might make me feel better."

Again, say it out loud three times, massaging your chest sore spots with the first phrase and using the Heart Chakra hold with the second. Your tapping phrase can then be along the lines of *"Simple exercises to help with my depression"* or simply *"Willing to be surprised."*

A challenge in this phase is that people who are depressed often fail to notice small gains. So even if the energy techniques do their job, you may not notice the relatively subtle changes. Yet knowing that simple techniques can bring about shifts in a favorable direction, even small ones, begins to build confidence that you can impact your depression by taking actions that are available to you.

Self-help programs for treating depression, such as the approach explained in the book *Mind Over Mood*, train people to register even minimal improvements and to take in the little lifts life provides.[18] They identify a wide range of experiences where improvements may occur: better sleep, more conversations with others, feeling more relaxed, smiling more often, getting your work done more efficiently, handling disagreements better, losing your temper less often, hearing others say you seem better, feeling more confident, standing up for yourself, seeing hope for the future, enjoying each day more, feeling appreciations and gratitude, and seeing improvement in your relationships.[19] Whatever the therapy, noting improvements will be of value. One change that is hard to deny is when your breath capacity increases after a simple tapping exercise. You might want to return to page 33 and repeat that exercise.

What we might call the "energetic signature of depression" includes:

A. Sluggish movement in the meridians and chakras

B. Energies not crossing over to support integration of the brain's right and left hemispheres

C. Energy blockages where stress has accumulated

D. Depletion of energies in vital areas

E. Energy disruptions that cause clouded thinking

The following simple techniques can give a boost in each of these areas, lettered below to correspond to the area.

A. Sluggish Movement in the Meridians and Chakras: The Four Thumps. You have already been using these points. For this subset, you won't be combining them with words. You will simply tap on each for two or three deep breaths (in through the nose and out through the mouth). Tap firmly (but never so hard as to hurt or bruise yourself) on each. Combined, they address the first part of the energetic signature of depression, giving a boost to the sluggish movement in the meridians and chakras.

- **Stomach-1.** Tapping on your cheekbones beneath your eyes (the first pair of acupuncture points on Stomach Meridian) sends the energy down to below your feet in a manner that merges with the energies of the earth and draws those energies up your body, which serves to sustain, nourish, and ground you.

- **Kidney-27.** When you are exhausted, the energies in your body literally reverse the direction of their flow for the purpose of getting you to stop and rest. But if this gets habitual,

it becomes a force that keeps you depressed. Tapping on the points under your collarbone (the 27th pair of acupoints on Kidney Meridian) flips the energies so they go in the proper direction.

- **Heart Chakra.** Tapping on the Heart Chakra in the center of your chest activates the chakra's energies, and all the other chakras resonate with this powerful force. Meanwhile, this tapping also invigorates the energies in the blood, stimulating the whole body as the newly enlivened blood flows through it.

- **Spleen-21.** Tapping on the 21st pair of acupoints on Spleen Meridian (under your arms) helps to disassemble and process, at the energetic level, the negative thoughts that are involved with depression, leading to a sense of greater peace and safety.

You can do the Four Thumps several times a day. They take only about a minute and can be done while you are doing other activities, such as watching TV, taking a shower, or going on a walk.

B. Energies Not Crossing Over to Support Integration of the Brain's Right and Left Hemispheres: The Crossover Shoulder Pull. The crossover motion in this procedure repatterns energies that are meant to cross over from one side of the body to the other but aren't. When you are depressed, the energies in your body don't cross over from the left side to the right or the right side to the left. Known as "homolateral patterning," this condition not only restricts a free flow of physical movements but also impairs communication between the left and right brain hemispheres, making it more difficult to think clearly.

Donna has seen homolateral patterning in the energies of every person she has worked with who was depressed. To correct this pattern, place one hand on the shoulder that is opposite of that hand, gently dig your fingers into the back of that shoulder, and drag them with some pressure over the top of your shoulder. Then gently pull with an open hand down and across your body diagonally to your opposite hip. Repeat on the other side. Do this several times. It is a quick way to get the energies of the opposite sides of your body and your brain flowing in harmony.

Repetition is important in changing longstanding energy habits. If you do the Four Thumps several times daily, as suggested earlier, you might immediately follow it with the Crossover Shoulder Pull. It requires less than a minute.

C. **Energy Blockages Where Stress Has Accumulated: The Hook-Up.** This simple technique helps the body process stress wherever it is stored by creating a circuit between the meridian that goes up the front center of the body (Central Meridian, also known as the Conception Vessel) and the meridian that goes up the back (Governing Meridian, also known as the Governor Vessel). The strengthened circuit radiates energy throughout the body that breaks up packets of accumulated stress.

To do the Hook-Up, place the middle finger of one hand on your "third eye" (between your eyebrows above the bridge of your nose) and the middle finger of your other hand in your navel. Gently press both fingers inward, pull them upward, and hold there for at least three full, deep breaths.

D. **Depletion of Energies in Vital Areas: The Triple Warmer Smoothie.** Triple Warmer is an energy system that governs the body's response to internal invaders (the immune system) as well as external dangers (the fight-or-flight response). When it detects a threat, it is able to "conscript" energies from every meridian (except Heart Meridian). A prolonged threat or *perception* of threat keeps Triple Warmer in a state of heightened alert, depleting energies from other body parts. Many psychological problems involve a sustained internal sense of danger. With depression, this may be so persistent that the imagined danger isn't even consciously registered, yet it may keep Triple Warmer on alert. When this occurs, Triple Warmer continues to collect energies from the meridians. If it doesn't use them for fighting or fleeing, they accumulate, resulting in an overall sense of heaviness in the body and depletion of energies in vital areas, both of which play into depression. By calming Triple Warmer, the energies it has conscripted from other meridians return to these areas.

One of the simplest yet most powerful ways to calm Triple Warmer is the Triple Warmer Smoothie. Lay your middle fingers across your closed eyelids. Take a deep in-breath. On the exhale, slide your fingers out to your temples. Then with another deep inhalation, slide your fingers around your ears, down your neck, and hang your fingers on your shoulders. With your next deep breath, drag your fingers down to the center of your chest. Place your open hands over your Heart Chakra. Hold there for three deep breaths, in through your nose and out through your mouth.

E. Energy Disruptions That Cause Clouded Thinking: The Wayne Cook Posture. As we will further explore in the next section, negative thinking and self-limiting beliefs are hallmarks of depression. While some of this may be due to cognitive distortions that can be corrected with logical analysis or tapping on internal contradictions, cognitive distortions may also be fueled and maintained by energy disruptions. The best single technique we know for remedying this type of energy disruption is called the "Wayne Cook Posture." Like the Crossover Shoulder Pull and the Hook-Up introduced above, it has many uses and is demonstrated in Donna's YouTube video of the Daily Energy Routine (der.energytapping.com).

3. Negative Thoughts and Beliefs

Whatever the physical and energetic components of depression, negative thoughts and beliefs generate a depressed mood.

Continually ruminating on what's wrong can simply collapse your energy levels. At the same time, depression intensifies negative thoughts and beliefs. It's a powerful but immobilizing circular relationship.

Negative thinking keeps your focus on limitations rather than possibilities. It distorts your perceptions and experiences in ways that are disempowering. It maintains self-defeating behavioral patterns. Negative thoughts and beliefs energetically resonate with depression, and depression energetically resonates with negative thoughts and beliefs.

Challenging one's negative thinking is one key to overcoming depression. While we can't address every possible negative thought here, we can identify three of the most common issues that lead to negative thinking and provide some methods to counter each with acupoint tapping. They include:

A. Diminished sense of self-worth

B. Jumping to false disempowering conclusions

C. Believing you are genetically destined to be depressed

To apply tapping to each, use the tools presented in Chapters 2 and 3. To get you started, we will discuss the dilemmas in these issues and formulate sample Reminder Phrases, Acceptance Statements, and Choices Statements. As you proceed, you will also note any Psychological Reversals or disruptive aspects. Going through the Basic Tapping

Protocol can thoroughly address your negative thoughts and beliefs one by one. While this may take some time and effort and require several sittings, overcoming depression deserves this investment.

A. Diminished Sense of Self-Worth. Depression is hard on your self-assessments. Because of low motivation and difficulties with taking care of even life's basic requirements, people with depression often feel they aren't useful, that their lives are meaningless, or that they don't really matter to anyone. This is often accompanied by shame—a sense that they simply aren't good enough—which also makes it hard to mobilize and take the steps that would lead them out of depression. To begin to apply the Basic Tapping Protocol to a sense of worthlessness:

Reminder Phrase: *"I don't deserve to feel good!"*

Acceptance Statement: *"Even though I don't deserve to feel good, I deeply and completely accept myself."*

Choices Statements: *"Even though I don't deserve to feel good,*

- *I choose to find the strength to wrestle with my despair."*

- *I choose to register that I have some good moments."*

- *I choose to recognize my value to those who love me."*

Notice how the Choices Statements begin to challenge the limitations of the negative thinking, as the second phrase becomes increasingly believable.

B. Jumping to Self-Limiting Conclusions. One of our own guiding models is that every human being has inherent value, and thus deciding one is worthless requires colossal cognitive distortions. Plus, a diminished sense of self-worth isn't the only area of distorted thinking that tends to accompany depression. "Automatic thoughts," as they are known in CBT, frame situations you face in ways that predict failure:

"I'll never be able to succeed at the things that matter most to me."

"I'm not smart enough to meet these challenges."

"I've failed at this before, and I'll fail again."

"I'll never get the love I need."

"I mess up whenever I try something new."

Automatic thoughts that immediately judge your efforts in highly critical ways can be particularly disempowering, undermining your inner resources and keeping you trapped in a cycle of negative thinking and depressed feelings. They also lead to falsely believing that others are judging you in the same harsh ways you are judging yourself.

CBT counters self-limiting thoughts and beliefs by having the person gather evidence that refutes them. It uses various approaches, from introspection to journaling to mini experiments to asking friends for their perceptions on the matter of concern. While approaches that apply logic to changing negative thoughts and beliefs can be effective, tapping is faster and more direct. It is one thing to know that the tendency to judge yourself harshly isn't a great strategy and to chip away at it with experiments, observations, and reason. It is quite another to quickly and efficiently shift the energy pattern and brain chemistry that is fueling negative thinking. That is what acupoint tapping can accomplish.

The process still requires some introspection and self-assessment. What automatic thoughts or ongoing beliefs limit you? Describe them in your journal. Select one to focus on first. Create a Reminder Phrase and an Acceptance Statement. As the SUD decreases, replace the Acceptance Statement with a Choices Statement. For instance:

Reminder Phrase: *"I'm a loser at love!"*

Acceptance Statement: *"Even though my intimate relationships have never worked out, I deeply and completely accept myself anyway."*

Choices Statements: *"Even though my intimate relationships never work out . . .*

- *I choose to recognize that intimate relationships are challenging for everyone."*

- *I choose to recall the positive ways I've contributed to my past relationships."*

- *I choose to figure out how to make my closest relationships more gratifying."*

Tapping to overcome depression generally includes a substantial focus on shifting negative thoughts and beliefs. Particularly attend to patterns of responding to life events in self-defeating ways, such as when a small setback causes you to want to give up.

C. Believing You Are Genetically Destined to Be Depressed. Viewing depression as a brain disease is another negative belief that often accompanies depression, particularly recurrent or longstanding depression, and it is more than understandable. While more than 40 gene variants raise the risk of depression,[20] the expression of those genes depends largely on lifestyle, thinking style, stress, and trauma. Plus, the role of genetics in depression is only part of the story. While it is true that 20 to 30 percent of people who have a parent or sibling with major depression are likely to develop the disorder, it's a slippery slope to go from that statistic to believing you are helpless. After all, 70 to 80 percent don't go on to develop it.

Nonetheless, some people with family members who are depressed assume after a bout of depression: "Something is wrong with my brain, and I'll always be depressed." Depression becomes part of their identity, and they act accordingly. Approaches such as CBT, meditation, and tapping teach you to step back and disidentify from your emotions and thoughts. They lead to recognitions such as "I am not my anger," "I am not my anxiety," "I am not my depression." This allows you to relate to difficult feelings in a manner that is more inquisitive and creative rather than defining yourself by them.

It is, however, also important to know your vulnerabilities. While defining yourself by them limits your vision of what is possible for you, understanding them allows you to take corrective and preventive actions. For some people, medication that decreases depression works, and they may fully accept that they will need to use medication for the rest of their lives, much as someone with type 1 diabetes needs insulin. Meanwhile, controversy exists about whether more natural approaches can bring about the desired changes in a seriously depressed brain without medication (and its stigma or side effects).

The predominant opinion is that for severe or persistent depression, a combination of medication and therapy is usually the best approach. However, for mild to moderate depression, research shows that psychotherapy can be as effective as medication.[21] The benefits of psychotherapy also tend to persist beyond the end of treatment. With or without medication, however, key issues such as self-worth, negative thinking, unresolved grief,

formative experiences, and relationship difficulties need to be addressed. Therapy, particularly approaches that have a somatic component such as tapping, combined with commonsense steps such as adequate sleep, nutrition, exercise, and support from family and friends, is often effective without the use of medication. If, on the other hand, people believe they are helpless to fight their depression, they will be. Here are some tapping phrases to get started, so that having had episodes of depression doesn't become your identity:

Reminder Phrase: *"My brain chemistry keeps me depressed."*

Acceptance Statement: *"Even though my brain chemistry prevents me from overcoming my depression, I deeply and completely accept myself."*

Choices Statements: *"Even though my brain chemistry prevents me from overcoming my depression . . .*

- *I choose to recognize that depression is a state that can be influenced."*

- *I choose to figure out how to deal with my tendency toward depression more effectively than ever."*

- *I choose to appreciate the positive steps I've taken."*

4. Formative Experiences

Difficult childhood experiences that have not been adequately processed may fuel depression. In exploring such experiences, look for early losses of parents, other loved ones, pets, self-esteem, safety, or security in its many manifestations. Any of these can have an enormous impact on your spirit, but you can use the Basic Tapping Protocol and related detective work to begin to heal whatever you identify. You saw how Margaret's depression traced not only to her divorce, as she had assumed; it also had roots that went all the way back to her father having abandoned the family when she was four. Here is how she began to work with that facet of her depression:

Reminder Phrase: *"I had to grow up without a dad."*

Acceptance Statement: *"Even though I had to grow up without a dad, I accept the lingering wounds this caused me."*

Choices Statements: *"Even though I had to grow up without a dad . . .*

- *I choose to know I have a right to all this anger that's coming up."*

- *I choose to recognize how well I've done without the love, support, and guidance I wish a father had given me."*

- *I choose to use the loss of my husband as a way to come to terms with my father's abandonment in new and empowering ways."*

More recent losses, such as of one's home, job, health, or an intimate, may also instigate depression. As a result, an important component of effective work with depression is grief work. We all have had losses, and emotionally processing them allows us to move on without unnecessary emotional baggage. Much of this occurs organically, without therapy or even without consciously taking oneself through the steps of grieving. But what of those experiences that have not been resolved and continue to drain you? How do you emotionally process them? Again, the steps in the Basic Tapping Protocol and subsequent detective work can be powerful antidotes to unresolved losses that may underlie depression. To get started, here are some sample phrases:

Reminder Phrase: *"I miss Ryan terribly."*

Acceptance Statement: *"Even though I can hardly bear how deeply I miss Ryan, I love and deeply accept myself."*

Choices Statements: *"Even though I can hardly bear how deeply I miss Ryan . . .*

- *I choose to honor the love I have had for him."*

- *I choose to recognize that he would want me to move forward."*

- *I choose to savor what I gained from this relationship and to use it as a resource for the rest of my life."*

5. Positive Exposure

What you do and where you go impacts your energy and mood. A challenge for many people is the amount of time they spend in front of electronic screens. Alarming increases in teen depression and suicidal behavior since 2010 seem to correlate with increasing amounts of screen time during that period,[22] though the strength of that correlation is still being debated. In any case, it is fair to say that a healthy balance between screen time and activities such as positive face-to-face time with family and friends, adventures in nature, or enjoyable physical activities are going to counter tendencies toward depression.

Beyond the actual hours of screen time is of course the content shown on the screen. Keeping yourself informed about local, national, and international news is very different from binging on depressing events from every corner of the world, imprinting themselves on your brain day after day. The simple fact is that what we expose ourselves to has an impact on our brains, energies, and mood.

If you are concerned about depression, be discerning about your digital media diet. Uplifting or inspiring content has a different impact than sources that provoke anxiety, fear, or hopelessness. Stories of people who overcome difficult challenges provide models. One of Donna's favorite scenes from a movie is in the historical drama *Amistad*. As Cinque fights for his life in a court of law that seems stacked against him, he confidently calls upon his African ancestors:

> I will call into the past, far back to the beginning of time, and beg them to come and help me at the judgment. I will reach back and draw them into me. And they must come, for at this moment, I am the whole reason they have existed.[23]

What inspires you? What strengthens you? Be steadfast in choosing uplifting activities rather than those that feed depression. Cultivate thoughts and images of hope and optimism. Build into your life new activities and pursuits that will help you feel better and more motivated. While these are hour-to-hour choices you make every day, you can use tapping so those choices are more likely to enhance your outlook and frame of mind. To begin:

Reminder Phrase: *"I am drawn to [an activity that brings you down]."*

Acceptance Statement: *"Even though I am drawn to [this activity], I deeply accept myself."*

Choices Statements: *"Even though I am drawn to [this activity]...*

- *I choose to recognize that my choice of activities will impact how I feel."*

- *I choose to steer away from activities that bring down my spirit."*

- *I am increasingly choosing activities that are uplifting and inspiring."*

6. Social Connection

A family member, a good friend, or a caring therapist can be a lifeline in pulling a person out of depression. Depression, however, does not make it easy to engage with others. Martha Manning, who provided the vivid account of depression described earlier, offers her experiences during visiting hours on the psychiatric ward where she was hospitalized for a major depressive episode:

> During visiting hours, I was always struck by the one-way conversations up and down the halls. As much as I cared for my family members, it was hard to tolerate their visits. Even with clinicians whom I judged warm and competent, it was difficult to share the same space. The only exception was my uncle, who was no stranger to depression. After a few fruitless questions, he became silent. In the silence, he began to cry. I felt my hand moving over his. We said nothing more for the entire visit.

It was the first time in a long time that I'd had a real conversation with someone.

You can teach those you are close to what you need from them when you are depressed. It may be space. It may be to pull you into conversation. Or it may be to honor the silence. It may be to take on an important task you don't have the energy to complete. It may be to quietly watch a movie, listen to music, or take a walk in nature with you. The more you can relieve them of the responsibility of trying to figure it out, the more likely it is that their caring will translate into ways of being that are truly supportive.

Cultivating a network of friends who know how to be there for you can be a golden step in building a lifestyle that counters depression. Depression correlates with a sense that no one cares about you or that people judge you or don't like you. If your actions toward them reflect these beliefs, you will be reinforcing such feelings in them. If forming fulfilling relationships has been a consistent area of frustration for you, you may wish to give special attention to the guidance in Chapter 8 for using tapping to improve your relationships at their psychological foundations.

In short, if you tell the people who care about you how you hope they will express their caring, that caring will be reinforced. Be mindful that what you convey shapes how you will be treated. While these are, again, hour-by-hour choices, you can program yourself to approach your relationships more constructively using the Basic Tapping Protocol. You might begin with statements such as:

Reminder Phrase: *"I want people to just leave me alone when I'm depressed."*

Acceptance Statement: *"Even though I want people to just leave me alone when I'm depressed, I deeply accept myself."*

Choices Statements: *"Even though I want people to just leave me alone when I'm depressed . . .*

- *I choose to appreciate that it's hard to entertain others when I'm depressed."*

- *I choose to recognize that positive connections with others will be good for me."*

- *I choose to take steps so those who care about me know how I need them to be with me when I'm depressed."*

- *I choose to cultivate relationships that bring out the best in me."*

7. Relapse Prevention

Some 50 percent of people who have had a major depressive episode will have a second one, and 80 percent of those who have a second one will have a third.[24] People who have a history of depression tend to have between five and nine full-blown depressive episodes in their lifetime. Other factors that play into relapse are the severity of the depression, genetics, thought patterns, and self-destructive habits such as substance abuse. Is there anything you can do to prevent a recurrence?

Marian Sandmaier, a writer who specializes in the workings of the human mind, describes what it is like to have had multiple depressive episodes. She writes, "Whenever I recovered from a particular bout, I was sure it was my last one. Then, when it wasn't, I was horrified."[25] Because of this terror, she developed a prevention plan, which she refers to as "depression-proofing." At the core of her plan is to develop confidence that while depression may return, there are specific ways to increase the odds of heading it off. These are tailored practices that, Sandmaier says, have brought her "back from the cliff" several times since her last depression three years earlier.

Part of Sandmaier's depression-proofing includes maintaining some of the practices that helped her recover from depression in the past. Staying vigilant about challenging negative thinking patterns and retaining good social support were paramount. Her other regular mood-boosters included avoiding overwork, participation in a weekly leaderless support group, walking in a garden, singing Motown, and listening to programs she finds soothing or inspiring. Periodic tune-ups with a therapist who has helped in the past may be useful. Other mainte-nance approaches may include regular exercise, meditation, or yoga. Building time into your life for periodic tapping sessions to address any of the issues dis-cussed in this chapter as the need arises can be a potent way of keeping yourself on a positive track.

The bottom line is to recognize that depression may return, to know the signs, and to take determined steps to head it off rather than to assume you are a help-less victim. One of these steps may be to return to therapy before waiting too long. Just keeping the mindset that you are not a victim is often not enough. It is not a failure to seek help when it is needed, which can be the most constructive step available at certain points.

A strategy Sandmaier uses to head off negative thinking traces to a method called "Focusing," developed by the phi-losopher Eugene Gendlin in the 1960s. Sandmaier describes how the technique quietly reshaped her "inner landscape":

> The approach centers on locating a *bodily* sense of whatever difficulty I'm struggling with, rather than my customary approach of inspecting the contents of my mind. It works something like this: once I find and name a felt sense—"a constriction in my throat" for example, or a "hot stone in my stomach"—I greet it. It can be just a few words, like "Hello I know you're there." Then I wait.

> Often, before long, my tight-ened throat or roiling stomach begins to morph into a visual image of a small, cowering girl. Guess who. She occasionally asks for wisdom or validation, but usu-ally she just wants a loving arm wrapped around her by the adult, compassionate part of me. Until I started this practice, I didn't know I *had* that part. But she emerges, readily, in response to this small girl. I feel about this child the way I feel about my daughter or my granddaughter—wanting fiercely to protect her and make sure she feels loved. As I continue to sit with that little one, I typically experi-ence a shift in my body, a less bur-dened, more spacious quality. . . . It gets me in touch, quickly and pow-erfully, with this stringy-haired little kid who doesn't deserve my depression-inducing scorn—only love and listening.[26]

You are already familiar with a form of focusing. Tuning in to your body's "felt sense" is part of how you create your SUD rating. For Sandmaier, the process also involved a spontaneous Affect Bridge (p. 109), where she went back in time and contacted the "stringy-haired little girl" who was once her. From there, a number of steps are possible. Sandmaier men-tions two of them that you have already witnessed: starting a conversation where your compassionate adult self shares the wisdom accumulated over the years *or* simply showers the child with love. Tapping during such imaginary exchanges embeds the benefits into your body. Tapping protocols also allow you to focus on other unresolved issues from that period of your life and systematically bring emotional resolution to them.

LETTING THE SUN SHINE THROUGH

This chapter has shown how to apply tapping in seven key areas that will have a cumulative effect in overcoming depression. It opened with ways for using tapping to meet sadness constructively. It then moved into depression. Depression adds energetic and biological components to sadness that make it much more problematic and often crushing. We reviewed the symptoms and causes for depression. We explored five dimensions of depression in the body's energy system and energy techniques for making adjustments in each of them. We also showed how to use the Basic Tapping Protocol to counter some of the biggest challenges in working with depression, such as a lack of energy for taking constructive steps, the belief that nothing is going to work, negative thinking, unresolved formative experiences, and preventing relapses. We want to close with one additional reflection.

While you may feel that your spirit is diminished when you are depressed, that isn't quite what is going on. Our colleague João Pestana, a psychologist in Portugal, explains, "What I've found for myself and with my clients is that we don't need to make the sun brighter. It's already bright enough. What we need to do is take the clouds away so the sun can shine through. That's how we discover how bright the sun within us really is, and it is exactly what tapping does. It removes the clouds, one by one!"

CHAPTER 6

Habits and Addictions

Change is hard. Negative thoughts, beliefs, and behaviors often continue
as if they have a life of their own.... By freeing the flow of energy in
the body, longstanding psychological issues can be eliminated.[1]

—Mary Sise, LCSW
President, Association for Comprehensive Energy Psychology, 2004–2006

SO FAR IN PART II, we've concentrated on using acupoint tapping to overcome everyday worries and sadness as well as more deep-rooted psychological conditions such as anxiety, depression, and PTSD. This chapter moves from exploring internal psychological states to establishing *behaviors* that can improve your life and eliminating behaviors that are interfering with your well-being and effectiveness in the world. We will start with *habits* that maintain behavior in ways that may be constructive or self-defeating and then move on to *addictions*, which are generally more harmful than simple habits and more deeply embedded in your nervous system.

HABITS

Donna's type in ancient Chinese medicine is called a "fire element." She is ebullient and full of enthusiasm. This carries into the tone and vibration of her voice and leaves a positive imprint on her clients and students. It doesn't, however, have such a desirable effect in one situation. If we are going somewhere and David is driving, it's not unusual for Donna to joyfully utter something like, "Look! There's the restaurant where we learned about Tiernan's first step" or "Oh! I just remembered who I have to call." Within the first syllable of these eruptions, David starts to hit the brakes, assuming from Donna's fiery tone that she is alerting him to an emergency on the road. It's a dangerous but habitual reaction.

David winds up being distracted at the wheel and then embarrassed. Donna is thinking, "What's wrong with this guy!" Meanwhile, the car behind hopefully didn't rear-end us. Recognizing that there is nothing he can do to change Donna from being a fire element, nor would he want to, David decided to use our work on this chapter as an opportunity for changing his habit of going for the brake in the first milliseconds of hearing Donna's excited utterances. He followed the steps outlined in the "Eliminating an Unwanted Habit" section below. Particularly useful was to tap while imagining himself driving and hearing the start of one of Donna's fiery exclamations. As David succeeded, our driving excursions became less vulnerable to these unexpected moments of tension.

Creatures of Habit. The saying "We are creatures of habit" applies to habits that help us as well as those that harm us. The same brain wiring that causes us to automatically brush our teeth when we get to the sink in the morning also prompts us to mindlessly turn on the TV the moment we get home. Whether for better or worse, habits are enormously efficient compared to figuring out how to handle every situation as it emerges. They are activated in the brain in milliseconds, thousands of times faster than conscious decisions. Nearly half of what we do is on autopilot, orchestrated by habitual behavior while our minds are occupied elsewhere.[2]

Because good habits were so useful for your ancestors—such as checking for the scent of a predator before stepping into an exposed area—your brain evolved to be quite adept at creating habits that stick. In a modern version, we teach young children to look both ways before crossing a street, a habit that serves them for the rest of their lives. However, the collateral damage with this arrangement is that habits you *don't want* are also hard to break. Good intentions and willpower for changing a deeply entrenched habit collide with the neural pathways maintaining it.

Beyond New Year's Resolutions. Most people find that the "New Year's resolution" approach to habit change is not very effective. You identify an area to better yourself and promise to make a decisive change, and you've forgotten the whole routine by January 4.[3] What we will show you here is more complicated than a New Year's resolution. On the other hand, it works. Long-standing habits that have become wired into your nervous system do not disappear just because you are suddenly inspired to eliminate them.

Habits are so important to the quality of our lives that they have been studied extensively, and a plethora of self-help books teach how to establish good habits and break bad ones. Among the best of these are Charles Duhigg's *The Power of Habit*, B. J. Fogg's *Tiny Habits*, and Stephen Covey's *The 7 Habits of Highly Effective People*.[4]

James Clear is probably the most widely consulted expert on habits. Clear's 2018 book *Atomic Habits* has sold more than 10 million copies and has been translated into over 50 languages.[5] He has worked with many Fortune 500 companies, universities, and professional athletes. We'll present the central features of his model and show how tapping can be applied to make them even more effective. While successfully installing a habit that is good for you or eliminating one that is detrimental frees and empowers you, we'll repeat that it also requires effort. If this is not the right time for you to take this on, you can skip this section and jump to "Addictions" (p. 227) if that is of interest to you or move on to another chapter. The instructions for building a desirable habit or eliminating one that harms you will still be here when you want them.

How Habits Develop

You were not born with habits. Every habit you have has been learned. The path from a need to a habit is quite predictable. Habits start with a need. The need motivates an action. If the action satisfies the need and the outcome has been pleasing, the action is more likely to be repeated the next time the need is felt. If the action doesn't meet the need or meets it but also creates new problems, the action is less likely to be attempted the next time the need is felt. Habit formation begins with this trial-and-error process—feel the need, try doing something to satisfy it, experience the outcome, evaluate, and remember what happened. If the problem keeps emerging and an action that satisfies it is repeated, the brain automates the process. A habit is born.

The need that motivates the action may be based in your body—hunger, an itch, an anxious feeling in the pit of your stomach—or it may be based on a problem in your life, such as improving your performance at work or responding more effectively to your child's angry outbursts. Many life challenges require us to devise strategies to bring about satisfying outcomes or to find ways of mitigating or preventing outcomes that are unsatisfying, painful, or costly.

At their best, habits simplify your life. A myriad of daily needs are addressed without your conscious attention. As Clear emphasizes, the conscious mind is the "bottleneck" of your brain.[6] Because your mind can only focus on a very limited number of issues at one time, your brain constantly strives to safeguard your conscious attention for what is most important. So your brain delegates automatic tasks to areas that can operate without conscious monitoring.

That is how habits are established neurologically. Research bears this out. While activity in the relevant brain regions is inevitably high during the process of habit formation, it is low once the habit has been established.[7]

The Components of a Habit: Cue, Craving, Response, Reward

Once a habit has been formed, Clear explains that a *cue* activates it. A cue may be a sensation within your body, such as your stomach gurgling to initiate a craving for food; or something external, such as seeing that 56 non-spam emails have come in since the last time you checked.

The cue activates a *craving*. Cues may, however, be interpreted in a variety of ways, depending on the thoughts, feelings, and history of the person experiencing the cue. Seeing 56 new emails might create a craving that involves curiosity and a desire to knock them out, with each response producing a slight ping of satisfaction. Or seeing those emails may lead to feelings of overwhelm and a craving to feel settled, without demands, and in control. These different types of cravings, though generated by the same cue, may lead to very different responses. What you crave, however, is not the action associated with the habit (e.g., answering the emails) but the change in your internal state that your response to the craving will bring about (e.g., the satisfied curiosity as you read each and then a feeling of accomplishment as you answer it). Clear gives several other examples:

> You do not crave smoking a cigarette; you crave the feeling of relief it provides. You are not motivated by brushing your teeth but rather by the feeling of a clean mouth. You do not want to turn on the television; you want to be entertained. Every craving is linked to a desire to change your internal state.[8]

The *response* to the craving is the third step in creating and maintaining a habit. The response to the craving to free yourself from a long list of unanswered emails might be to set aside other priorities and tackle the list. Or, as Clear points out, the response to seeing the list, feeling overwhelmed, and craving to regain a sense of control might be to bite your fingernails. You are taking control of your internal state by reducing your discomfort, even in this entirely tangential way.

Either tackling the list *or* biting your fingernails may produce a *reward*, different as those two rewards may be. In either case, the reward is the fourth and final step in building a habit. The *reward* is the outcome of the *response* that was designed to satisfy the *craving* that was initiated by the *cue*. The reward brings about an internal state that produces satisfaction or relief from the craving, at least for the moment.

If completing the emails leads to relief and satisfaction, that reward will further ingrain the habit of putting everything else aside to respond to your emails. If biting your fingernails reduces the stress of encountering the list, biting your fingernails becomes associated with seeing a long string of emails.

These four components of a habit also map the necessary steps for *establishing* a habit. They are, in this order:

- *Cue*: a trigger

- *Craving*: a desire triggered by a cue

- *Response*: a behavior initiated by a craving

- *Reward*: the outcome when a craving is satisfied

If any of these steps are missing or of insufficient strength, the habit will not be created.

We have built upon these four natural steps in habit development in designing tapping protocols for creating desirable habits and breaking undesirable ones. We will ask you to identify one "good" habit you would like to develop and one "bad" habit you would like to eliminate. We will take you step by step through creating or breaking these habits by adding tapping to leverage each of the four natural components of habit development.

CREATING OR STRENGTHENING A DESIRABLE HABIT

Begin by selecting or envisioning a habit you wish to create or strengthen. You may already know exactly where you would like to focus. If you are not sure, consider changes you would like to see in your life. You may desire to be more fit; to have greater success in your work; to have greater intimacy in your marriage; or to be a better pianist, cook, or tennis player. Choose an area that matters to you. In reflecting on this area, what is a behavior that, if done regularly, would begin to bring about the desired change? *That* is the habit you can cultivate. You may want to journal various possibilities before settling on your choice for the first time through this process.

As you begin establishing even the most important habit, Clear advises, start small! The new habit should be a modest step toward the desired change. If you want to get fit, the habit might start with walking up the stairs instead of taking the elevator at work. If you hope to have greater intimacy, the habit might start with expressing an appreciation for your partner each day. Identify small steps. They will have a cumulative effect. You can introduce larger steps once the small steps have become ingrained. At this point, you are looking for building blocks, not the whole building. When a small habit becomes routine and relatively automatic, expanding on it becomes easier. Trying to do it all at once is a path toward discouragement and failure. Take all the time you need to identify the habit you wish to build, then proceed through the following four steps. But first, to get into the zone, begin with the following "Quick Fix."

Quick Fix: Establishing a Desired Habit

Bring to mind a behavior you would like to do or do more frequently. Give an SUD rating to the amount of distress you feel in your mind and/or body when you think about not yet having established this habit. Say out loud the first statement below as you tap on the Top-of-the-Head Point. Then say the next statement while tapping on the next point. Go through each statement, cycling through the 12 tapping points as you move from one statement to the next. Skip any phrases that don't fit for you.

"I want to establish or strengthen a habit that [name desired habit].

Even though I have some resistance to building this habit,

I accept this resistance.

Even though I'm not sure I'll be able to pull this off,

I'm willing to focus on my abilities rather than my fears.

I want to start this new habit, but [name a concern].

I accept this concern.

I recognize that I may have some ambivalence.

Maybe I haven't succeeded when I've tried to establish this habit before.

Maybe I expect to fail.

Establishing this habit matters to me.

But I haven't really been able to get the ball rolling yet.

It's hard to make this change.

It doesn't come automatically.

But I know deep down I want this new habit.

I choose to take action and get started.

I choose to release my doubts.

Past failures don't define the outcome here.

This new habit is worth my time and effort.

I can imagine all the good that will come from it.

I'm choosing to be open to a new level of confidence.

And I choose to enjoy the process.

I choose to anticipate the accomplishment.

I appreciate my efforts.

I choose to realize that this deserves my effort.

I'm happy to be feeling more inspired.

I'm encouraged as I begin to feel more confidence that I can do this."

After going through this sequence two or three times, you will probably find that the new habit is seeming more possible. Gauge this with another SUD rating on your distress about the habit not yet being fully established. You have also been preparing yourself to go deeper into establishing it by next combining tapping with James Clear's approach, as shown in the next part of the chapter.

Two Ways to Proceed

You can approach the program presented in the remainder of this section in either of two ways. You can read the text as it is written and apply each of the four "Your Turn" instructions as you come to them. Or you can skip most of the text and jump to the four headings describing the experience of the test driver (in this case, Rianna) and then carry out the instructions that follow. The practice instructions alone will build your habit, but we have found Clear's model and the theory backing it to be so useful that we have described it in some detail.

Step 1: Make the Cue Obvious

Cues initiate the four-part process of *cue*, *craving*, *response*, and *reward*. Approaching the door to your place of work might be a cue to fix your hair. We have hundreds of simple mini habits. Seeing an open bag of potato chips on the counter might be a cue for craving something salty. We also have many habits that are more complex. Having your partner express irritation with you might be a cue for escalating the exchange or withdrawing, two common but ineffective habits for fielding conflict.

The first step for developing a habit is to make the cue obvious. For some habits, a minor shift in your environment is the simplest way to do this. Clear offers examples such as:

- To remember to take your medications each night, put your pill container where you will see it before you go to bed.

- To practice guitar more regularly, place your guitar stand where you regularly need to detour around it.

- To drink more water, place full water bottles throughout your house.[9]

In many situations, however, creating environmental cues to initiate the habit isn't possible. A second way to cue a habit is to make an *existing habit* the cue for the new one: *"When I've finished my last bite of dinner, I take my vitamins." "When I come home in the evening, I immediately go to the chair by the window and meditate for five minutes." "After I put on my shoes in the morning, I open my journal and begin to write." "As soon as I finish my morning emails, I do a one-minute stretching routine."*

A third strategy Clear suggests is based on the fact that the two most common cues in everyday life are *time* and *place*: *"It's 7 am, so I start getting ready for work." "I just got to my workstation, and I look for the report from the previous shift."* Even though many daily habits are not related to a specific time or place, you can often use the power of time and place to set a firm mental intention so that a particular time and/or place becomes the cue: *"Whenever I approach the front door of my house, I stop for a moment and take a deep calming breath."*

"Before I begin a meal, I tune in to something I am grateful for and put it into words." You are setting an intention that a particular time or place initiates the habit you want to establish.

Each of these approaches has two parts. The first involves identifying the cue (your front door, 8 pm on weekdays, a meal) or creating it (an alarm, leaving the guitar where you will notice it, water bottles throughout the house). All these make the cue more "obvious." The second part involves mentally pairing the cue with the desired behavior. You can combine both parts into a single affirmation or statement of your intention, such as *"When I see my guitar, I pick it up and practice for 10 minutes."* You can use tapping to empower this strategy.

As you've seen throughout this book, when an intention or affirmation is stated while stimulating selected acupuncture points, the desired outcome is more likely than when the intention or affirmation is stated without stimulating the acupoints. Once you've formed this Intention Statement, you can use tapping to energize it.

Introducing Rianna

Rianna is a busy executive in her early 50s. During the pandemic, she started working mostly from home. The habit she wished to establish was to take time to exercise. She wanted to start with five minutes daily and ultimately increase that to 20 minutes. The cue she selected was time: *"When I see 3 pm on the clock, I am ready to exercise, and I begin."* She also had an alternative that if she wasn't home (she still had some meetings at the office), she would exercise as soon as she got home. She gave a believability rating as to how likely she was to follow through. It was only a 2. After a few tapping cycles, visualizing herself happily exercising, she got it up to a 5, but it seemed to settle there.

Rianna realized she was up against a Psychological Reversal involving guilt about taking time for herself. She always felt behind in both her work and family obligations. She formulated an Acceptance Statement: *"Even though I feel guilty about taking time to exercise, I deeply and completely accept myself."* That led to this Choices Statement: *"Even though I feel guilty about taking time to exercise, I choose to recognize that the best thing I can do for everyone who cares about me is to take care of myself."* She then tapped on a series of statements, first around *"Feeling guilty about exercise"* and progressing to *"Everyone who matters to me wants me to take care of myself."* This got the believability up to a 7. While she might have gone into the childhood roots of the guilt, this was not calling to her, and she proceeded to the next section.

Your Turn: Getting Started

Follow these 8 steps and record pertinent parts in your journal. Doing them shouldn't take much longer than reading them.

1. Describe the habit you wish to establish. Remember to start small. You are not playing Vivaldi's Guitar Concerto in D or James Taylor's "Fire and Rain" every time you pass the guitar. You are rehearsing a passage or practicing a scale. You can adjust the specific behavior as you wish, such as increasing the time you will practice.

2. Identify or create the cue you wish to make obvious, whether an item you put where you will see it, an already established habit that will become a cue for the new habit, or a time or place that will serve as the cue.

3. Create and record an Intention Statement along the lines of *"When [describe the cue that occurs], I [describe in the present tense the specific behavior that will follow]."* If your goal is to carve out time to read uplifting material before going to sleep, your Intention Statement might begin: *"When I get in my pajamas, I read a passage from [an inspiring book]."* You can expand the behavior over time to reading one page from the book to two pages to an entire chapter. But first establish the habit in a simple form you are likely to be able to implement.

4. Give an SUB rating (Subjective Units of Believability) to your Intention Statement, where 0 means "No way, not going to happen" and 10 means it is totally believable that the cue will prompt the desired behavior.

5. Create an Acceptance Statement, particularly if the believability is low. For instance, *"Even though it's only at 3 that I believe I will [state your intention], I deeply and completely accept myself."* State it three times, rubbing your chest sore spots with the first phrase and holding your hands over your Heart Chakra with the second phrase.

6. Repeat your Intention Statement out loud as you tap on each of the 12 tapping points. You can tap on one point while saying the first part of the statement and tap on the next point while saying the second part of the statement, or you can say the entire statement at each tapping point. To the extent you are able, also visualize the cue while naming it and see yourself doing the behavior while describing it.

7. Take another SUB rating. If the believability number is not increasing, be alert for any unresolved aspects or Psychological Reversals and address them. Follow with another round of tapping and another SUB rating. Do the Integration Procedure when you feel overloaded with these steps.

8. As soon as the believability begins to rise, convert your Acceptance Statement into a Choices Statement (in the form of *"Even though . . . , I choose to . . ."*), state it three times while rubbing your chest sore spots with the first phrase and holding your hands over your Heart Chakra with the second phrase. Proceed through another round of tapping on your Intention Statement.

Once you have taken this as far as you can—that is, to the point that the SUB is not increasing—you are at a decision point. If the SUB is at an 8 or above, that indicates that your intention is likely to translate into your behavior. Having a highly specific cue that leads to an immediate action may be enough to set your new habit into motion. See what happens over the next few days without trying too hard or judging yourself. If these steps have established your habit to your satisfaction, we suggest jumping to the fourth step (p. 213), which presents ways of maintaining the new habit.

If the SUB is still below 8, or if your habit isn't getting established, your efforts likely need more support. This is where making the craving attractive, the second step, comes in. The cue captures your attention. The craving motivates you to carry out the habit.

Step 2: Make the Craving Attractive

You may not crave the action you are trying to establish habitually. While some desirable behaviors are immediately reinforcing, such as taking a deep relaxing breath before you open the door to your home, many are not. You may not crave 10 minutes of meditation or exercise, at least not until the habit is already in place. Eventually, however, once you have formed a healthy habit, you will miss it if you don't do it. But to get to that point, you need to know that creating a desired habit often requires actions that aren't comfortable.

Clear summarizes this irony: "With our bad habits, the immediate outcome usually feels good, but the ultimate outcome feels bad. With good habits, it is the reverse: the immediate outcome is unenjoyable, but the ultimate outcome feels good."[10] The extra dessert tastes good, but the long-term effects on your health, weight, and appearance feel bad. Taking that extra lap feels bad, but having increased endurance feels good. Meditation builds new neural circuits that promote peace and clarity of mind, but not instantly.

Reframing. *Immediate* rewards are our strongest motivators. Healthy nutrition simply may not be as appealing in the broccoli-versus-french-fries wars, even though the long-term outcome is more desirable. However, because language is powerful, it is possible to shift the way you think about any ultimately beneficial activity, even though it may be less appealing because of the effort, time, or discomfort required.

Clear points out that changing a single word in the way you describe your desired habit to yourself can shift your emotional response to the whole endeavor. "I *have* to cook dinner for my family" becomes "I *get* to cook dinner for my family." "I *have* to go to bed earlier" becomes "I *get* to go to bed earlier." "I *have* to babysit the grandkids" becomes "I *get* to babysit the grandkids." While both versions are true, one brings up a sense of duty and drudgery, the other a sense of anticipation and possibility. Reframing is a core technique in CBT (p. 102), and simple reframes can shift your relationship to any activity. Among Clear's examples:

- A man who was asked if it is difficult to be confined to a wheelchair answered, *"I'm not confined to my wheelchair; I'm liberated by it. If it weren't for my wheelchair, I'd be bed-bound and never be able to leave my house."*

- An athlete or performer can reframe nervousness to *"I'm excited, and I'm getting an adrenaline rush to help me concentrate."*

- The ubiquitous wandering of the mind that frustrates meditators can be reframed as *"another chance to practice returning to my breath."*

- Instead of telling yourself that you need to go run in the morning, you can say, *"It's time to build my vitality and endurance."*[11]

One of our friends tells his wife when he is faced with a new challenge, *"Another damned opportunity to grow!"* In brief, a quick and easy way to reprogram your mind and make a habit seem more appealing is to reframe your desired habit to emphasize its advantages rather than its disadvantages. And, again, combining the reframed statement with acupoint tapping embeds it more deeply into your psyche and nervous system.

Social Reinforcement. A second way Clear suggests for making the craving more attractive is to become involved with others who also value the desired behavior. Social reinforcement is a powerful motivator. Habits that receive approval, respect, and praise are attractive to us. Say that you want to develop a habit of practicing the piano so you will be sought as a performer. Hanging out with other musicians and discussing your progress is going to increase your motivation to practice. If you participate in a support group or an online community that values the behaviors you are trying to establish, you will have another source of reinforcement for those behaviors.

Strategic Pairing. A third strategy for making the craving triggered by the cue more appealing is to routinely follow the desired behavior with something you already crave. Pairing the cue with a craving that is already attractive associates the cue with pleasure. *"After I have finished [my exercise, my meditation, doing the dishes], I will [put on the headphones and listen to my favorite music, play with Fido, enjoy my garden, eat that snack, log onto Facebook]."* You are pairing the desired behavior with an experience you already crave.

The neurochemistry behind this strategy is worth understanding. The neurotransmitter dopamine is the most powerful brain chemical involved in motivation. The classic experiment demonstrating this relationship was published in 1954 when scientists blocked the release of dopamine in rats. The rats lost all motivation. They ignored food and water that was readily available, showed no interest in courtship, and within a few days had died of dehydration.[12] At the other extreme, mice who received a release of dopamine when they poked their nose into a box developed such a strong craving that they began poking their nose into the box 800 times per hour. While we may find this humorous, Clear points out that humans are not wired so differently. Slot-machine players have been known to spin the wheel 600 times in an hour.[13] Perhaps closer to home for many readers is that "adults in the US spend an average of two to four hours per day tapping, typing, and swiping on their devices."[14] The relationship between our devices and our dopamine cravings is well established.

Using Anticipation. A surprising principle for reshaping behavior is that far more dopamine is released when you *anticipate* a reward than when you *receive* one. A tiny shot of dopamine is released *before* you open each email with an intriguing subject line. The real estate in your brain that is dedicated to pursuing a goal is far larger than the circuitry involved with enjoying having attained the goal. We evolved to be motivated to *get* what we want more than to *enjoy* having attained it. Notice the ways this plays out in your life. Clear uses the example that it is often more exciting for a child to anticipate Christmas presents than to play with them. You know people whose love lives are dominated by the passion of the chase rather than savoring the relationship. The takeaway from this principle is that *anticipating the pleasurable experience* that will follow the habitual behavior you are cultivating releases large quantities of dopamine and is a powerful motivator. Knowing you will get to go back to working on your painting after you've reconciled the day's business receipts creates dopamine-driven anticipation.

To review, you can move into this second step by reframing your relationship with the desired habit, engaging social support that makes the craving more attractive, following the desired behavior with something you crave, or building anticipation into the mix. Any or all of these can be bolstered by tapping.

How Rianna Made Her Craving More Attractive

Rianna changed her evolving Intention Statement from *"I take the time to exercise—without guilt"* to *"I hunger to exercise, and it's a pleasure to do this for myself."* Another way of making the craving more attractive was to promise herself that after each workout, she could sit on their massage chair for five minutes, a luxury she enjoyed but rarely indulged. For social support, she knew her husband was always pleased to see her taking better care of herself, and she vowed to turn to him whenever she needed support in establishing her new habits around exercise.

Your Turn

Describe your desired habit in your journal, framing it in the most positive and appealing language you can find. Next, see if you can identify a pleasurable activity to follow the desired behavior routinely.

Then consider whether there is a way you can get social support for building the habit. Finally, see if there is a way to build anticipation into the arrangement. The appeal for implementing the habit will likely become stronger by doing any of these. Now, having made these adjustments, go through the eight steps in the "Your Turn" instructions under "Make the Cue Obvious" (p. 203). They will very likely take you further in increasing your SUB and your confidence about establishing the new habit.

Again, give yourself a few days to see what happens without trying too hard or judging yourself. If your new habit has been spawned by taking these first two steps—great; jump to Step 4. If the new habit has not yet been established or is fragile, no worries. Continue to Step 3, which corrects for the most common error in attempting to establish a new habit.

Step 3: Make the Behavior Easy

This third step is based on what Clear calls the "Law of Least Effort."[15] Making the desired behavior easy to do means it is more likely that you will do it. We need to recognize that habits we want to replace have been established after hundreds, maybe thousands of repetitions. Clear invokes the neuropsychologist Donald Hebb's famous dictum that "neurons that fire together wire together" by explaining that every time a habitual action is repeated, the associated neural circuit gets activated.[16] Repetition is necessary for forming a new habit, and the way to get yourself to repeat an action is to make the action easy.

The "Two Minute Rule." This is one of Clear's strategies for making a desired behavior easy when initiating a new habit. Twenty minutes of yoga may be a lot for a beginner. But spending two minutes seeing a posture demonstrated on video and briefly practicing it begins to set the habit in motion. Most important is that it is easy enough for you, whatever your mood. You must establish the habit of *showing up* before you can improve on the habit. Improving on it can be gradually introduced once the basics of the habit have been set into place.

Path of Least Resistance. Another way to make the new habit easier is through small adjustments in your environment. You saw how simple changes in your surroundings, such as leaving the guitar in a conspicuous spot, make the cue more obvious. To make it easier to follow the cue and craving with the desired response, put that desired behavior on the path of least resistance. For instance, if you set out the yoga mat and load up a yoga video after breakfast, you will have an easier path to the desired behavior when you return home from work. Take whatever practical steps you can devise so that when the cue appears, the desired response will be as easy as possible.

Other Practical Steps. Additional practical steps can make the new habit almost automatic. If your desired habit is to take breaks to refresh rather than stay glued to the computer screen for your entire workday, setting an hourly chime can remind you to pause and spend a minute looking out the window or stretching your body. Other examples from Clear include:

- To reduce your calories when you eat at restaurants, ask the server to pack half your meal to go rather than serving you the full meal.

- To get to bed early, use a timer that turns your router off at 10 pm so you won't be tempted by the internet.

- To interact more with others, hang out in places where it is easy to be sociable.[17]

The need for the response to be easy may seem like laziness, but Clear points out that laziness can be a smart strategy because the brain is wired to conserve its precious energy.[18] He also proposes that the most effective form of learning for embedding a new habit is not planning but practice. Consistent practice of even the easiest actions causes, through repetition, the behavior to become progressively automatic.

How Rianna Made It Easier to Exercise

For Rianna, the five minutes of exercise wasn't the hard part, so she didn't need to dial that back. She needed to continue tapping on the guilt. She updated her Acceptance and Choices Statements and continued to address her guilt:

Updated Acceptance Statement: *"Even though I'm still finding it difficult to exercise without guilt, I appreciate my efforts and I recognize that a change like this is hard to implement."*

Updated Choices Statement: *"Even though I'm still finding it difficult to exercise without guilt, I choose to focus on the way my body likes moving and stretching."*

After implementing these and further tapping on the guilt, her image of exercising without guilt had reached a believability level of 9.

Your Turn

You've already done tapping to make the cue obvious and the craving more attractive. If these two steps haven't led to the desired habit change, consider dialing back on what you were initially trying to accomplish or finding another way to make it easier. Also, review your Acceptance and Choices Statements and consider updating them. Imagine the desired behavior as becoming easier to carry out as you go through the tapping routine. Does the believability increase? Again, watch what happens over the next few days with these additional simple adjustments, staying alert for unresolved aspects or Psychological Reversals. Address any that emerge.

Step 4: Make the Reward Satisfying

This final step helps not only to establish a new habit but also to maintain it over time. A way to make activities that yield long-term rewards more satisfying on a daily basis is grounded in Clear's insight that making progress is the most effective form of motivation.[19]

Tracking Your Progress. Moving forward toward a goal is satisfying in itself. Tracking your progress each day for simply carrying out the desired behavior is reinforcing, even if the behavior itself isn't immediately reinforcing. Clear cites studies showing that people who keep track of their progress toward health-related goals are significantly more likely to improve than people who skip that step.[20] For instance, in a study of more than 1,600 people, those who kept a daily food log lost twice as much weight as those who didn't.

Making It Vivid. Simply keeping a journal or habit log can be a satisfying way of tracking your progress when establishing a desired habit. However, visual feedback such as charts on your refrigerator may be even more reinforcing. Ideally note the outcome immediately after the behavior, though a nightly review of your list of cues may be more workable. A principle that can also guide you is that you are more likely to remember the final part of an experience. So if the ending moment of your habit-building for a particular day is to put a green mark on your refrigerator chart, which is satisfying, you are increasing the chances of repeating the habit the next time the cue appears.

Enlisting an Accountability Partner. While journals, habit logs, and colorful visual progress records are all reinforcing, one of the most effective ways to motivate your new habit is to appoint an "accountability partner." Knowing that someone who cares about you is watching can be a powerful motivator. To use this approach, you would enlist one or two people and make a "habit contract" with them. A habit contract is a verbal or written agreement that specifies the intended behavior and the "punishment" if you do not follow through with it.

Making It Compelling. You can build in compelling consequences for your successes or lapses. The consequence might involve money, time, inconvenience, or embarrassment. An example provided by Clear is a man who needed to be up by 5:55 each morning. If he wasn't up to stop it, a tweet would automatically go out to a selected group of his friends indicating that he had failed to be up in time and that five dollars would be added to the PayPal accounts of the first five people to reply. In another example, when a man didn't carry out the exercise required by his contract, he had to dress up more than required for work (e.g., no jeans, T-shirts, hoodies, or shorts) and wear the hat of a rival sports team.

According to Clear, the underlying principle operating here is that when a failure is painful, it effectively teaches you a new habit. Without any tough consequences, you are more likely to ignore your commitment to a new habit.[21] Beyond a contract with an accountability partner, the principles suggested earlier for making a craving more attractive will also help make the reward more satisfying: become involved with others who also value the desired habit.

Stay Focused and Consistent. Additional hints from Clear include: Don't work on too many habits at once. Keep your focus on a limited number of goals. Most importantly, stay consistent. No matter how busy you are or even if you are discouraged with your progress, Clear advises, "Don't break the chain. . . . Never miss twice. If you miss one day, try to get back on track as quickly as possible."[22] Let the first time be a cue to double your efforts to follow through the next day. Otherwise progress gained can be quickly lost.

How Rianna Made It More Satisfying to Exercise

Rianna recognized that exercise was already satisfying in two special ways: her body felt better after exercising, and she started to lose unwanted weight largely because the exercise reduced her appetite. She also created a seven-day chart on her refrigerator and indicated with a smiley face or a frowning face whether she had exercised each day. She chose her husband to be her accountability partner. While it is not always a good idea to have accountability partners who might have their own agendas for how you should change, in this case it worked.

At the beginning of each week, she got him to agree on a reward if she had exercised at least five of the seven days. One reward was a special dinner at a favorite restaurant. Another was that she and her husband would go to a play that he wasn't particularly eager to see. Another was bringing someone in to clean the house. The punishment was simply not getting these rewards. After the first week, she only had three smiley faces. Still, her husband decided to take her to the restaurant since she had at least been conscientious in filling in the chart all seven days (the fact that it was one of his favorite restaurants of course had nothing to do with his decision). The second week, she had six smiley faces. On the third week, she had five. Even after her exercise habit was well established, she decided to continue with the charts, partly because she knew they reinforced the exercise, which had grown to 20 minutes each day, and also because she enjoyed the rewards. Even deciding on them was fun.

Your Turn

Using Step 4 to implement and maintain a new habit, decide how you will track your progress. Make it as vivid and as much fun as your creativity allows, but at a minimum, use a journal or a log to record your actions. Consider whether to involve an accountability partner. With or without a partner, a contract that specifies the desired behavior, as well as a consequence for not doing it, uses the goal-setting principle that tracking measurable objectives makes them much more likely to be implemented. Focus on a very limited number of goals, and "never miss twice." Periodically do the tapping routine you used to initiate the habit to support your progress.

ELIMINATING AN UNWANTED HABIT

Given that our brain chemistry is designed to create habitual behaviors, and the principles are the same whether it is establishing good habits or bad habits, most people find themselves carrying desirable as well as undesirable habits. Common harmful habits include eating unhealthy foods, eating more than your body wants, eating too fast, eating late at night, not drinking enough water, over-consuming alcohol, staying up when you need to be sleeping, not exercising, channel surfing, spending too much time on social media, biting your nails, not picking up after yourself, always carrying too much in your purse, being negative in your responses to others or in your self-talk . . . the list could go on and on.

You will choose an undesired habit for this section and tackle it, again using Clear's model, augmented by acupoint tapping. Breaking even a small negative habit is empowering. Note that the flip side of eliminating a bad habit may be developing a good habit. You can word it as *"Staying up when I need to be sleeping"* (bad habit) or *"Getting enough sleep"* (good habit). If you want to focus on the negative qualities of the habit (which may be more motivating), stay with this section (e.g., *"Staying up"*). If you want to focus on the benefits, use the previous section (e.g., *"Getting enough sleep"*). To get started here, begin with the following "Quick Fix."

Quick Fix: Eliminating an Undesirable Habit

Bring to mind a behavior you would like to eliminate. Give an SUD rating to the amount of attraction you feel in your mind and/or body toward the habitual behavior. Say out loud the first statement below as you tap on the Top-of-the-Head Point. Then say the next statement while tapping on the next point. Go through each statement, cycling through the 12 tapping points as you move from one statement to the next. Skip any phrases that don't fit for you.

"I'm tired of [name the habit].

But I'm conflicted about letting it go.

Even though I have this uncertainty,

I completely accept this dilemma.

Even though this habit has served me in some ways,

I'm tired of being controlled by it.

I feel the strength of the habit in my [name body part].

I'm tapping to reduce that feeling.

I know this habit isn't good for me.

I want to let it go.

Even though I'm conflicted about letting go of this habit,

I understand that it's no longer serving me.

I know that life will be better without it.

So I choose to be open to letting it go.

Even though it may mean letting go of some things that make me comfortable,

I see how it's been holding me back.

I'm ready to release this habit and let it go.

And I choose to do it with ease.

This habit has controlled me for too long.

It's not serving me anymore.

And I'm ready to take back control.

I'm ready to let it go.

I'm releasing the tension and conflict.

I'm ready to set myself free.

I appreciate that I'm feeling more ready to let it go.

I am letting it go with ease and grace."

After going through this sequence two or three times, you will probably find that the texture of the habit is already softening. Gauge this with another SUD rating on the amount of attraction you still have toward this habit. You have also been preparing yourself to go deeper into overcoming it by combining tapping with Clear's approach.

Four Steps for Breaking a Habit

The four steps for eliminating a habit are similar to those for establishing a new habit, except the principles are now reversed:

Step 1. Make the cue *invisible* instead of more visible (e.g., hide the candy where it is inconvenient to get to it).

Step 2. Make the craving *unattractive* instead of more attractive (e.g., stay informed about the health costs of excessive sugar).

Step 3. Make the undesired behavior *difficult* instead of easier (e.g., don't keep the candy in your house).

Step 4. Make the reward *unsatisfying* instead of more satisfying (e.g., use an accountability partner).

Building on the earlier discussion of Clear's four steps of behavior change, our focus here will be on how to use each step, again incorporating the use of acupoint tapping for the purpose of breaking an undesired habit.

As in the earlier section, you can read this and do the procedures as you come to them. Alternatively, scan down to the test-driver excerpts and then do the "Your Turn" instructions that follow them, referring to the longer discussion as you wish.

Step 1: Make the Cue Invisible

Avoiding temptation is easier than resisting it. Cues activate temptation. If you don't see a bag of Doritos every time you open the kitchen cupboard, you are less likely to open it. If you remove the TV from your bedroom, you are less likely to stay up watching *Seinfeld* reruns. Reducing exposure to a cue that causes temptation is one of the most practical ways to eliminate an unwanted habit.

Clear suggests that a secret of people who appear to be highly disciplined is not so much in their self-control but rather that they are good at setting up their lives so that they don't have to call upon heroic willpower and self-control all the time.[23] As a result, they spend less time in situations that tempt them into unwanted behaviors. Self-restraint is easier when it isn't needed. Eliminate the cues and you reduce the need. Clear emphasizes this with two stories that, from opposite directions, illustrate the same principle.

During the Vietnam War, an estimated 20 percent of service members were addicted to heroin. Because of the compelling physical properties of this addiction, the common wisdom was that they would not be able to break their addiction when they came home. Yet only 5 percent resumed the use of heroin within the first year after their return. This challenged just about everyone's beliefs about this drug. Clear understands this surprising finding through the lens of changes in environmental cues. While in Vietnam, the soldiers were surrounded by triggers that made them want to use heroin. The drug was easy to get. The soldiers were in the continual stress of the war. Their friends included other soldiers who used heroin. And they were thousands of miles from home. Once they got back to the United States, however, they were in a place where none of those triggers were present.

This plays out in a reverse manner in the high relapse following residential treatment for heroin addicts. Clear again attributes this to the power of cues. A person gets addicted to heroin; receives treatment at a clinic where the people, places, stresses, and other cues that made them want to use are not around; and then goes back to their old neighborhood where they are surrounded by everything that originally led to their addiction. It's not surprising that 90 percent of heroin addicts start using again once they get home from rehab.

Whether for addictions or everyday habits, brain research suggests that once a habit has been established, the urge to repeat the behavior is felt whenever the cues for the habit appear. When addicts were shown a picture of cocaine for just 33 milliseconds, faster than the brain could consciously register, reward centers that generate desire were activated.[24] Eliminating cues is a more effective strategy than simply resisting temptation. While it may be obvious that removing an addict's exposure to the drug of choice, associated paraphernalia, and addicted friends is a good plan when starting to

tackle an addiction, what can be done with less formidable habits? Among Clear's suggestions:

- If you are easily triggered into feeling you're not good enough, stop viewing social media accounts that make you feel jealous or envious.

- If you're putting too much money into tech gear, quit reading reviews of the latest releases.

- If you're spending too much time playing video games, put the console into a closet after each use.

Tapping. While these steps for eliminating the cues that trigger unwanted habits can be effective, many cues can't be evaded. An irritating coworker may cause you to stew in resentment about your job and become less efficient. The empty space at your dining room table that had been filled by a child or life partner, now deceased, may lead to binge-eating to comfort your grief. The continual march of "new and better products" makes the appeal of shopping and its attendant drain on finances and accumulation of clutter hard to resist. Website clickbait may take you into time-consuming, mind-numbing rabbit holes. Even if you can't eliminate a cue from your life, you can greatly reduce its influence through tapping.

Here is an example of using tapping to change your response to a cue. If, for instance, your organization keeps a tray of tasty chocolates set out for customers in a spot you always walk by, you can imagine seeing them as you tap along with phrases like:

"I crave that chocolate."

"I want it so much."

"I can't help myself."

"I accept this craving."

"The temptation is there every day."

"It's hard to stop myself."

"But I'll feel bad about myself."

"I'll feel I failed."

"Having that chocolate every day isn't good for my health or my weight."

"I choose to let this craving pass."

"I choose to do what's best for me."

"This craving is leaving my mind and body."

"Tapping is dissolving my craving."

"Seeing that tray is an opportunity to affirm my commitment to my good health."

"I'm feeling calm and at peace about having to see those chocolates every day."

Notice how the statements build from acknowledging and accepting the craving to recognizing its costs to releasing it. You can move back and forth to each of these themes about any craving as feels right. And it's not that you have to tap on these words every time you pass the tray. If you tap on them a few times at home while imagining the chocolates, the feeling of having released the craving will start to come up when you pass the tray. You are building a new response to the cue.

Sometimes working with a cue will uncover other aspects of the habit. In David's focus on his hair-trigger response to hitting the brake, he created a driving scenario in which he imagined suddenly hearing Donna's excited voice and tapping on it so it wouldn't trigger a threat response. In the process, however, an aspect emerged involving feeling judgmental toward anyone who raises a false alarm. He flashed on a time he had accidentally set off a fire alarm as a teenager, resulting in a full response by the fire department. He had never come to terms with that experience. After the tapping neutralized his guilt about it and he returned to the driving scenes, he experienced an interesting combination of decreased alarm yet greater alertness. This transferred over to actual situations when they were driving together.

Ericka's Unwanted Habit and Cues

One of our colleagues was concerned about her driving. Ericka resorted to speeding when late for work, and it is a habit she definitely wanted to break. She lives two hours from a job she does three days a week. On a day that she must commute, she often leaves her house too late to arrive at her workplace on time. This is the *cue* that has her spending her drive in a tense, anxious state, frequently driving over the speed limit and constantly watching her mirrors for the highway patrol. She had already received a speeding ticket and knew that if she got another one, her insurance rates would go up; and if she got two more, her license could be suspended.

The power of Ericka's cue—leaving home too late to get to her job on time—was 8. Her Acceptance Statement was *"Even though I drive too fast when I'm late for work, I fully accept myself."* The first tapping cycle, using the Reminder Phrase *"I drive too fast when I'm late for work,"* got the power of being late for work down to 6. This brought up several memories of when she had been reprimanded for being late. After tapping on these, the power of the cue of being late on her way to work had dropped only slightly, down to 5. But her focus changed to ensuring she would give herself enough time so she didn't have to rush. The new cue was seeing that she had enough time to squeeze in one more task before leaving for the drive. It was for this urge to do "one more task" that she used tapping to turn into a cue to "just say no."

Your Turn

Describe a habit you would like to eliminate and identify the cues that activate it. Make a plan that reduces your exposure to these cues as much as possible. If one or more are unavoidable, use tapping to reduce their power.

Select the most powerful of any unavoidable cues you have identified. Give it an SUD rating. Note that we are back to a measure of distress—or in this case, powerlessness—instead of believability, so a rating of 0 is the ideal. You are rating the amount of influence the unavoidable cue has over you, with 0 being no influence at all and 10 meaning that you find it irresistible.

Create an Acceptance Statement and say it three times while rubbing your chest sore spots with the first phrase and placing your hands over your Heart Chakra with the second. The statement can be along these lines:

Acceptance Statement: *"Even though [name the cue] causes me to want to [name the behavior], I love myself and accept my desires."*

Next, go through the 12 tapping points, naming the cue out loud at each point. Continue through the Basic Tapping Routine, doing the Integration Procedure and following it with another trip through the 12 points while repeating the cue. Remember, you are generating signals that reduce your brain's response to the cue. Give another SUD rating to the cue's power.

If the SUD has gone down, change your Acceptance Statement to a Choices Statement, as usual saying it three times while rubbing your chest sore spots with the first phrase and placing your hands over your Heart Chakra with the second. The statement can be along these lines:

Choices Statement: *"Even though [name the cue] causes me to want to [name the behavior], I choose to reduce its influence over me."*

Go through the 12 tapping points, again naming the cue out loud at each point and changing the statements as modeled in the chocolate temptation example above.

If your sense of powerlessness regarding the cue is still relatively high, tap on any unpleasant sensations associated with the cue and any objections (Psychological Reversals) to being free from the cue's appeal. Continue with this detective work until the SUD won't go down any further. Even if you have reduced the SUD just a little, the cue has that much less hold on you.

Step 2: Make the Craving Unattractive

A craving is generally an expression of a deeper need or motivation. Clear's list of these more fundamental motives includes the need to obtain food and water, conserve energy, find love, reproduce, connect and bond with others, win social acceptance and approval, lower stress, reduce uncertainty, and achieve status and prestige. A new habit doesn't usually create a new motivation but rather attaches itself to basic human drives.[25] The same drive can be addressed in many ways. One person might reduce stress by watching TV; another by going to the gym.

Subjectively, a craving is a desire to "change your internal state" based on the sense that "something is missing."[26] You anticipate that the behavior will supply what is missing, changing your internal state in a way that is satisfying. A habit is built around your past successes with that prediction. A long-standing habit may not, however, be the best way to supply what is missing or change the internal state. And it may keep you from discovering better ways.

To make a habit less attractive, you can reflect on its unintended costs. For instance, if TV binge-watching or channel surfing is the habit you want to break, consider that long periods with little movement promote lethargy and listlessness. Binge-watching also does little toward accomplishing what is important to you or completing tasks that are weighing on you. What are the other costs? Another way to get at the costs of a habit is to highlight the potential benefits of ending the behavior. What else could you do with your time if you weren't in front of the screen? These reframes make the craving to settle in front of the TV for long sedentary hours less attractive. Our work with clients has shown that tapping on well-crafted statements that acknowledge the costs, rather than making the person feel guilty, give such reframes more teeth.

Another question to ask yourself: What deeper need does the habit fill? If zoning out in front of the TV reduces stress, what are more fulfilling ways of reducing it? Exercise, meditation, yoga, sports, and meeting with friends are popular and substantial solutions. Or maybe being glued to the TV is simply a way of passing time. What ways of passing time would be more gratifying? Right now we'll focus on making the habit less attractive, but knowing you have envisioned an alternative way of meeting the old habit's underlying need already begins to reduce its power. Later, if you wish, you can again go through the steps presented earlier for establishing a new habit to reinforce this alternative.

How Ericka Made the Unwanted Habit Less Attractive

For Ericka, speeding was an easy solution to make up time when she left the house late. But, of course, it might eventually lead to much worse consequences than getting a speeding ticket. She searched the web to find just how dangerous it is to go slightly above the speed limit. She discovered that the rationale for speed limits is based on the rates of likely accidents. Just a 10 percent decrease in average speed could result in a 20 percent decline in injuries and a 40 percent reduction in fatalities from car crashes. She allowed herself to imagine that by speeding, she was increasing the chances that she would injure herself or others, even causing death. She thought about how her car is potentially a lethal weapon, and she wanted to operate it in the safest way possible. This gave her much more motivation to commit to reducing her speed on the road and leaving plenty of time to get to her destination.

Your Turn

Reflect on the costs of the unwanted habit and the anticipated benefits of not having it. Make a list. Select one item that seems pivotal. You will be focusing on it. You can return later to any others that still seem pertinent. Give an SUD rating to the attractiveness at this point of the unwanted habit.

Based on the item you selected, create a new Acceptance Statement and say it out loud three times, again rubbing your chest sore spots with the first phrase and placing your hands over your Heart Chakra with the second. The statement can be along these lines:

Revised Acceptance Statement: *"Even though I have been willing to [describe the cost of the habit], I love myself and accept the choices I have made."*

Once the attractiveness of the habit begins to diminish as you tap on its costs, convert the Acceptance Statement to a Choices Statement. For example:

> **Choices Statement:** *"Even though I have been willing to [describe the cost of the habit], I choose to remember this cost when I have an impulse toward the habit."*
>
> You are associating the cost with the habit, making the habitual behavior less attractive. Continue the tapping cycle until the attractiveness of the habit stops going down. As usual, if any aspects or Psychological Reversals appear, address them as they emerge.

Step 3: Make the Undesired Behavior Difficult

The best way to break a habit, according to Clear, is to make it impractical to do.[27] Social media companies work this in reverse. Their systems are designed so that greater effort is required to *stop* looking at the screen than to continue looking. For instance, rather than actively clicking to advance to the next Netflix or YouTube episode, all you have to do is keep your eyes open and it will appear in front of you.

For Clear, social media had become such an obstacle to his usual high productivity that he devised an elaborate scheme to counter it. He instructed an assistant to reset the passwords on all his social media accounts every Monday. This kept him logged out of social media on all his devices through the week, and he couldn't do anything about it. On Friday, his assistant would send him all the new passwords. This allowed him to do all the social media he wished on the weekends. He reflects,

> One of the biggest surprises was how quickly I adapted. Within the first week of locking myself out of social media, I realized that I didn't need to check it nearly as often as I had been, and I certainly didn't need it each day. It had simply been so easy that it had become the default. Once my bad habit became impossible, I discovered that I *did* actually have the motivation to work on more meaningful tasks. After I removed the mental candy from my environment, it became much easier to eat the healthy stuff.[28]

While it may take some planning and effort to make the undesired behavior difficult, it can be done for virtually any habit. If staying within your budget is an issue, you can set limits on your credit cards. This doesn't make it impossible to have some flexibility, but it will force you to go to the bank to withdraw cash when you exceed your budget. If reading every word in *People Magazine* is your vulnerability, cancel your subscription. Temptations for junk food are thwarted when you have to go to the store each time you have a craving. While these are structural rather than psychological shifts, they can be quite effective.

How Ericka Made the Undesired Behavior More Difficult

Once Ericka absorbed the substantial increase in the possibility of injuries or fatal consequences caused by speeding, she became more committed to changing the way she drove. She decided to cue some new habits around her commute that would make speeding much less likely. First, she set alerts on her phone for one hour, 30 minutes, and 10 minutes before her ideal departure time. Then she set up a cue that once she came onto the freeway, she would set her car's cruise control at exactly the speed limit so that she wouldn't have to maintain her speed manually. While it may have been overkill, she also set up a news alert for her email so that she would receive all reports of traffic accidents on the freeway that she drove. She wanted regular reminders of the dangers of speeding to make her new habit stick. Meanwhile, she continued to tap on leaving home with enough time for a relaxed drive.

Your Turn

A simple energy protocol can help you devise your plan. In fact, the same basic strategy can be used to generate new ideas any time you need them. Create a statement such as *"Even though I'm drawn toward [describe the habitual behavior], I choose to find creative ways to make it harder to do."* Say it out loud as you rub your chest sore spots with the first phrase and place your hands over your Heart Chakra with the second. Repeat it until an idea comes to you about making it harder to do. Have your journal handy so you can write it down. Continue until you have at least one way to make the behavior harder. Implement it. You are finding ways, in Clear's terms, to "increase the friction," which multiplies "the number of steps between you and your bad habit."[29]

Step 4: Make the Reward Unsatisfying

The key in this fourth step of breaking a habit is to do the opposite of what you do to create a habit. Rather than connect the habit with an immediate reward, you put the emphasis on the long-term rewards for avoiding the undesired behavior so it overshadows the immediate rewards of doing it. Tracking your progress each day that you avoid the habitual behavior is reinforcing. Again, "the most effective form of motivation is progress."[30]

How Ericka Made the Reward Less Satisfying

Ericka wanted a visual way to track her progress around not speeding. She made a calendar that noted her commute days and put it on the back of her front door. She hung a marker next to it so that before she left, she would mark down whether she drove the speed limit on her previous commute and if she arrived at work on time. Soon, the calendar dates she had colored in as successes became a visual reminder to keep up her progress.

Your Turn

Using this fourth step to eliminate a habit, decide how you will track your progress. Make it as vivid and as much fun as your creativity allows. This can be done in a journal or through visual feedback such as charts on your refrigerator or putting a colored marble in a jar each time you succeed with the habit you are developing and a different color marble each time you don't. An accountability partner can also be a powerful motivator. For breaking a habit, the "habit contract" would specify the behavior you are avoiding as well as the consequences for not following through.

Remember that the consequences could involve money, time, inconvenience, or embarrassment, such as the man who tweeted whenever he failed to honor his contract that his friends could reply and have five dollars added to their PayPal accounts or the man who had to go to work wearing the hat of a rival sports team. The same principles are at play. If doing the behavior has an undesirable consequence, you are less likely to repeat it. If the consequences are relatively painless, they will have little influence in preventing the behavior. Keep your focus on a minimal number of goals. Periodically do the tapping routine you used in Step 1 for eliminating a habit (p. 217) in order to support your progress. With or without an accountability partner, a contract that specifies the undesired habit as well as a consequence for repeating it is a potent tool.

ADDICTIONS

Acupoint tapping is one of the primary treatment modalities at the Avery Lane Addictions Clinic in Novato, California. Its clinical director, the psychologist Adriana Popescu, reported in a peer-reviewed journal that she and her staff have found energy psychology to be "a powerful, evidence-based approach that sets the standard for effective addiction treatment."[31]

While the four steps for changing a habit can be applied to overcoming an addiction, addictions are a feistier animal to tame than mere habits. The renowned Swiss psychiatrist Carl Jung held that "every form of addiction is bad, no matter whether the narcotic be alcohol or morphine or idealism."[32] Addictions, like habits, are maintained by triggers, rewards, and repetition, but more is going on.

Subjectively, the cravings are usually more intense. With everyday habits, the cravings may be compelling but not so compelling that they dominate your life. Whether or not you carry out the habitual behavior to satisfy the craving is a matter of will and conscious choice. You can abstain without becoming obsessed with the craving or risking withdrawal symptoms if you don't gratify it. As habits move into addictions, however, willpower and choice have diminishing influence, and the behavior continues even as the costs begin to outweigh the gratifications.[33]

The biochemistry of addiction is not fully understood, but we know that by the time a habit has moved toward the addictive end of the spectrum, the following changes are occurring in the brain:

- Thoughts about the addictive substance or activity cause dopamine to flood the brain, triggering pursuit of the pleasurable substance or activity with increasing strength.

- The brain's reward centers also become overstimulated with these quantities of dopamine, so the brain simultaneously attempts to reduce dopamine production and receptivity.

- This reduced sensitivity results in greater amounts of the substance (or a greater intensity of the activity) being required to feel pleasure. Known as "tolerance," the amount of the substance or intensity of the activity that previously brought substantial pleasure is now producing less pleasure.

- The ability to feel pleasure in other areas of life without the addictive substance or behavior is also diminished as the addictive behavior attaches itself to a wider array of experiences. You can't enjoy a walk in the park without a cigarette. You are fidgety through dinner if you've not checked your Facebook feed.

- Discontinuing use of the substance or the activity leads to withdrawal symptoms, which—depending on the nature of the addiction—may include anxiety, depression, fatigue, sweating, vomiting, or even seizures or hallucinations.

- Continued overuse of the substance or repetition of the addictive behavior leads to changes in the neocortex. The neocortex orchestrates problem-solving and other processes involving reasoning and deliberation. These changes result in compromised judgment, impaired decision-making, and diminished self-control in relation to the addiction.[34]

The good news is that most of these brain changes are reversible if the addictive behavior is discontinued.[35] Just as we chose James Clear to be our model for the best practices outside of energy psychology for establishing new habits and breaking old ones, we have chosen an approach developed by the psychologist Tom Horvath as our reference for treating addictions. It's not that we ourselves don't have some experience and credentials bringing energy methods to working with addictions,[36] but we want to frame acupoint tapping within the best practices of the broader field of addictions treatment.

Dr. Horvath is a past president of the American Psychological Association's specialty division on addictions and the founder of an addictions treatment system called "Practical Recovery." Of the dozens of highly credible books on overcoming addictions, we chose his *Sex, Drugs, Gambling & Chocolate: A Workbook for Overcoming Addictions* because of its authoritative pedigree, practical instruction, and focus on all types of addictions, not just drugs and alcohol.[37] In fact, in the book's opening, he lists 111 types of potential addictions, including shopping, watching sports, collecting things, gaming, grooming, lotto, and chocolate. You probably have a few that are on his list. The point is not to pathologize everyday addictions but to understand them and choose to free ourselves of any costs they may be insidiously extracting from our lives.

Many less severe addictions will respond to the steps already presented for breaking habits. In this section, our focus is on how to apply tapping protocols to more serious addictions, such as drugs, alcohol, smoking, gambling, eating disorders, irresponsible sex, shoplifting, pornography, or taking progressively dangerous risks, which are some of the most common addictions that might lead a person to seek help from a therapist. As with the approach we used for addressing severe anxiety, PTSD, and depression, our primary orientation shifts at this point in the chapter from self-help to offering guidance for therapists and people working with a therapist in applying acupoint tapping protocols with addiction. If your self-guided efforts are not getting you what you need, we encourage you to enlist a competent professional to help you address your addiction. When we use the word *you* in the following sections, we are referring to the person who is using therapy to overcome an addiction.

THE STAGES OF RECOVERY

Dr. Horvath's program is designed to take you from "I can't live without it" to "I live even better without it."[38] While special considerations are often needed based on the type of addiction, Dr. Horvath believes the same underlying principles and treatment strategies can be applied to all addictions. Studies have shown that changes in behavior related to health and mental health, whether self-guided or with professional support, tend to go through seven predictable stages.[39] These include:

1. Precontemplation

2. Contemplation

3. Determination

4. Action

5. Maintenance

6. Termination

7. Recovery if a relapse occurs

Dr. Horvath points out that while most of the material available to help people overcome addictions is oriented toward the fourth, or "action stage," most addicted individuals have not gotten that far. Mismatches between the individual's stage and the treatment offered are one of the main reasons for treatment failure. We will organize the remainder of this chapter around these seven stages and show how the procedures Dr. Horvath recommends during each stage can be augmented by acupoint tapping. Addictions are among the most intransigent conditions therapists treat, and tapping can change a person's neurological landscape in ways that deepen and accelerate the therapeutic process.

1. Precontemplation

In the first stage, precontemplation, the person doesn't view the addiction as a problem and is not interested in bringing about a change. If therapy is sought at all, it is for different reasons than the addiction or it is forced upon the person by a spouse's threat to end a marriage or a court order after a DUI or shoplifting arrest. Besides an underlying dread of the overwhelming effects that withdrawal might cause, the precontemplation stage may be afflicted with errors in reasoning. People in this stage often overestimate the benefits of continuing the addiction and underestimate the harm the addiction is doing to their bodies, relationships, and future. Advice or efforts at persuasion only echo what everyone else has most likely been telling the person and is likely to increase resistance and distrust rather than produce the intended effects. Dr. Horvath doesn't expect people who are in this stage to be reading his book, but therapists often find themselves face to face with addicts who have no interest in ending or even fully acknowledging their addiction.

In this stage, a therapist can foster engagement and rapport with open-ended questions, active listening, and nonjudgmentally reflecting back the person's feelings. Tapping can be introduced and established as a viable treatment in the client's mind at the start of treatment. The therapist may, for instance, apply tapping to issues that are of immediate concern to the person, such as situations that trigger unwanted anger or jealousy, or frustrations with relationships or work. Tapping on the stressors the person has identified and seeing them diminish is persuasive. Establishing the effectiveness of the therapist's tools makes it easier to draw on that trust if and when the person becomes ready to examine their addiction critically.

2. Contemplation

A person in the contemplation stage is thinking about quitting or at least about cutting back on the addictive behavior. Still, the rewards and pleasures provided by the substance or activity may continue to promote at least some minimization of the problems the addiction is creating in the person's life. The costs may be getting more difficult to ignore. But the time, energy, and emotional loss involved in overcoming the addiction may also seem daunting. Many people have spent years in this contemplation stage, and they may also revert to it even after starting to make progress in moving to subsequent stages.

During this stage, Dr. Horvath focuses on the rewards and costs of the addiction, weighing them against one another. Trusting the person to recognize the implications of this cost-benefit analysis often increases motivation to overcome the addiction. Success in overcoming previous addictions is also reviewed to identify resources for the work that is to follow.

After selecting a single addiction for the initial focus, the client reflects on the benefits and costs, often journaling, and is also instructed to discuss them with the therapist or a trusted friend. Identifying the benefits includes remembering how the addictive behavior once felt, even if it no longer provides the same high. Dr. Horvath's list of potential benefits of an addiction, whether the early benefits or the current ones, includes:

- **Generating positive emotions** such as pleasure, self-confidence, worthiness, euphoria, feeling fully alive

- **Coping with negative emotions** such as fear, anxiety, sadness, depression, anger, shame, guilt, boredom, and loneliness

- **Social benefits** such as sharing a special activity or belonging to a group; or rebelling from people who want to control you or escaping from your spouse, parents, or children

- **Physical benefits** such as satisfying the craving, reducing physical pain, boosting energy, increasing enjoyment of sex, or getting better sleep

- **Intellectual benefits** such as thinking more clearly or creatively

To get at the costs of their addiction, Dr. Horvath has people reflect on a typical experience with the addiction, focusing on what seemed uncomfortable, painful, negative, or dangerous. Again, discussing these costs with a therapist or trusted friend may deepen your acknowledgment and understanding of them. Among the downsides to consider are:

- **Emotional costs** include fear, anxiety, sadness, depression, anger, shame, guilt, disgust, loneliness, emotional instability, pessimism; feeling worthless, crazy, or suicidal

- **Social costs** include no longer fitting in, increased conflict with others, spending time with people you don't respect or like, spending less time with people you care about, or disrupting your central relationships

- **Physical and health costs** such as diminished overall health, physical problems caused by the addiction, lowered energy and endurance, poor sleep, less enjoyment of sex, or withdrawal symptoms

- **Intellectual costs** such as hampered ability to think clearly, delusions, diminished creativity, poor memory, or hallucinations

- **Work and productivity costs** such as decreased effectiveness and output, excessive time missed from work or school, accidents caused by the addiction, impaired abilities, or having less time for hobbies or personal interests

- **Financial costs** such as money spent directly on the addiction, money spent on coping with the consequences of the addiction, money lost because less was earned or opportunities were not taken, or savings spent

- **Time lost** directly on the addiction or coping with the consequences of the addiction

- **Legal costs** based on arrests, fines, lawyers, or jail time

- **Reductions in personal integrity** such as being dishonest with others and/or yourself, lowering your self-respect, being irresponsible, letting down people who matter to you, or acting in conflict with your deeper values

The purpose of all this reflection is to address the ambivalence that characterizes the contemplation stage. Dr. Horvath explains:

> This issue can be difficult because you are really "of two minds" about change: you love the pleasure of the addiction and what the addiction does for you, but you also hate the trouble your addiction causes you. . . . It's not hard to change a behavior that only causes pain. It's hard to change your addiction because it causes both satisfaction and pain.[40]

Getting Your "Two Minds" to Communicate. By articulating the benefits and costs of the addiction, you are preparing your "two minds" to engage with each other constructively, which is exactly what is required during the contemplation phase. While friends or even a therapist might be tempted to "lead the witness" *away* from accepting the addiction, having people recognize and accept each element of their addiction supports them in making a clear-headed, life-affirming decision they will ultimately abide by. Energy psychology protocols are well-suited for this. A core principle we've discussed in previous chapters is to help the person (1) *accept themselves* and (2) *embrace both sides of an internal conflict with deep acceptance* before proceeding to resolve the conflict.

Built into the structure of the Basic Tapping Protocol is the Acceptance Statement. You are looking your dilemma squarely in the face, appreciating the challenges, and accepting that this is where you are in your life right now. This also acknowledges and accepts the reality that you are still undecided about how much effort you want to put into overcoming your addiction. Doing the routines that stimulate energy centers along with saying statements such as *"Even though I am struggling with this addiction, I recognize and accept the benefits it has brought me"* puts your psyche at ease. Nothing will be taken away before you are ready to eliminate it.

The person designs statements to rouse both sides of the dilemma: *"I want to give up my addiction **and** I don't want to give it up!" "Even though I love going out with my drinking buddies [benefit], I'm here paying good money for help getting over my addiction [cost]."* Bringing both sides to mind so starkly creates tension in the body. Tapping on the 12 acupuncture points while alternating between the first phrase of the statement and the second phrase reduces that tension.

Reducing the tension between the benefits and costs or opposing desires allows you to address the conflict with greater clarity. It also opens the way for a more constructive enactment of a dialogue between the "two minds," as introduced on page 113. The use of tapping during the dialogue helps bridge the emotional gap between the two sides. By working with the energetic underpinnings of the conflict rather than trying to resolve it with logic or willpower, acupoint tapping can usually quickly bring the two sides within speaking distance.

3. Determination

After a clear intention to overcome the addiction is in place, the next stage is to work with that determination and translate it into effective preparation. Here, you create a game plan to prepare for the challenges ahead. You envision and articulate the desired changes and how they will be accomplished. What will be the role of therapy? What other resources will you need? Perhaps a support group or medication to ease withdrawal would be useful? What immediate behaviors, even if in small steps, will take you toward the goal?

This might involve becoming less available to friends who share the addiction or practicing greater restraint even while the addiction is still active. A smoker might remove triggers like ashtrays and lighters. A drinker could clear the liquor cabinet. Another important element in this preparation stage is deciding what to tell family and friends about the intention to overcome the addiction. This admittedly tricky step can solidify your resolve to overcome the addiction and pave the way for the action stage.

Meeting the Need Without Incurring the Cost. Dr. Horvath identifies the major task in this stage as mapping out new ways to meet the *needs* the addiction satisfies in a manner that doesn't carry its costs. He identifies numerous activities you might consider for learning new coping methods: individual therapy; group therapy; peer support groups; coaching; discussions with others; observing models of success for overcoming addictions; working out new models in your imagination; pursuing inspiring books, movies, plays, lectures, or educational programs.[41] While some of these resources can only be pursued solo, Dr. Horvath emphasizes the value of connecting with others as you learn new coping methods to meet the needs that had been satisfied by your addiction.

Dr. Horvath's overriding principle for creating a plan during this stage is that your "day-to-day choices [will be] based on your ultimate goals and values."[42] This requires candid self-reflection, recognizing ways your addiction doesn't fit your deepest goals and values and formulating a new vision that does. Considerations for your plan might include initiating adjustments in your life that will help you succeed in overcoming the addiction, deciding on which resources to use for learning new coping skills, or dealing with any resentment you hold about giving up the addiction. It can also involve choosing to aim for moderation or total abstinence, anticipating circumstances that might make you feel out of control, and envisioning how you will meet them.

Using Tapping During the Determination Stage. Tapping protocols can augment the inner work required as you build your determination during this stage. For instance, internal blocks to proceeding may arise and dilute your determination to the extent that you are thrust back into the contemplation stage.

When these setbacks occur, address them with tapping, along with the use of Acceptance Statements. Nonetheless, wrestling with internal blocks is often inescapable and is best anticipated and met with patience rather than taken as a sign of weakness or failure. The desire to change a longstanding pattern always collides with the forces keeping that pattern in place. To complicate the process, with an addiction, some of those forces may involve changes in the brain caused by the addictive behavior, such as habituation and the need for increased amounts of dopamine to obtain the same amount of pleasure. You may find yourself returning to the inner dialogue of the contemplation stage many times, again augmented by the tapping. Each time, it is likely to take on new texture and produce new insights about how to succeed.

Although tapping can reduce the distress involved in recognizing the costs of an addiction, this might not seem a good strategy. It may seem that it would be better to *increase* the distress evoked by statements such as *"The hangover the next day is terrible," "I fight with my wife when I'm wasted," "My kids get disgusted with me,"* or *"I could lose my job."* However, reducing your anxiety about such statements by tapping on them doesn't diminish your awareness of their costs. Rather, it gives you greater mental acuity to navigate inner conflicts and make a plan.

During this stage, you might also find yourself returning to basics, rating the intensity of a statement such as *"I don't want to give up [the addiction]"* and tapping on it. As the tapping sends calming signals to the areas of the brain activated by the thought, the neurological intensity of the charge diminishes. More positive wordings supporting your determination can be introduced at that point, such as *"I choose to be free of [the addiction]."*

Not surprisingly, it isn't usually a straight line to the positive affirmation because other aspects—feelings, thoughts, sensations, beliefs, memories—often arise. For instance, a person considering giving up a highly addictive drug such as methamphetamine might experience panic, sadness, positive memories of being high, a loss of the assurance that extra energy is available at will, or memories of terrible, painful sensations rooted in a previous time of going into withdrawal. Such aspects then become the focus of the tapping until their arousal power is reduced to as low as you can get it. Fluctuations in these ratings inform the therapist about the next direction to take the wordings. Along with the acupoint tapping, this stage of building determination and envisioning a plan still requires attuned inquiries, active listening, and the other bedrock qualities of psychotherapy, but by helping people dismantle inner resistance to the changes they desire, the steps taken during this phase become more potent and congruent.

Formulating a detailed vision about how life will be when you are completely free of the addictive behavior can be motivating in the action stage and beyond. Being sober often involves an entire shift in one's identity and lifestyle. Tapping on a few phrases that spell out that vision imprints it into body and mind. Noting and addressing inner objections to the desired vision and examining any such Psychological Reversals also paves the way toward successful action.

4. Action

Dr. Horvath identifies this as "the stage of major effort and behavior change."[43] The pivotal concept during this stage involves cravings. Clinical trials that used tapping protocols in treating substance use disorders found cravings to be significantly reduced.[44]

Managing Your Cravings. How you manage the deeply subjective experience of cravings has many dimensions, and a spectrum of new coping skills and shifts in emotional reactions and thought patterns may be built during the action stage. Tapping can be used to:

- **Change how you respond to the internal and external cues** that trigger the addictive behavior. This is where your behaviors conform to or begin to overcome your addiction. Tapping itself can reduce the strength of a craving and its association with the cues that have triggered it.

- **Develop skills in the self-management** of pain, stress, and anxiety. This may increase resilience when cravings tied to the addictive substance or behavior emerge, opening alternative ways of providing relief and comfort.

- **Address unresolved emotional issues** that increase vulnerability to craving harmful substances or activities. Trauma and other adverse childhood experiences are frequent precursors that can be revisited, defused, and often healed by tapping that concentrates on emotional wounds from the past.

Progress in these three areas may be important in the recovery process. Here we will explore them in detail and show uses for acupoint tapping in each.

Reprogramming Responses to Cues That Trigger the Addictive Behavior. In a landmark series of studies on food cravings and weight management conducted at Bond University in Australia, individuals receiving four 2-hour group tapping sessions showed dramatic reductions in cravings. Significantly, fMRI readings of the participants' responses to images of high-caloric "junk" foods showed substantial deactivation in brain areas associated with rewards.[45]

Cues that generate cravings—people, places, or things connected with the addictive behavior—are obvious *external* triggers in an addiction. Other external triggers that are not directly related to the addiction but can still rekindle addictive patterns may include work pressure, relationship difficulties, social isolation, transitions in job or home, and holidays or anniversaries. Where these external triggers involve concrete situations, *internal* triggers may include thoughts and emotions such as anxiety, stress, fear, anger, loneliness, grief, memories, guilt, futility, or a sense of emptiness.

While some external triggers can be physically removed, many can't be. However, you can unlearn the *responses* that have been conditioned to these triggers and pair more adaptive responses with them. Acupoint tapping protocols use similar desensitization and reconditioning strategies for addressing internal and external triggers. Changing your responses to either type of trigger is an inside job.

Most of the triggers involved with addictions are learned associations. For instance, the conditioning that connects the sight of a cocktail glass with pleasant memories and the craving for a drink is formed in memory centers in the amygdala and hippocampus. The Basic Tapping Protocol can be applied to send deactivating signals to the amygdala and hippocampus that weaken the association and the craving. We will briefly review the entire Protocol here as it can be applied to addiction. Whenever we refer to the Basic Tapping Protocol throughout the remainder of this chapter, we are thinking of this sequence:

- Give an SUD rating to the strength of the association between the trigger and the craving or the amount of distress or difficulty the issue causes.

- Formulate Acceptance and Choices Statements and repeat them while stimulating energy points.

- Tap on the 12 acupoints accompanied by phrases that address the issue, at first simply naming it.

- Do the Integration Procedure and another round of tapping.

- Take a new SUD. If the SUD is going down, the phrases that accompany the next rounds of tapping may become increasingly strategic or assuring—for instance, from *"I want a drink when I see a cocktail glass"* to *"Cocktail glasses don't trigger me"* (when that has become the subjective truth).

- If the SUD becomes stuck, identify aspects and Psychological Reversals and focus on them for another trip through the Basic Tapping Protocol.

- Continue until the original SUD is down to 0 or near 0.

- Challenge your results.

All of this is detailed in Chapters 2 and 3. When the deactivating signals generated by the tapping reach the brain areas maintaining an outmoded pattern, changes in that pattern are initiated. In this stage of working with an addiction, the association between the trigger and the craving and the strength of the craving are weakened. It's that simple! And it isn't *always* that simple (as shown later in the discussion of the maintenance stage of overcoming an addiction).

Developing Skills for Better Managing Pain, Stress, and Anxiety. Dr. Horvath emphasizes, "You are not responsible for the existence of craving, only for your response to it."[46] Applying the Basic Tapping Protocol to a craving may dismantle the core of an addiction. Still, additional skills for managing pain, stress, and anxiety can equip you to more effectively manage your life without the addiction.

Physical pain lures many people into substance abuse. More than a million people in the US have died in the past two decades from a drug overdose, and 75 percent of those overdoses involved opioids, which are often prescribed for pain management.[47] Of course, if you are plagued by agonizing pain and your doctor offers a medication, it is an appealing option, but alternatives to medication for pain management are also available. The effectiveness of acupuncture in treating pain is well established,[48] and the manual stimulation of acupoints by tapping or holding them has been shown to be effective in the self-application of pain reduction techniques.[49]

Energy psychology protocols for chronic pain typically address emotional and physical dimensions of the experience of pain, but energy psychology tools for rapid relief can be readily taught focusing on the pain alone. For instance, a "Brief Energy Correction" technique that involves holding a series of acupoints while thinking about one's pain was presented via Zoom to 39 subjects reporting pain levels that averaged 5.53 on a 10-point scale. More than two-thirds of the participants were working with a pain that had been present for over a month. Following a 90-second procedure, the average pain level score was 1.58, amounting to a 71 percent reduction, which is astounding for such a brief intervention.[50] Substance abuse counselors who offer such tools to people with chronic pain are empowering them during all stages of recovery, and these tools provide added confidence during the action stage. Energy psychology protocols have also been successfully used on a self-help basis to manage anxiety[51] and stress,[52] sometimes supported by mobile apps.[53]

Addressing Unresolved Emotional Issues That Increase Vulnerability to Serious Addictions. Reducing the intensity of a craving inevitably also involves working with the emotional drivers fueling the craving. As you begin to make gains in overcoming the addiction, issues that are more fundamental may emerge, and they may require your attention before further progress can be made. Again, in the tapping world, this is called "peeling the layers of the onion." If you reach a point where the SUD on the intensity of the craving won't go down any further, it is often a sign pointing to deeper layers of emotional distress that need to be addressed if the addiction is to be permanently overcome.

These unresolved issues reveal themselves as aspects (p. 67), which may involve feelings, thoughts, sensations, beliefs, or memories. Suppose you've been making progress on reducing the intensity of an addiction, and the next time you turn inward to take an SUD reading, you suddenly see a blue wall. You don't know what it means, but as you sit with it, a memory emerges. When you were 14, you had to sit in a small room as punishment for bullying other kids in your class, and during that time you stared at a blue wall. You promised your parents, your teacher, and yourself that you wouldn't do this anymore. But a week later, you were there again for the same reason, staring at the blue wall and feeling shame and unworthiness about another angry outburst that hurt one of your playmates.

As an adult, as you tap on that shame and sense of unworthiness, you realize that it was in that room with a blue wall that you decided you could not control your impulses. This belief has carried into your attempts to break your addiction. As you realize it is a self-defeating and irrational belief (you have a lifetime of evidence that you have learned to control angry impulses), you use the tapping approach to overcome irrational beliefs (pp. 104-108). As you transform the belief, you eliminate another cog in the machine that drives your addiction.

You don't necessarily need to pursue every unresolved issue that makes you more vulnerable to the addiction. But unresolved trauma, abuse, or neglect may demand attention before an addiction can be completely overcome. What you can do, in an atmosphere of safety that invites sensitive issues to emerge, is to be alert for whatever comes into your awareness when you are having difficulty reducing your craving.

Clues like the blue wall are particularly likely to reveal themselves when you are taking the SUD rating. When they do, apply the Basic Tapping Protocol to them. To move into this territory, you might also begin with a Choices Statement such as *"Even though that was a great solution for when I was eight, I choose to recognize that I don't live in that family anymore"* (rubbing your chest sore spots on the first phrase and placing your hand over your Heart Chakra with the second). Exploring your history as it relates to the current addiction can, at one point or another, become a central (though temporary) focus of the treatment.

Increasing Self-Esteem and Confidence. Low self-esteem often has a circular relationship with addictions. Simply recognizing the damage the addiction has been causing can be an assault on your sense of self-worth. An overzealous inner critic can be another drain on your self-respect as you attempt to put your recovery plan into action. Guilt and/or shame almost always play a role in the problems caused by a serious addiction.

Limiting beliefs such as "I am not worthy unless [fill in the blank]" may greatly diminish self-esteem. In fact, the addiction itself may have become a way of trying to escape from the feelings of unworthiness. Many substances and mind-numbing activities can temporarily mask a person's insecurities and, when the addictive behaviors are curbed, those insecurities can rise to the surface and arrest progress. Again, tapping on these types of issues initiates neurological mechanisms that defuse their emotional charge. For instance, in working with the roots of low self-esteem, the tapping might be accompanied by statements such as "I needed to get straight As to feel worthy" or "Dad sure taught me how to be hard on myself."

As your confidence about overcoming the addiction begins to grow, this confidence can also be reinforced. Progress builds on progress. Identify the steps you have taken toward recovery; even tiny steps can be amplified with recognition, self-appreciation, and tapping. Tapping on positive states and statements such as "I can now handle my life without engaging in [the addictive behavior]" further embeds the suggestive power of the statements into your nervous system.

5. Maintenance

Dr. Horvath opens his chapter on maintenance, which he calls the "relapse prevention stage," with this quip: "It's easy to quit. I've done it dozens of times."[54] In this stage, the new behaviors and coping methods need to be reinforced so that returning to the addiction becomes less desirable and less likely. A danger here is to prematurely jump, in your mind, to the termination stage, where you begin to consider yourself free of the addiction. It's necessary, rather, to recognize the tendency to become complacent when the focus on overcoming the addiction has lost its intensity. You may even think that a small setback doesn't really matter, rather than interpreting it as a sign to double down on your efforts. When things start to go well, it is also easy to underestimate the ways that new life challenges and stressors may cause you to revert to old ways of seeking relief or escape.

The good news is that you can always return to issues that had seemed resolved and approach them with greater understanding and skill. As the American industrialist Henry Ford is often quoted as having said, "Failure is merely an opportunity to more intelligently begin again." New skills for dealing with pain, stress, or cravings can be revisited and practiced during this maintenance stage.

Triggers not directly related to the addiction may also provoke a relapse. For instance, tensions that erupt in a person's marriage after several months of sobriety might trigger renewed cravings. Some detective work (Chapter 3) may be needed to know where to focus the tapping. A thorny scenario might be that due to their childhood experiences, the partners needed the emotional distance created by the addiction. With the obstacle to intimacy removed—in this case, the addiction—they may unconsciously introduce other ways to maintain distance. This new marital strife might itself then become a trigger for relapse.

For instance, Emery, a returning client, had gone several months without drinking when his marriage to Talia became tense. His tapping phrases to focus on the newly emerged marital discord included *"I hate it when Talia yells at me," "The tension when I come home from work," "We argue about everything now," "The silent dinners."* After tapping on every aspect of the situation that Emery could identify, the threat response to each diminished. He could visualize each of the scenes without explosive reactions or escape fantasies. The tension with Talia was still problematic, but Emery wasn't being hijacked by his limbic system into stress reactions that ultimately triggered cravings for a drink. From there, he was able to use tapping to establish more constructive responses to the marital conflict and finally to focus on his difficulties with intimacy.

If a person has been in treatment for anxiety and then relapses, the therapy can usually pick up from where it left off. If a person with a substance use disorder, a gambling habit, or other disruptive addiction has a major relapse, however, significant parts of their life may need to be rebuilt. So the maintenance stage should not be rushed, regardless of how much optimism may seem warranted

following the action stage. At the same time, and somewhat paradoxically, the capacity for self-reliance should also be reinforced.

Another strength of energy psychology during the maintenance stage is that as you anticipate difficulties, you can take immediate steps to shore up internal strengths and reduce vulnerabilities. The last part of the Basic Tapping Protocol is "Testing Your Results" (p. 74). With an addiction, this can involve imagining situations whose intensity makes it likely for the old emotional and behavioral responses to reemerge. Any difficulty with the scene is tapped down until various plausible scenarios have been tested. For instance, you have fallen off your bike, have agonizing knee pain, and you never got rid of your last bottle of Demerol. Or you just found evidence that your wife is having an extramarital affair when you receive a call from an old crack buddy who is in town and wants to share some "good stuff." Deeply feeling into the most challenging situations you can imagine and tapping to reduce the impulse to abuse helps prepare you for whatever circumstances may arise.

6. Termination

A point comes when people are ready to test their wings and move on. To a sufficient degree, you have neutralized self-defeating responses to triggers; healed major childhood wounds; adopted new strategies for dealing with pain, stress, anxiety, and cravings; enhanced your self-esteem; strengthened your confidence; and implemented changes in your lifestyle. You have not repeated the addictive behavior for a long enough period to inspire hope that you have adjusted to abstinence and can stay the course even when addiction triggers are present. Many people get to the point that their risk of abusing is no greater than it is for someone who has never had the addiction. What you anticipate is also an important framing. Some think of themselves as being in an unending recovery process, which keeps them on alert. Others frame it that they are completely free of their addiction.

In the termination stage, you take steps so that slips don't become relapses. Dr. Horvath explains that coping with a craving is a skill that will atrophy if you don't practice it regularly. If you slip back into an addiction, this is not a disaster. It gives you the opportunity to shore up gaps from the previous round.[55]

But even success has its hazards. Living without the addiction may feel strange or even empty. Steps should be taken in the final phase of treatment to anticipate the possibility of relapse. This is often a theme in the closing sessions, along with reviewing the support systems put in place during the therapy and determining which of them are still needed and how they will be maintained. Because clients have already been applying energy psychology as homework, acupoint tapping can be used to make mini-corrections that prevent relapse.

This skill has been developed throughout the treatment and can be part of the post-treatment plan.

7. Recovery If a Relapse Occurs

Dr. Horvath notes that while stopping the addiction completely is the goal of the change process, the reality is that most people cycle through the stages any number of times before the addiction has been conquered.[56] So it is best to frame relapses as learning experiences rather than to allow them to reinforce shame, guilt, hopelessness, or a sense of failure. If the relapse brings the person back into treatment, an analysis of what occurred can show which of the above stages the person has reverted to. (Fortunately, relapses almost never catapult you back to square one.) More important, a relapse highlights what is needed to help prevent future relapses. Tapping can be applied in the ways discussed above on whatever issues still require attention.

THE STAGES IN ACTUAL PRACTICE

Of course, human experience never conforms to neat stages, however carefully formulated and logical they may seem in the abstract. The following case history, provided by our colleague, Robin Bilazarian, LCSW, a highly regarded energy psychology practitioner and trainer, illustrates how the stages may come out of sequence, overlap, or not all appear. Yet the basic principles remain.

The case illustrates the winding road that may need to be followed in working with an addiction.

CASE HISTORY PROVIDED BY ROBIN BILAZARIAN

Michael was 42 when he entered therapy with me [Robin] for anxiety. He was also feeling overwhelmed following a divorce, insecure about a new girlfriend, and hoping for a closer relationship with his children, who painfully preferred to be with their mother. A police officer for 18 years, he was feeling "jumpy" and hyperalert, often with buzzing feelings throughout his body. He was having trouble concentrating, and he was making trivial mistakes at work—losing his pens, forgetting his phone, or heading in the wrong direction—that while noticeable only to him, were of substantial concern.

In our first session, I asked him about alcohol and drug use, which he minimized. He explained that as a cop, he would occasionally drink with his fellow officers after hours to debrief or commiserate. He denied anything more than occasional social drinking, perhaps a few beers during the week and no drugs whatsoever.

History-taking revealed that Michael had been extremely shy as a boy and that by his teens, he had developed severe social anxiety and a sense of inferiority. He was comfortable in his job because the required behaviors were structured, scripted, and clear. Out of uniform, however, he felt socially unsettled and awkward, with his body occasionally buzzing into what he called "mini panic attacks." Aside from being on the job, he generally wasn't comfortable in his own skin. His explanation for the divorce was simply that his wife "wanted more out of life" than he could offer. Previous marriage counseling with another therapist had failed, and they ultimately decided that they had irreconcilable differences.

I introduced him to EFT tapping in our second session. He liked it immediately because he felt an instant release of his overwhelming anxiety-based physical and emotional discomfort. Michael's tapping in the early sessions focused on his difficulties with his ex-wife, his upset about his children not wanting to take overnights with him, and his losses following the divorce. He also seemed to worry about almost every aspect of his life: time, money, friendships, work, family, logistics, and so forth. In a basic energy psychology technique called "Tell the Story" (p. 166), Michael would describe to me the upsetting, anxious, and concerning worries of his week while we continuously tapped. Then we would go back to the story to pull out the salient parts and therapeutically tap on the emotion about that issue. Here are some examples of the wordings he used and the before-tapping and after-tapping SUD scores:

"Devastated that my children will not spend the night with me." SUD: 8 → 1

"Annoyed that I don't have a pool in my new condo." SUD: 5 → 0

"Jealous that my ex-wife is dating." SUD: 7 → 1

"Angry that I looked foolish to [his ex-wife] when Paul [his son] didn't want to go to the circus with me." SUD 8 → 0

When the emotions and physical discomfort were calmed and desensitized, he usually had a spontaneous insight—a cognitive shift such as:

"The children need time to get used to my new condo, and this will get better as they age."

"I can join a gym with a pool."

"It is okay that she is dating because I am too."

"It's a divorce. She isn't going to support me. It's my kids that matter."

Every session included at least one tapping sequence. Whenever we hit a "wall" or a concern that seemed a key to a deeper issue, I'd say, "Let's treat that," meaning let's use tapping. The frequent tapping during our sessions also taught Michael how to use tapping on his own whenever he was upset or anxious.

The treatment of Michael's generalized anxiety disorder seemed to be going well when, after eight weekly hour-long sessions, he received a DUI. He at first minimized the seriousness of the incident. He told me he was unlucky to have been caught this one time, but that because he was a cop, it would go away, as he'd seen in other police districts. But it didn't go away.

He was suspended from work with a mandate that he had to go into inpatient rehab or lose his job. He considered quitting or taking an early retirement, but that would mean losing the substantial full benefits that a few more years on the force would bring. Still, he felt he could never go into rehab because that would be a public admission that he had failed to maintain the standards expected of a police officer. Here are some of the wordings we used to tap on this dilemma:

"Embarrassed that my colleagues will see me as a failure." SUD: 8 → 1

"Deep hidden shame that my children will know I am a nothing." SUD: 10 → 2

"Worried my ex-wife will use this to further restrict my visitations." SUD: 10 → 2

"Terrified that my advancement at work is now dead." SUD: 6 → 0

"Angry that cop gave me a DUI!" SUD: 10 → 2

Michael had to get ready to go away for weeks of residential rehab. He knew that confidentiality could never be maintained. "Cops talk," he said. Besides inviting the judgments of others, it would be an admission to himself that he had a serious alcohol problem, and he wasn't there yet. At this point, I checked in on suicidal ideation, which he promised he would never do, mentioning the permanent harm it would cause his children.

In the same session, Michael began to reveal parts of his story he had initially concealed. He had been drinking heavily since he was 18 to self-medicate his anxiety—social anxiety in particular—and a deep inferiority complex. Like many young men, his drinking started with anxiety about speaking to women, where "a drink or two, or seven or eight, loosened me up." He was even a funny drunk back then, not a trait he had when he was sober. He particularly liked the "courage" drinking gave him in social situations.

He admitted he had driven drunk too many times to count and was lucky not to have harmed anyone or been caught before. His drinking had progressed to nightly. After scolding his kids, he would drink because scolding them brought up memories of the harsh corporal discipline he got from his father.

Tapping helped him accept what he believed was a public admission of weakness to his children, family, and coworkers as he made the difficult decision of going into rehab. The rehab facility was known for treating first responders and provided AA and NA groups specifically for them, which he continued to attend after discharge, along with returning to our weekly sessions. Michael was suspended from his job for six months, and he also lost his driver's license for six months. He was able to obtain marginal work in a local grocery store he could walk to during this six-month period, and he got rides to therapy.

As Michael acknowledged to himself that his drinking was creating serious problems, the tapping began to reach deeper. The basic rhythm started by tapping on a current concern, reverted to past history to clean up old triggers and unresolved issues, and then moved into future performance and fears. A major theme was his social anxiety, which was the reason he started drinking in the first place. He described the mini panic attacks he had in social situations and how he never knew what to say. I had him attune to every present, past, and imagined future social situation we could think of: a group of three, a group of 10, a party, walking into a room of strangers, a work gathering, and more. Each time we would first tap on how his body felt—typically pressure in his chest, tightness in his throat, a queasy stomach, or tightness in his shoulders. We would tap until the intensity level dropped to 0. Then we tapped on emotions about the issue, such as *"Terrified of walking into a room of strangers."*

We also focused on a variety of situations from his past where he felt picked on and bullied. The tapping calmed his bodily responses and the intensity of his upset about the memory. From there, we imagined future situations and tapped down his anxiety as he practiced icebreakers and small talk until his nerves settled and his confidence grew. He also needed to come up with a reason for refusing to drink in social situations. We tapped on his being worried about how others will react to him turning down a drink. At first he used the alibi of claiming to be on antibiotics that couldn't be mixed with alcohol, but later he wanted to tell the truth, and we tapped on his feelings around that.

Finally, we tapped on the inevitable truth that because of his alcohol transgression, he was sad that he "would not be considered for promotions again." With that tapping, he reached a place of gratitude that he still had a job, was still respected by his colleagues, and perhaps more respected for "taking care of his business." He decided to stay the two more years to reach full retirement benefits. Ironically and appropriately, he became a mentor and advisor when other officers were having trouble with alcohol.

After six months of weekly treatment following his month in rehab, we reduced visits to biweekly sessions, which we continued for another year and a half. After no slips, we graduated him from treatment. Three years later, he returned for six sessions because his new girlfriend was having conflicts with his children, who now had a close relationship with him. At that point, he had been sober for five years, had retired with full benefits, and was working another job. He had continued with the first-responder AA meetings and was still using the "Tell the Story" tapping technique when he became upset or anxious. He was proud that his old department still called him for advice about officers with substance abuse problems.

CONCLUSION

At the start of his treatment, Michael was deeply entrenched in his alcoholism and in even deeper denial about it. His journey toward sobriety, and then being recognized as an expert in overcoming addictions, shows both the challenges and the reasons for hope. Addictions are defiant. We do not mean to imply otherwise. But bringing tapping protocols into the process of overcoming an addiction gives you an edge in meeting the challenges and hastening your way back to a more clear-headed and fulfilling life.

CHAPTER 7

Peak Performance

EFT won't teach you how to play a Bach fugue or hit a
baseball. But it may help you maintain mental presence
and focus to such a degree that the fastball seems to "slow
down," permitting you to hit it with exceptional ease.[1]

—Patricia Carrington, PhD
Psychologist and widely loved EFT pioneer

GREG WARBURTON IS ONE of the first sports performance trainers to have systematically used acupoint tapping to help individual athletes and entire teams perform more consistently at their best.[2] This chapter will address a wide range of activities in which you might wish to excel, but we are starting with sports performance because it is easy to see progress—in scores, standings, and statistics.

Warburton began his career as a counselor at a camp for troubled teens.[3] He loved working as a therapist with young people but found that "talking wasn't enough." After learning to integrate tapping into his counseling, he used it as "a creative and effective language" that goes beyond the reach of just talk. Meanwhile, he struck up a friendship with Dan Spencer, the pitching coach for the local college in Corvallis, Oregon, when they would run

into each other while working out at the gym. It occurred to Warburton that he could apply the same principles that were proving so valuable with his young clients to help athletes. It took two years for Spencer to warm up to the idea, but finally he courageously allowed Warburton to introduce the strange-looking technique to the pitchers and catchers for whom he had direct responsibility.

Spencer's team, the Oregon State University (OSU) baseball team, was already nationally recognized. The previous year, they had made it to the College World Series, a Division 1 tournament in which the country's eight top college baseball teams face one another, but they were quickly eliminated. After Warburton's training in 2006, the OSU team not only returned to the College World Series, they also won it. And they won it again the next year. In that year, 2007, freshman pitcher Jorge Reyes was seen on national television (ESPN) tapping acupoints in the dugout between innings, leading to puzzled commentary by the sportscasters. Reyes won two games and Most Valuable Player of the series. Coach Spencer was named National Pitching Coach of the Year and observed that to get "to the 'promised land,' which in college baseball is the World Series in Omaha, Nebraska, coaches have to adapt and be willing to experiment with new methods and techniques." Bringing in Warburton was an experiment for him. His conclusion: "The acupoint tapping added another piece to the championship puzzle. It's been a great tool for us."

In 2010, the head coach of the OSU wrestling team invited five of his starting wrestlers to work with Warburton. Most athletes are more interested in physical rather than mental training, and only one of the five invited—Chad Hanke— contacted Warburton. The next year, Hanke made it to the University Nationals and won six consecutive matches to take the championship. He defeated six All-American wrestlers, including the previous year's national champion. Of the five OSU wrestlers originally referred to Warburton, only Hanke went on to excel, winning two University National Championships and later wrestling for Team USA in the Olympics. Did tapping make the difference? Hanke believes it was a critical element in giving him an

edge, stating in a televised interview that his work with Warburton "helped me achieve at the next level."

As Warburton became better known beyond Oregon, he was invited in 2012 by the head coach of the University of Arizona varsity baseball team to work with some of the pitchers who were having control problems. Warburton soon found himself introducing acupoint tapping to the entire team. They took the College World Series that year, winning all 10 postseason games.

Warburton's services are not only sought by colleges. For instance, in 2018 he worked with rower/sculler Catherine Widgery, who went on to win the single scull US National Rowing Championship, placing second (by less than one second) at the Euro-Nationals Rowing Championship, and winning the World Championship. Four years later, Widgery contacted Warburton again, just before competing in the 2022 World Championships. She let him know she was caught up in "thought attacks." She said that trying to "think my way to a good place" wasn't working. She was just days away from competing in the 2022 World Championships. During renewed training with Warburton, she said in an email,

> I can feel a palpable shift in the way energy is moving through my body. I would hardly have believed it was possible to feel such a change. No worries about my hip. Though I've had a couple of moments when it

seemed terrible, I just worked with my tapping and consciously allowing my body to relax and heal.

Widgery went on to win three gold medals in the World Championships. In a note of thanks, she said, "I've been doing a LOT of tapping. . . . Once again, thank you so much for your great work with me!"

Of course, in all four of these vignettes, acupoint tapping was only one part of an effort that included exceptional innate ability, dedication, training, and coaching. But in each case, Warburton was called in to bring an individual or team with great potential to exceed their past achievements. As all athletes and coaches know, that does not happen automatically. In each case, tapping was the new piece that elevated their performance. The athletes' innate abilities, strong determination, cutting-edge training, and superb coaching stayed relatively constant, yet in each case, after introducing tapping, they exceeded their past performances significantly. These vignettes are consistent with most of the stories Warburton has accumulated during his career. He has, over the years, been connected to 11 national championships, a level of consistent success that few, if any, sports mental performance coaches can claim.

In this chapter you will see how acupoint tapping can be combined with other psychological methods to measurably boost your ability in any skill you choose. Reports of tapping bringing about superior achievement have been appearing since Gary Craig's 2010 *EFT for Sports Performance*,[4] but the technique is not limited to athletic achievement. You can select an activity in which you wish to "up your game"—whether in sports, singing, acting, dancing, parenting, painting, public speaking, writing, teaching, or managing a staff—and discover how tapping changes your nervous system and can uplevel your performance. Because Greg Warburton is the most accomplished practitioner we know of who is using acupoint tapping to generate top performances, we will build on his methods throughout the chapter.

TAPPING INTO GREATER CONFIDENCE

Whatever issues might be addressed by training and practice, confidence is a fundamental quality that always affects performance.[5] Realistic confidence in your abilities leads to better concentration, sounder decisions, and a more positive outlook. Confidence may be enhanced or impaired by many factors, from early triumphs or disappointments—and the guiding models that grew out of them—to more recent experiences. In the only study to date that specifically examined the relationship between tapping protocols and confidence, a standardized measure of "performance confidence levels" showed significant improvements after a single tapping session with each of 10 female college athletes, gains that were maintained on a two-month follow-up.[6] We'll review several cases that show how tapping protocols were used to increase confidence.

Brayton. Brayton was admired among his friends for the way he could describe the world's wrongs in rap. He would size up a situation and come out "freestyling" the words, rhymes, tone, and beat that nailed injustices with perfect irony and sarcasm. One of his friends started recording these on his cell phone whenever Brayton would come up with his gems, often never to be repeated. Brayton's friend knew Joseph, who worked for a record label. Joseph was impressed with the informal recordings and set up an audition. On the day of the audition, Brayton woke up with a sore throat and had to cancel. The audition was rescheduled, but Brayton became confused and missed it. Meanwhile, Joseph had a sense that he was on the trail of a new talent and took it upon himself to drop in on Brayton.

With a few routine questions, Joseph quickly ascertained that Brayton was terrified of putting his songs out in the world. He loved his spontaneous creations, and he found it gratifying when he would memorize and refine one of them. But he had a lifetime of not meeting his parents' and teachers' expectations, and his music was the one place he could shine without their judgments, largely because they didn't understand it. Joseph told

Brayton he would like to visit him again with a friend who he felt could give him confidence about the audition. The friend had helped some of Joseph's other clients using the odd-looking procedure of talking and tapping. In that visit, Brayton was guided to tap on several of the most painful memories from his childhood when he had disappointed the adults in his life, on his sensitivity about expectations, on how good it felt when his friends were captivated by his impromptu performances, and finally on seeing himself nail it at the audition. By the end of an hour, Brayton was feeling confident about bringing his talent to a larger audience. His guiding model related to performance had been transformed.

Mario. Even guiding models built on a lifetime of positive experiences with a given skill can be undermined by a recent experience, such as an injury or major setback, receiving a negative review, or blowing an exquisite opportunity. Mario was a chef at a prominent Chicago restaurant where he was known for his innovative cuisine and creative chef's specials. He was selected to be on the culinary competition television program *Chopped*, which features the best chefs in the world. Mario was excited as the big day approached. He would get to show off his talents to millions of viewers. On the day of filming, however, he absolutely bombed. He summed up his performance as "mortifying." After that, everyone— from his customers to the kitchen staff to the restaurant owner—noticed that Mario's special recipes had lost their creative edge. The guiding model that had served him so well no longer supported his signature flair.

In working with Mario, David focused not only on the distress, regret, and humiliation Mario felt in the months following the TV appearance but also on the early experiences that had led Mario to his confidence and mastery. It turned out that these had become difficult to access after his public disgrace, and it was clear that an irrational belief had taken hold, which was that he was a mediocre cook who had simply been enjoying good luck in the kitchen. They tapped on all the ways that Mario had established personal mediocrity in his life—he was a mediocre singer, a mediocre athlete, a mediocre writer: *"Even though I'm a mediocre singer, athlete, and writer, I deeply and completely accept myself."* When we got to *"a mediocre cook,"* we both had to laugh, and he was back on track. The "spell" was broken.

Ghalen. Ghalen was a talented high school basketball player, but in the heat of a game, he would lose his confidence and perform far beneath his abilities. As his coach tried to understand the reasons, Ghalen described how everyone in his family believed he would never be as good as his big brother. To make matters worse, most of his early experiences with basketball were in pickup games with his brother, where Ghalen was usually the youngest and often the shortest one on the court. The guiding model that he wasn't very good compared to other players was deeply ingrained, and recent successes weren't changing it. While he was able to make affirmations about confidence, all the encouraging self-talk in the world wasn't going to do much for his performance until his early experiences had been addressed.

Independent of Ghalen's challenges, the coach brought in a tapping practitioner to work with the team, and Ghalen was one of the demonstration subjects. Asked to choose a basketball memory that carried a negative charge, Ghalen recalled a close game in a tournament at the local Y where he had a chance to make the game-winning shot. He glimpsed his older brother peering at him, got set, and shot, only to have the ball blocked by a taller defender. His brother yelled for everyone to hear, "Why didn't you pass it?" After tapping down the charge on that experience, Ghalen took up the invitation to do more work with the tapping practitioner, and his confidence took large leaps as the painful emotions and negative beliefs from that and similar past experiences were neutralized and memories of more recent successes were tapped into his nervous system.

Nine-Year-Old Jane. A common challenge in many sports or other activities in which participants stretch themselves beyond the usual limits of the human body involves concern about performing at one's upper limit while avoiding injury: "If I lift that much weight, I will stumble"; "If I try to keep up with the fastest hikers, I'll pull a muscle." While a realistic assessment of physical capacities is critical for any athlete, dwelling on what can go wrong is a confidence buster. Denise Wall, a tapping specialist, describes a session with Jane, a nine-year-old girl who had become a local star gymnast after six years of training and practice, starting at age three. Jane had suddenly become fearful and refused to return to practice. Wall discovered that the fear began when Jane was learning to do a handstand backward on the balance beam. Jane was afraid that "her hands did not know what to do" and that she didn't know how to fall if she had to. Wall continues,

> We tapped on her fear of falling, not knowing how to fall, fear of being hurt, fear of having people watch her fall, and fear of letting her team down. Then, after the tapping, I asked her to see herself moving backward on the beam, see herself knowing how to fall, knowing where her hands could go, how her knees could bend, how she could land and remount. She mentally practiced falling skillfully and remounting. She practiced having her hands know where to go. She practiced her feet landing on the sweet spot of the beam.

The problem was gone. I asked her mom to have her review falling safely with her coach and to walk it through on the grounded balance beam. Jane returned to her gym and moved up to the next level. I met her mom several months later and she said that only one other time did they need to tap, and Jane has been fine ever since.[7]

Jane's guiding model for six years had supported her success with gymnastics, but with one new routine, her shattered confidence stopped all progress. A single tapping session, albeit applied with a sophisticated understanding of a gymnast's skills and fears, reinjected confidence into her guiding model.

Team Confidence. The most effective way to develop confidence is to build the skills needed to succeed. This can occur at the individual level or can permeate through an entire team. The Southern Oregon University women's softball team in Ashland, Oregon, is another college team whose leap to a national divisional championship corresponded with the introduction of Warburton's training. In 2018, the team made it to the National Association of Intercollegiate Athletics (NAIA) World Series but did not win. In 2019, Warburton received a call from the head coach, Jessica Pistole, inviting him to work with the team.

Coach Pistole included her entire staff and team in learning acupoint tapping to help the players consistently perform at their best while competing in a relaxed body and calm state of mind. The team won the national championship in 2019 and again in 2021 (following the suspended season of 2020 due to COVID-19), and again in 2023. The players who had worked with Warburton the most closely had remarkable years. One was selected as the NAIA World Series Most Valuable Player. Another was awarded Player of the Year after breaking the division's career batting average record. A third was honored as the division's Pitcher of the Year. The NAIA 2022 Player of the Year, Riley Donovan, texted Warburton that his methods "have helped me get through so many tough innings." Coach Pistole, herself a two-time NAIA National Coach of the Year, commented to Warburton, "Those tools were huge for us!"

Brayton, Mario, Ghalen, Jane, and the Oregon women's softball team all found tapping to be an effective way of enhancing or restoring confidence. Whether focusing directly on confidence or developing the skills that engender confidence, the steps are reasonably straightforward and build on techniques you've already been using.

Energy psychology offers powerful tools for cultivating a desired skill. So far in this book, you have seen how acupoint tapping can be combined with other psychological methods for overcoming unresolved childhood experiences, worry, anxiety, panic, post-traumatic distress, sadness, depression, self-defeating habits, and addictions. Here we focus on enhancing your skills in an area of your life that you are likely to find gratifying. To get started, begin with the following "Quick Fix."

Quick Fix: Peak Performance

Bring to mind an area where you would like to be at your best, whether at an upcoming event such as a talk or competition or a general skill such as cooking, writing, speaking, coaching, or boundary-setting. Give an SUD rating to the amount of distress you feel in your mind and/or body when you think about needing improvement in this area. Say out loud the first statement below as you tap on the Top-of-the-Head Point. Go through each statement, cycling through the 12 tapping points as you move from one statement to the next. Skip any phrases that don't fit for you.

"I want to be better at [name desired skill].

I am open to releasing what's holding me back.

Even though I know I could improve,

I deeply accept where I am with this ability.

Part of me wants to improve.

But I'm feeling held back.

Maybe it's fear or doubt.

Maybe it's other people's expectations.

I can feel the resistance and conflict in [name body part].

I'm tapping to reduce this feeling.

I don't want to be in my own way anymore.

I choose to release whatever is holding me back.

I choose to open myself to my best performance.

I can envision what will help me improve.

I choose to follow that vision.

I'm capable of getting very good at this.

I'm ready to move forward.

I'm ready to stretch my abilities.

I'm ready for success.

I'm open to learning and improving.

I enjoy that process.

I'm sensing how I will savor having this skill.

I'm grateful for the opportunity to move toward my best.

I release any tension or resistance.

I feel the excitement."

After going through this sequence two or three times, you will probably find that you are already feeling more encouraged and maybe inspired. You have also prepared yourself to go deeper into developing this skill by applying the guidance offered in this chapter.

A FIVE-STAGE ACUPOINT TAPPING APPROACH FOR BRINGING OUT YOUR BEST IN AN AREA THAT MATTERS TO YOU

Vivid imagery, mental rehearsal, affirmations, and confronting self-limiting beliefs have all been shown to be effective techniques for changing guiding models, emotions, and behavior.[8] To help turn tapping into a personal power tool that has few rivals among existing self-help strategies, combine acupoint tapping with the following:

1. Formulating a performance goal you care about

2. Identifying and neutralizing internal objections

3. Creating "Power Phrases"

4. Expanding your Power Phrases into vivid imagery and mental rehearsals

5. Increasing the impact of your mental rehearsals

Many of the techniques you will be using here were first introduced in Chapters 2 and 3, but you will see how this chapter expands on them and orients them toward peak performance.

Step 1: Formulating a Performance Goal You Care About

When President John F. Kennedy said to America in 1962, "We choose to go to the moon in this decade,"[9] he was setting an intention that soon became a major component of the nation's guiding model. It was consistent with larger models within the national psyche at the time—that the United States is a leader, an innovator, an inspiration—but it expanded this into a new and previously uncharted area. This goal, he said, "will serve to organize and measure the best of our energies and skills." That is precisely what effective guiding models do. With the moon speech, Kennedy concentrated the nation's guiding model into a highly specific area. In the remainder of this chapter, you will be developing a guiding model to bring about a new level of achievement in an area that matters to you.

Guiding models tracing to childhood provide a context for everything that follows (as we saw in Chapter 1). They give definition and texture to your relationship with any activity you seriously pursue. They answer questions such as: "Are my aspirations worthy?" "Do I expect to succeed with a challenging task?" "Am I willing to work hard for a goal or am I more inclined to simply flow with what comes easily?" "Does competition stifle me or invigorate me?"

In September 2022, Donna was literally taken off the stage while teaching in Ohio and rushed to the Cleveland Clinic hospital where cardiologist Aaron Weiss undoubtedly saved her life.[10] Dr. Weiss had known he wanted to be a heart surgeon since he was just a boy. He writes in his formal bio statement, "I was six years old the first time I said I wanted to be a heart surgeon.

I am fortunate now to wake up every day and do just that." This guiding model from his childhood led him to undertake the tremendous challenges required to get a degree from a top medical school and secure a position as a top surgeon in the world's foremost cardiology hospital. Even though we were beneficiaries of all those efforts, Dr. Weiss would never take a compliment from us. He would always deflect our appreciation to his team of anesthesiologists, other physicians, nurses, physician assistants, physical therapists, orderlies, and on and on. But now we have him cornered. Thank you, Aaron Weiss!

Many people at the top of their profession—from healers to teachers to actors to athletes—had a comparable vision of themselves during childhood and followed it to achieve exceptional success. Yet even those who don't rise to the top of their field will fare better in their special calling when an internal model guides them to take the required steps along the way. And for most people, the experiences that shape their pursuit of a profession or pastime don't coalesce until after childhood. No matter where you are in your life, it's not too late to identify an activity in which you would like to excel or at least approach your full potential. You don't have to reach for the moon, as Kennedy got the country to do, but that doesn't mean you can't make a sizable leap forward.

In fact, research on goal setting shows that the more ambitious and specific a goal—within the person's ultimate ability to attain it—the higher the level of subsequent achievement. More than 1,000 studies have shown that "setting high and specific goals is linked to increased task performance, persistence, and motivation, compared to vague or easy goals."[11] Simply setting a goal puts you on a path toward improving your abilities, circumstances, or state of mind. Goals serve the function of focusing your attention and directing your efforts toward behaviors related to reaching the goal. They marshal your motivation. They also make you more willing to persistently pursue your intention despite setbacks. A goal differs from a desire or a momentary impulse in that you commit thought, emotion, and behavior to reach it. Yet even with that commitment, many goals go unmet.

Here we will take principles from sports psychology and business practices and integrate them with Warburton's acupoint tapping approach so your efforts for improving an area of your life will be well rewarded. You may elect to reach a higher level of performance in an activity you already do reasonably well, select a skill in which your performance to date has been disappointing, or decide on a pursuit that is entirely new to you. Recall that effective goals are *ambitious* and *specific*. At this point, the intention you will set for yourself can be quite general—we'll get to specifics later—but we encourage you to make it reasonably ambitious.

An ambitious goal simply means it will involve some difficulty to attain what you want. Kennedy's wording, "We choose to go to the moon," is a good model. "*I choose to be a better parent." "I choose to write my best song ever for my upcoming performance." "I choose to finish the county triathlon." "I choose to learn* Fortnite *so I can communicate better with my grandson."* When Warburton begins to work with an accomplished athlete or team, an ambitious goal is already assumed: consistent top performance.

Kennedy said, "We choose to go to the moon in this decade [and accomplish related goals] not because they are easy but because they are hard." He understood that ambitious goals not only aim for a higher payoff but they are also more motivating than easy goals. For now, your task is simply to *look* at your goal and imagine a future in which it has been accomplished. It is the six-year-old Aaron Weiss choosing to be a heart surgeon. It is you today, envisioning where you are headed, naming a specific way your future will be different from the present. Later in the chapter we will detail the steps for getting there, but for now, your focus is on a broad goal.

Ben's Goal

Our test driver for this chapter, Ben, is a 52-year-old psychologist who specializes in working with troubled teens. He is a colleague who was going through an earlier draft of this book to learn tapping. He had been invited to give a keynote address at a major conference on the alarming increase in suicides among youths. The invitation was a career landmark, and he wanted to deliver on it well. The conference was coming up in three months when he got to this chapter. He stated his goal as *"I choose to make this the best talk I've ever given."*

Your Turn

Select an area of your life in which you would like to see improvement. It might involve a performing art (e.g., singing, acting, dancing); an athletic activity (e.g., basketball, tennis, golf); another competitive activity (e.g., chess, poker, gaming); an interpersonal skill (marriage, parenting, leadership, sales); or a solitary activity (carpentry, gardening, cooking, sewing, web design). Form an intention statement that sets your sights on improvements you would like to initiate. You can use the *"I choose to . . ."* format or any other wording that describes an ambitious goal. For instance, *"I choose to beat my sales record next month." "I see myself on the list of top players in the local pickleball senior division."* Record your goal in your journal. Forming a goal you will be committing yourself to is an important choice, so give it the time and focus it requires. For now, that is enough. Tapping will begin with the following step.

Step 2: Identifying and Neutralizing Internal Objections

When President Kennedy announced that the United States would be shooting for the moon, he inspired millions of people. But he also catalyzed strongly voiced public objections: "It's not possible." "It will cost too much." "It's too dangerous." "It's a quixotic mission." "It's a waste of resources." Objections to a desired goal, what we have been referring to as Psychological Reversals, are not just the province of personal psyches. Personal or social, some type of reconciliation between the goal and the objections is necessary if the goal is to be wholeheartedly pursued. In the case of the moon mission, all of these objections were debated. None of them broke the will of those charged with carrying out the mission, but they weren't ignored, ultimately informing and refining the initial vision with the realities of the tasks ahead.

Peak Performance and Psychological Reversals. At the individual level, Psychological Reversals are *internal*

objections or conflicts about reaching your goal. They often reveal why that goal isn't already a reality. They may be at the forefront of your awareness or operate in the more distant regions of your psyche. Some Psychological Reversals, when processed, lead to useful adjustments to the goal itself. But a surprising number of inner objections to well-formulated goals are distractions that can be dissolved at the energetic level using tools you have already learned. In any case, pursuing even a beautiful goal will be less successful if a contradiction exists between your self-image or core beliefs and the intended change. If your overriding guiding model includes messages involving expectations of failure or that your efforts don't really matter, your aspirations may keep hitting an invisible ceiling. As we saw in Chapter 3, the seven most common types of Psychological Reversal involve:

- **Desirability:** a conflict between *wanting* and *not wanting* to reach the goal

- **Plausibility:** a belief that it is *not possible* to reach the goal

- **Safety:** a sense that it is not emotionally or physically *safe* to reach the goal

- **Worthiness:** a conviction that you don't *deserve* to reach the goal

- **Sacrifice:** not wanting to *give up* something that would be necessary to reach the goal

- **Courage and determination:** not being willing to *do what is necessary* to reach the goal

- **Identity:** a concern that reaching the goal is *not compatible* with who you are

Some Psychological Reversals emerge from recent experiences, as we saw with Mario, the chef, and Jane, the young gymnast. Warburton is always alert for recent setbacks that turn into Psychological Reversals, diminishing the person's sense of capability. For instance, he told us of Peyton Souhrada, a 14-year-old high school freshman who was asked to pitch for the varsity softball team. In her first game, she was so nervous that she pitched balls into the dirt or out of the catcher's reach, leading to several of what Warburton calls "thought attacks" in the coming days: "I can't pitch for varsity," "I'm not good enough," "I'm afraid to embarrass myself again." These were reflected in her performance.

Warburton taught her how to take these worries and fears as a starting place, tapping on thoughts such as *"I'm afraid to try pitching again"* and *"I don't know if I can regain my control."* By reducing the charge on this negative self-talk, she could persuasively initiate positive self-talk, such as, *"Control is my natural gift."* These phrases became internalized through tapping. She went on to pitch for the varsity team for the rest of the season. She wrote to Warburton, "Self-talk really helped me relax and pitch up to my capabilities. I could use it at any time to help calm me down and focus. The tapping was also great for me . . . it made me calmer and more confident." By her junior year, she was a First Team All-State player.

Reversing Psychological Reversals. Whether based in childhood experiences, self-defeating beliefs, or recent setbacks, Psychological Reversals can be energetically addressed using the following steps. This is often enough to be able to proceed with a focus on the original goal without progress being further impeded. In other cases, the goal may need to be adjusted.

1. Identify a Psychological Reversal (if several are at play, address them one at a time) and give it an SUD rating on how strong it feels.

2. Create an Acceptance Statement focusing on the Psychological Reversal, using the familiar format: *"Even though I don't believe it is possible to achieve this goal [or resolve this problem], I deeply and completely accept myself."*

3. Say the Acceptance Statement out loud three times while rubbing on chest sore spots with the first phrase and holding your hands over your Heart Chakra with the second.

4. Go through a tapping cycle (SUD rating, Acceptance Statement, the 12 tapping points while stating the Psychological Reversal as your Reminder Phrase, the Integration Procedure, another trip through the 12 points, and another SUD rating).

5. If the SUD has not gone down, repeat this process. Stay alert for any aspects that emerge (sensations, emotions, memories, or beliefs that are pertinent to the Psychological Reversal) and focus your tapping on them.

6. Once the SUD has gone down, substitute the Acceptance Statement with a Choices Statement (in the format of *"Even though I don't believe it is possible to achieve this goal [or resolve this problem], I choose to [describe a positive action or change in attitude or beliefs]."*)

7. Go through another tapping cycle, revising your description of the Psychological Reversal to a more empowering statement.

8. Continue until the SUD is at 0 or will go no lower after three tapping cycles.

Aspects That May Emerge. When an aspect appears (Step 5 or beyond), if it is a sensation, tapping while naming or simply focusing on the sensation is usually all that is needed. If it is a memory, belief, or intense emotion, you may need to go back to the experiences that give it a charge or shaped the belief, and focus on them. Self-talk reflects the guiding model that is in control during a given activity, and if it is harshly judgmental, everything that follows will be in its shadow until it is addressed.

Steven Ungerleider, a leading sports psychologist who has served as a consultant to the US Olympic Committee, notes that for peak performance, it may be necessary to go back and explore "childhood concerns, fear of failure, embarrassment, humiliation among friends and family, and childhood trauma."[12] These may all be aspects of the current challenge. Self-talk that frequently evokes emotions such as fear, shame, disgust, anger, or contempt signals a need for revising the roots of the model that governs the activity.

From Disempowering to Empowering. For many people, regardless of the activity, much of their internal chatter when facing a new challenge emphasizes weaknesses, doubts, and self-criticism. This often traces to less-than-skillful teaching methods during the person's childhood, often from well-meaning adults: "Megan, you always buckle under pressure!" "Ricardo, why are you so clumsy!" "Sally, you say such stupid things!" Many Psychological Reversals boil down to hearing an inner voice that keeps your attention on your weaknesses or mistakes. Tapping on such memories is the quickest and most effective way we know for putting them behind you.

While the above process for reversing a Psychological Reversal may seem complicated, remember that it only takes about a minute to go through the Acceptance Statement or Choices Statement procedures and another minute to go through the 12 tapping points with the verbalizations, so it can all be done quite efficiently. Because Psychological Reversals can torpedo progress, it is well worth the effort to eradicate them as you change a response pattern or pursue a goal. Consider any Psychological Reversals that may undercut your efforts to reach your goal. You will follow the steps outlined above and briefly illustrated by this glimpse into Ben's work.

Ben's Psychological Reversals

Ben's objections/conflicts about his next talk being his best ever were largely about whether that hope was possible. These included:

"I'll forget to keep eye contact with the audience."

"The dynamics are so complex that people won't be able to follow them."

"I can't memorize a 90-minute talk."

"The topic is so emotionally intense it will trigger the audience."

"My PowerPoint slides will prevent me from connecting with the audience."

For each, he made an Acceptance Statement using the familiar format: *"Even though I'll forget to keep eye contact with the audience, I deeply and completely accept myself"* (while rubbing chest sore spots with the first phrase and holding his hands over his Heart Chakra with the second). Addressing a Psychological Reversal in this manner not only reduces the power of the reversal but it also often opens new insights for resolving the conflict. For instance, "I can't memorize a 90-minute talk" led Ben to finally learn how to use a "presenter's monitor" to accompany his PowerPoints. The tapping and the insights that followed it worked to reduce the strength of each concern except the one about eye contact. After several cycles of tapping on *"Difficulties keeping eye contact with the audience,"* the SUD simply wasn't going down. In fact, the process brought up memories of his having been criticized for being so glued to his notes that he came off like an automaton.

Ben gave some creative thought to this issue and changed his Acceptance

Statement to this Choices Statement: *"Even though I forget to keep eye contact with the audience, I choose to practice keeping eye contact with at least five people when I speak at meetings in these coming weeks."* Just the thought of doing this gave him confidence, and he changed his tapping statement to *"I keep eye contact easily and naturally."* This got his concern about possibly forgetting to keep eye contact down to 4. Experimenting with his plan to keep eye contact when speaking in meetings, he found he could do it and that he was establishing the habit. His concern about not keeping eye contact became a nonissue.

A Psychological Reversal not on Ben's list emerged later. It had to do with a feeling of it being emotionally unsafe to excel. Rather than anticipating a great talk generating respect and admiration in his colleagues, Ben feared it would cause them to be jealous or shun him. Doing an Affect Bridge (p. 109) to explore the roots of this problem brought him back to a time in high school when he won a district-wide math contest. Another top math student who always seemed competitive with Ben began telling others that Ben cheated on the test. Others believed it, though it was a total lie. Known as the "tall poppy syndrome," this is the tendency in some cultures or social groups to discredit or disparage those who have achieved notable success, as if "cutting the tall poppy down to size." Ben carried this fear from that point on, and it emerged vividly when working on his talk. Tapping on his experience following the math contest was the first step toward removing it as a psychological block.

Your Turn

Review your initial goal and the types of Psychological Reversals listed above (desirability, plausibility, etc.). Sense into any that might interfere with your reaching your goal. Or, from another angle, here are the questions you considered in Chapter 3 for identifying Psychological Reversals:

- The thing about me that makes it impossible for me to reach this goal is . . .

- If there were an emotional reason for me not reaching this goal, it would be . . .

- To reach this goal, I would have to . . .

- What I really want, rather than just this goal, is . . .

- Thinking about this goal reminds me of . . .

- I would be more willing to reach this goal if first . . .

Once you have identified any Psychological Reversals that might interfere with reaching your goal, describe them in your journal and go through the eight steps on pages 259–260 with each of them. Remember: combining words that evoke difficult or self-limiting emotions with the stimulation of energy points sends signals to the brain that defuse the emotion. You may also find yourself revising your goal along the way. If your goal is *"I choose to be a world-class surfer"* and your Psychological Reversal is *"But my balance is terrible,"* something has to give. By the time you have completed the above, you should have a goal that you can wholeheartedly embrace as you move through the remainder of the chapter.

Step 3: Creating Power Phrases

The sports psychologist Dorothy Harris taught that "the only difference between the best performance and the worst performance is the variation in our self-talk."[13] This is what the great Yankee catcher Yogi Berra was getting at when he famously quipped that "90 percent of the game is half mental."[14] Self-talk is the inner voice that accompanies you throughout the day, and it may be for better or for worse. In either case, it combines your conscious thoughts and beliefs with deeper beliefs and programs—what we have been referring to as guiding models. You are actually talking to yourself any time you are thinking about something, which is much of your waking life. You may or may not notice your self-talk, but it is almost always there, at least at a subliminal level, when you are doing an activity—even those that are largely automatic, such as putting on your shoes.

By identifying and defusing your Psychological Reversals, you have *already* been changing the kind of self-talk that was previously likely to interfere with the skills or outcomes you are pursuing. Once you've cleared the major Psychological Reversals that emerge when thinking about your goal, it becomes possible to craft self-talk that will actually help you achieve what you intend.

The Nature of a Power Phrase. Warburton emphasizes the value of creating "positive replacement phrases" in self-talk, an antidote to "falling back into the pit of negative, unproductive thinking." He notes that sustaining positive self-talk—which some of his athletes refer to as their "Power Phrases"—literally creates new neural pathways in the brain. He explains that "your words and thoughts go directly into your body as energy. So you want your words to build a championship vocabulary."

Warburton sees this as a "foundational mental and emotional training practice." Remember how Jane, the young gymnast, benefited from self-talk that included *"My hands know where to go," "I move backward with ease," "I know how to fall."* Ghalen, the high school basketball player, internalized Power Phrases such as *"I'm a great ball handler," "The hoop is huge," "I'm good at this game after all."* When Catherine Widgery, the sculling champion, would feel discouraged, Warburton taught her to fully immerse herself for several seconds in the accurate Power Phrase *"I'm still ranked as the world's fastest woman."* The OSU wrestling champion Chad Hanke focused on just one Power Phrase: *"Nobody holds me down."* This galvanized his mental focus. He started tapping on this Power Phrase early in his work with Warburton, said it to himself regularly during a match, and

continued to use it the following year as he again placed first in the nation.

In Their Own Words. Warburton pays close attention to the athlete's own words as they craft Power Phrases, and he challenges them to be sure the phrases fit them. Andrew Moore, a freshman pitcher at OSU, saw Warburton walking by the playing field after one of their sessions and called out, "Greg, I think I have it: *'Four pitches or less.'*" To get a batter out within four pitches means throwing mostly strikes. After a tapping session that focused on some unproductive self-talk about expecting to struggle after pitching five innings and on embedding the *"Four pitches or less"* Power Phrase, Moore pitched a complete 9-inning, 2-hit shutout game. He threw 87 pitches to 27 batters, averaging just 3.22 pitches per batter. In the third start after he created his Power Phrase, he pitched another complete 9-inning, 2-hit shutout, averaging 3.1 pitches per batter. In his following start, he again pitched a complete 9-inning shutout, with 107 pitches to 31 batters, averaging 3.45 pitches per batter.

Moore later wrote to Warburton about how the Power Phrase and tapping helped him stay in the "four-pitches-or-less frame of mind." He went on that year to tie OSU's single-season pitching record with 14 victories, and he was the first freshman in the school's history to be named a First Team All-American.

Champions develop self-talk that keeps their sense of mastery active and automatic. Often it involves bringing an awareness of their highly refined skills to the present moment. Babe Ruth, baseball's most famous slugger, used to tell himself after a swing and a miss, "Every strike brings me closer to the next home run." Power Phrases can help you stay present, focused on the task at hand, and they create positive self-fulfilling expectations, regardless of the activity.

Self-talk isn't just for athletes. The Power Phrases Mario generated after his realization that maybe he wasn't *just* a mediocre chef included *"The creativity that made me a great chef is still inside me," "People love my flavors," "I'm looking forward to what I can do with these new herbs."* Brayton, the rapper, would affirm to himself that others' expectations are no longer a problem for him. Characteristically, he did this in rap: *"Nothin's gonna get in my way / This gift of mine has the final say."*

Negative Self-Talk as a Cue for a Power Phrase. Self-talk can be cultivated to affirm your strengths and potential. You can use it to reprogram internal dialogue from self-defeating statements into positive statements and to instruct yourself through each action of a complex skill. For many activities, self-talk that gets you into the present moment or focused on the next step has the organic benefit of bypassing self-criticism. In fact, simply *noticing self-criticism can become a cue for a Power Phrase.* Dr. Ungerleider gives examples from famous athletes he has known or worked with. The tennis great Pete Sampras would combat distracting thoughts with self-talk such as:

"Get out of this mindset."

"Let go of that last point."

"Prepare for the next point."

Some negative self-talk can be readily converted into affirmative statements. Hearing unproductive words in your mind, such as berating yourself for an error, can become a reminder to pull up a Power Phrase you've practiced, such as *"Here comes my next opportunity."* In other instances, however, it may be necessary to first modify relevant guiding models by revisiting the experiences that shaped them.

Self-Talk Reveals Guiding Models. While guiding models often operate beneath conscious awareness, bringing them to the surface allows you to explore and alter them so they can better support your current needs and aspirations. Some of them may already be clear to you. Others can be brought into your awareness in many ways. Simply observing your self-talk is one of the most obvious and natural methods.

Some guiding models may never need to be examined until you push the envelope of your potential. If you are developing a new skill, they may loom large in your awareness. For instance, you may have never felt comfortable persuading people to adopt your point of view. The guiding model maintaining that discomfort may have been shaped by events or messages from your family, peers, or teachers during your early years. But now imagine that after years of success in civil service jobs, you are offered a position as the campaign manager for your local congresswoman.

You take it because you believe in her mission, but you suddenly find yourself needing to persuade others of the importance of her vision. You can certainly use acupoint tapping to reduce your nervousness and discomfort about making a strong case that is designed to persuade others to your point of view. But if you are going to become comfortable with your new responsibilities, you may need to revisit times where you might, for instance, have been given the message to never counter your parents' opinions. Once you've defused the emotional residue of such experiences and revised the part of your guiding model that prevents you from confronting the opinions of others, a Power Phrase such as *"I'm shining a light on the situation"* can be effective when self-doubts arise as you bring the congresswoman's message to the public.

Power Phrases can be formulated not only to address your primary goal but also for the many small steps required to achieve it. Ben's goal focused on a specific event—the keynote address he was going to deliver—but he had a variety of subgoals in preparing for it. He developed Power Phrases for many of them.

Ben's Initial Power Phrases

Starting with his Psychological Reversals, Ben created these Power Phrases:

"Eye contact is my new habit" (versus "I'll forget to keep eye contact with the audience").

"I make it simple" (versus "The dynamics are so complex that people won't be able to follow them").

"I will have an outline of the main points on the presenter monitor" (versus "I can't memorize a 90-minute talk").

"I lead the audience gently and with sensitivity" (versus "The topic is so emotionally intense it will trigger the audience").

"I am designing PowerPoints that will keep the audience engaged" (versus "My PowerPoints will prevent me from connecting with the audience").

"Everyone who really matters to me wants me to succeed" (versus "My colleagues will be jealous and find ways to put me down if the talk is a great success").

Ben tapped while saying each Power Phrase (the italicized parts), adding one a day and rotating among them so he was focused on no more than three a day. In a few instances he had to give further attention to the corresponding Psychological Reversal, but all six Power Phrases were readily available to him within a couple of weeks.

As Ben wrote an outline for the talk and created PowerPoints to reinforce the main concepts, phrases such as *"I make it simple"* and *"I'm designing PowerPoints that will keep the audience engaged"* guided him in his preparation. Once the outline and PowerPoints were reasonably well completed, however, he found himself resisting practicing the talk. He firmly believed that practice was the key to delivering a successful presentation, but he got bored and unmotivated after running through it a couple of times. He would let weeks go by without rehearsing. So, he developed a Power Phrase to help him with this too: *"I learn something new every time I rehearse."* And he indeed began to fine-tune the presentation with each rehearsal. Whether or not he had rehearsed on a particular day, he committed to doing a round of tapping each evening on that phrase. He was soon looking forward to the rehearsals as a creative activity, and he began practicing once each week leading to the talk and a few times the week before it.

Your Turn

Review the Psychological Reversals you identified earlier and select any that still carry a charge. For each one that does, formulate a Power Phrase that counters the message of the Psychological Reversal. Write it in your journal. Then repeat it as you tap on the 12 acupoints. Adding tapping to a Power Phrase helps embed it in your whole body-mind system. While you may not be able to tap *during* a speech or while in the heat of a soccer match, tapping as you practice a few Power Phrases helps make them more available at times that you can't tap.

Limit yourself to working on no more than three Power Phrases at a time. Once a Power Phrase becomes comfortable and established so you can call upon it when it's needed, you can move on to other phrases on your list. If you sense resistance to a Power Phrase, consider revising it *or* treating the resistance as a Psychological Reversal, using the procedures described in Step 2 (p. 258).

Step 4: Expanding Your Power Phrase into Vivid Imagery and Mental Rehearsals

Your Power Phrases build upon the strength of language. They become even more potent tools when you further charge them by adding *imagery* and *mental rehearsal* as well as *tapping*. When people think of an image, it is usually static, like a freeze-frame. This is useful for refining the image. But selecting an image is just the first step in creating your mental rehearsal. While we are teaching imagery, mental rehearsal, and tapping with mental rehearsal as three separate topics, you will see that they merge into a single practice—one smooth operation—that gives your Power Phrase a lot more juice. Selecting the image to build upon is an important starting point.

Imagery. Vivid imagery involves your mind and body in your Power Phrase in ways that just saying or thinking the words cannot. While athletes and performers are taught that imagery is a powerful tool, they are often not shown how to use it effectively. We introduce imagery to our groups with a simple experiment you can do right now:

Sit back and follow the instructions as you read along. Hold out one hand in front of you, imagine you are holding a lemon that has been cut into quarters. Use your imagination as vividly as you can to see the lemon's yellow skin and to feel its bumpy texture with your fingertips. Notice the indent marks on the peel and its juicy inside. Now bring the lemon up to your nose and sniff. Can you smell it? You are about to bite into the juicy pulp of one of the sections. Imagine you are chomping into it—not just a little nibble! Really bite it. Imagine chewing it. . . . Okay, remove it and place it in the composting bin. Take note of whether you salivated.

In our classes, most people raise their hand to indicate that they did salivate. Your body and neurochemistry undergo physical changes when you use your imagination. Your brain treated your mental lemon like a real lemon. It sent saliva to neutralize the sour acid even though a real lemon wasn't present.

When you repeatedly use a Power Phrase in conjunction with vivid images, you are training your body and mind to have perceptions, thoughts, and actions that are consistent with the Power Phrase.

Imaging Isn't Only a Visual Experience. Imaging is more than just inner seeing. It may include any combination of senses. In the lemon experiment, you may have seen the lemon, felt its texture and weight, experienced its sour taste, smelled its citrus aroma, felt drawn or repelled, or any combination. In fact, many people cannot see mental pictures, or what they can see is faint, vague, or fleeting. So when we say "image," we are referring to whatever the combination of sensory modes and emotions your mind uses to construct inner experiences.

Sources of Effective Imagery. Dr. Ungerleider points out that imagery and mental rehearsals are double-edged: "Although practice makes perfect, practice also makes imperfect if you are practicing the wrong imagery."[15] Replaying your mistakes can be useful when generating imagery for correcting them, but continually replaying them locks them into your nervous system. Where do you get the best images for your mental rehearsals? Major sources include watching masters, recalling your own best performances, or even watching a video of yourself at your best.

- **Watching Masters.** Much of our imagery traces back to what we have observed in others. Our internal processes are shaped in part by, as Dr. Ungerleider puts it, "the flood of new pictures from external experiences to our minds."[16] The neural mechanisms that orchestrate this involve "mirror neurons," which are brain cells that react when a particular action is performed and when it is only observed. Dr. Ungerleider recounts this story from the four-time Olympic pole vaulter Earl Bell: "I used to train in the winter, and we'd go to this indoor gym that was the same place our basketball team played. Part of our warm-up was to shoot some one-on-one and have some fun. My little three-year-old would come and watch us. A few months later, his grandma bought him a little basketball and a net—a little four-foot-high goal that had a little ball about five inches in diameter, so it fit nicely in his hands. She set up the hoop and put the ball in his hands, and he started to take a shot. But first he squared up in front of the hoop, flipped his wrists, and just took this beautiful little jump shot. This is the first time he had ever played ball. All he'd ever done was watch us, and already he has a great jump shot."[17]

- **Recalling Your Own Best Performances.** Success paves the way for future success. The positive images that are most attuned to your body, psyche, and sense of self are going to be based on your personal bests. A personal best is believable. It was accomplished before—by you! Therefore, your ability to succeed has already been proven. Everyone would, however, like to be able to *always* operate at or excel upon that level of performance, and recalling past successes or imagining going beyond them is a potent source for fruitful imagery.

- **Watching Your Own Best Performances.** It used to be mostly athletes, actors, and singers who had access to videos of their past performances. Even then, coaches and directors often used these to analyze mistakes or weaknesses. Today, nearly everyone carries a video camera in their ever-present cell phone. If the activity you are pursuing lends itself to video, it's easy to set up a tripod and record your practice sessions. You can use the recordings to smooth out rough spots, but for our purposes here, we want you to use them to galvanize into your mind your best moments. They can become sources for strong mental rehearsals.

Because athletes typically have ready access to video replays, Warburton urges them to review their top performances and tap while watching them. He emphasizes that this creates or reinforces neural pathways that pattern the desired sequence of actions. One athlete summarized the principle by saying, "Oh, I get it, you want us to soak in the good stuff!" Warburton worked with Tyler Malone, a top hitter on the 2018 Oregon State University baseball team. A key piece of the mental training was to practice imagery after watching his best batting performances and to tap on that imagery. Malone went on to hit home runs in five consecutive games that season, and he also hit three home runs during the national championships.

Once you have a single image that expresses a Power Phrase—whether that image is rooted in watching masters of your chosen skill, thinking of or watching videos of your own best performances, or simply generated from within—you are ready to expand the image into a mental rehearsal.

Mental Rehearsal. A classic study of the effects of mental rehearsal on developing a new skill was conducted using student volunteers. The study involved making basketball free throws. The volunteers, who were not basketball players, were divided into three groups. One group practiced shooting free throws every day for 30 days. The second group also practiced shooting free throws for 30 days, *but only in their minds*. They did not touch a basketball. The third group was not given any instructions related to basketball. After 30 days, all three groups came back to shoot free throws. The ones who did not practice at all showed no improvement. The ones who practiced with an actual ball improved 24 percent. The ones who practiced only in their minds improved 23 percent, which is statistically equivalent to those who practiced on the court.[18]

In a survey of 1,200 elite athletes, all of whom had made it to the Olympic trials, the factor that distinguished those who qualified for the Olympics from those who just missed was that the future Olympians put more effort into "mental tune-ups" in the final stages of preparation.[19] Dr. Ungerleider was one of the investigators. He explains that mental rehearsal can program the mind to respond in a specific way to a specific situation. He explains that "the brain uses the same pathways for *seeing* that it does for *imagery* [but] instead of processing visual information from the outside, a visual signal is processed from within."[20]

Dr. Ungerleider identified four areas in which mental rehearsal can be beneficial: (1) technique enhancement, (2) error analysis and correction, (3) preparation for performance, and (4) overall skill-building.[21] Mental rehearsals can be as effective as actual practice, in part because they allow you to break down an activity, figure out how to respond to each challenge, and then envision implementing the new action. And as you will see, combining tapping with mental rehearsals increases their potency.

Mental Rehearsals "On the Spot." Mental rehearsal is usually carried out as a part of preparation and training, but it can also be done just before the action. Before going onstage, a performer might take a couple of deep breaths and imagine the first 10 seconds of engaging with the audience. An executive might envision moving through the agenda just before opening a potentially contentious staff meeting. A tennis player could take a deep breath before each serve as she imagines the movements to speed the ball into the service box. Even if you can't bring a full rehearsal scene into your activity, you can use one of your Power Phrases at any point.

Adding Tapping to Your Mental Rehearsals. Warburton teaches his athletes to notice moments in their mental rehearsal when they become tense, anxious, or doubtful. He interrupts the mental rehearsal at these points and has the person tap to clear whatever triggered the tense response.

They then return to the mental rehearsal in a more relaxed body and calmer state of mind. Warburton has his athletes progressively intensify the competitive moments in their practice so they are rehearsing under the greatest pressure *before* they compete, again tapping at each step that causes tension. They not only begin the mental rehearsal in a relaxed state but they also end it in a relaxed state. These anticipatory steps while tapping pay off in a calmer performance, even in the highly stressful circumstances where it matters most.

The first published study of tapping with sports performance involved a single 10-minute tapping session conducted with a group of female soccer players.[22] A comparison group received a standard soccer coaching session. The tapping group's improvement in kicking a goal from 50 feet away was statistically superior to that of the comparison group. While this was an early and rudimentary study, it illustrates how even a bit of tapping can make a sizable difference.

While applying tapping to mental rehearsals may seem obvious for improving athletic skills, what about other activities? Take knitting, for instance. If your goal is to learn to knit beautiful sweaters, you may wonder what mental rehearsal has to do with you. You may find knitting itself to be a form of relaxation, not a stressful activity, and certainly not one performed in front of a crowd scrutinizing your every stitch. It might seem that learning to tap away the stresses involved in carrying out the skill may not apply to knitting (or many other solitary activities). On the other hand, developing the abilities of dexterity, creativity, planning, and following and deviating from patterns, as well as matters of aesthetics and audience reception, may be packed with stresses and challenges.

Using Rehearsals and Tapping to Pinpoint and Overcome Challenges. Whether knitting or pole-vaulting, every skill involves subskills, and each may pose its own challenges. If you lose your confidence and patience trying to knit into the back of a stitch; or if you tighten at critical moments when rehearsing a pole vault, song, or comedy act; or if you panic when your queen is threatened while envisioning a chess game, you have identified an area where mental rehearsal can be used for practicing more effective action. When you have difficulty with a specific skill, you can identify where you stumble and improve that smaller piece of the overall activity.

Warburton teaches his athletes highly focused self-talk and rehearsal techniques in areas in which they are having difficulty. He has had great success breaking down visualization practice into steps. For example, Warburton worked with the then upcoming professional baseball player, Wade Meckler, on fine-tuning his batting. Warburton asked Meckler to put his attention on the bodily experience of his entire swing motion. As Meckler did this, he noticed, "Okay, there is something wrong at my hip turn." Then he did a round of tapping, focusing on "*Something wrong at my hip turn*" to clear this block to the full and proper execution of his batting swing.

Once he was able to imagine the motion with his hip turns corrected, he could sense and tap on an ideal swing. Meckler started the 2023 baseball season in the minors, progressed through all levels of Minor League Baseball over that summer to play with the San Francisco Giants in September 2023, a rare professional baseball achievement.

Whatever the skill you are developing, if you do a mental rehearsal in slow motion while also tuning in to the bodily experience, you are likely to find areas that can benefit by making refinements. The specifics vary greatly depending on the activity, but the principle holds that what you rehearse in your mind impacts what you will do with your body.

In the following instructions, you will be mentally rehearsing the scene(s) you have selected while tapping through the 12 acupoints as many times as it takes. Similar to the "Tell the Story" technique (p. 166), this further empowers your imagery by sending signals to your nervous system via the acupuncture channels, which build neural pathways that correspond with the imagined activity.

Ben's Mental Rehearsal

Ben's rehearsal zeroed in on keeping contact with the audience, using engaging language, and conveying compassion. For his initial image, he had once spoken to his son's high school class on Career Day, and it was one of his favorite presentations ever. The students were so interested in hearing how a therapist helps teens with anxiety that it brought out Ben's playfulness and as good a rapport as he'd ever had with an audience. He expanded this into a mental movie of his anticipated keynote address and tapped on it. Note that this was very different from his much longer practice sessions, where he was rehearsing and further developing his talk in real time. Each of these mental rehearsals took only a minute or so.

Your Turn

Begin by selecting a single image that represents you performing at your best in the activity your goal focuses upon. The image will be like an *illustration* of your goal or one of your Power Phrases. It may be based on having seen a person whose skills you admire doing the activity, a memory or video of one of your personal bests, or a scene that simply emerges from your imagination. Next, expand the image into a mental rehearsal, essentially making an internal movie of you flawlessly carrying out the sequence. Your mental rehearsal can represent the entire activity or highlight a single part in which you would like to put more focus. Finally, play it like a movie in your imagination and tap as you rehearse, going through the 12 tapping points as many times as necessary to complete the sequence of skills you are rehearsing. If your mental rehearsal focused on a single trouble spot, you can also create additional mental rehearsals for other challenges.

Step 5: Increasing the Impact of Your Mental Rehearsals

Once you have created and mentally rehearsed a superb performance, the final step is to increase its impact on your psyche and nervous system. The principle is simple. The more believable the mental rehearsal is to you, the more impact it will have. You will be able to use procedures you have already learned to increase its believability and thus its effectiveness.

In the previous chapters you were shown how to imagine a desired response to a challenging situation. You rated the *believability* of this imagined response and took steps to increase that believability. The same process, which includes SUB (Subjective Units of Believability) ratings, can be used with a mental rehearsal.

How Ben Increased the Impact of His Mental Rehearsal

The first time Ben did the mental rehearsal, he enjoyed it, but the believability about pulling it off was only at 4 of the possible 10. His next Acceptance Statement was *"Even though it's only at a 4, I accept myself anyway."* One of the Psychological Reversals he identified was that he wouldn't be able to use simple language when expressing complex ideas about how thoughts of suicide affect the brain in ways that are different from anxiety alone. Having an outline on the presenter monitor rather than having to memorize his talk would allow him to ad-lib, which would make it easier to stay engaged with the audience. But going free-form could also be a trap for his tendency to become too intellectual.

Ben tapped on *"I'm afraid I'll find myself resorting to complex technical language,"* which started with an SUD of 8 but got down to a 2 after a few tapping cycles and a new Choices Statement: *"Even though I'm afraid I'll resort to complex technical language, I choose to rehearse and internalize simple phrasings for the technical material."* He also worked through several other Psychological Reversals in this manner, and he pushed the believability score up to 9 (recall that while you want to lower your SUD, you want to raise your SUB).

Your Turn

Begin by assigning a Subjective Units of Believability (SUB) rating to your mental rehearsal or any scene within it that has been or might be challenging. Proceed through the steps illustrated in Ben's account to increase the believability of the scene. You can do this with the mental rehearsal of your activity in its entirety as well as each segment you wish to give special attention.

CONCLUSION

Learning a new skill or improving an existing one enriches you. Whether it is for an activity that others will see or a solitary endeavor, efforts that expand you tend to be deeply gratifying and often exhilarating. Humans have always been seeking ways to maximize the results of their efforts. This chapter has introduced you to some of the most effective strategies to date for achieving peak performance, and it has shown you how to use tapping to further empower them.

CHAPTER 8

Relationships

Tapping balances a couple's energies for deeper levels of empathy, love, and playfulness. Having the partners mindfully tap during hard times also helps them step back from distressing thoughts and emotions so their communication becomes more creative and constructive.[1]

—**Fred Gallo, PhD**
The psychologist who coined the term "energy psychology"

IN HER FOREWORD TO our *New York Times* best-selling book on relationships, *The Energies of Love*, our longtime friend Jean Houston, the cultural historian and pioneering researcher on human capacities, wrote of us:

> When you first meet them, they seem an unlikely couple. Donna is exuberant, spontaneous, and intuitive. David is quietly reflective, studious, and always looking for deeper meanings. She is champagne; he is still water. She is of a tropical nature; he is most definitely northern. And yet, with all their contrasts, they have, through dint of unstinting effort and rich affection, cultivated a loving, creative, and exemplary marriage. He puts her feelings and intuition into words. She sees and orchestrates

energies that enable him to enter a different universe of understanding. Together, they have done the hard work of relationship, and we are their beneficiaries.[2]

We opened that book by admitting, "We often joke, or half-joke, that if we can make it, any couple can make it." Looking through the lens of our 46 years together at the time of this writing, our early years in particular were fraught with pain and disharmony. Friends who witnessed our friction firsthand doubted that we'd last through the month. Beyond our professional credentials of having helped improve hundreds of marriages, we must hold some distinction in the "bad to good" category of relationships. As Donna is fond of saying, "Thank god I didn't leave him when I should have!"

In the great tradition of teachers who teach what they need to learn, we began offering workshops early in our partnership, aptly named "The Relationship Rollercoaster." We were certainly becoming experienced experts on that topic. A key insight of the Relationship Rollercoaster workshops was that nature tricks us humans by arranging our biochemical and energetic responses so we are primed to become passionately attracted to one special other. For heterosexual couples, the design is to get a potential mother and father so deeply enmeshed with each other that they will stay together long enough to raise their offspring. However, the emotional resources expended for this "Romantic Love" stage are enormous. These resources soon need to go into raising and providing for a family. So, this compelling programming for starry-eyed passion has a definite half-life.

As it fades, the next stage is "Disappointment and Reckoning." Where did that passion and those idyllic perceptions of one another go? But if you can make it through the pain and disillusionment of this stage, the pot of gold that ideally awaits you is a "Deep and Flowing" stage that will last for the rest of your days. Of course, many other factors are also involved, but the trajectory from Romantic Love to Disappointment and Reckoning to Deep and Flowing is nature's urging.

Even in our roughest times, we had a sense that the Deep and Flowing stage was supposed to be our destiny together, and this got us through our turbulent early years. A relatively unique understanding we brought to our classes is that each stage has its own *energetic* frequency. A couple can navigate by exploring and working with this energetic foundation of their perceptions, feelings, and hopes.

One of the most frequent takeaways we've heard from couples who went through those workshops is that when they stopped judging their relationship through the lens of the early uber-passionate stage—or even through an uber-passionate stage they never actually had—the background tune of disappointment faded. This allowed the partners to do the hard work of reconciling differences (or parting) to get to a gratifying flow they might otherwise never have reached. They were glad they didn't leave each other when they "should have."

Psychologists use the term *companionate love* to describe this more mature type of love, which "is characterized by strong feelings of intimacy and affection for another person rather than strong emotional arousal in the other's presence."[3] Such relationships are "high in intimacy and commitment." It's not that we don't still have passion—we do—but the soul connection is what we cherish most.

YOUR GUIDING MODELS AND YOUR RELATIONSHIPS

Your guiding models are at the root of your ability to establish a nourishing partnership. They began forming during your infancy and continue to evolve throughout your life. Tapping protocols can be used to update these models so they propel you toward ever more fulfilling relationships.

Cultivating mutually supportive, emotionally enriching relationships is a key to success in almost everything you do. Our ancestors depended on one another to survive, and families and communities remain vital for our health and well-being. Hundreds of studies show that the quality of your connections with those you are close to determines a great deal about your resilience in the face of stress, your outlook when you meet a challenge, the effectiveness of your immune system, your health and longevity, and your overall happiness.[4]

What we present in this chapter may bring you to core issues from your childhood that are ready to be more fully resolved in a manner that will upgrade your current relationships. Personal evolution has, in fact, been compared to an upward spiral in which you keep circling back to the same issues over and over but at a higher level of psychological development, allowing you to address them in new and more decisive ways.[5] That's the promise of this chapter. The process, however, may be challenging. One of our test drivers wrote,

> This chapter was by far the most difficult for me. It opened huge areas that I realized are necessary for healing big parts of my life. Delving into the material, I often felt like I wanted to run. The chapter required me to be open, honest with myself, and precariously vulnerable with my partner. Many times I thought, "I'll skip the rest of the chapter." But I stayed with it. I'm THRILLED that I did! Thank you for this material. It has helped me navigate very stormy waters.

So be ready for the possibility that this chapter may take you into some "stormy waters." While it is more likely to be hopeful and inspiring, pace yourself as needed. You can take breaks. You can use your journal for reflection. You can enlist support from others. The deeper you go into the processes, the more transformative they are likely to be. To get started, begin with the following "Quick Fix."

Quick Fix: Relationships

Bring to mind a relationship in which you would like to improve communication, heal conflict, or go deeper. It can be your partner, your boss, your child, your parent, a friend, a colleague, an ex-spouse, or an imagined future partner. Give an SUD rating to the amount of distress you feel in your mind and/or body when you think about your desire for these changes. Say out loud the first statement below as you tap on the Top-of-Your-Head Point. Then say the next statement while tapping on the next point. Go through each statement on the list that fits for you, cycling through the 12 tapping points as you move from one statement to the next. Skip any phrases that don't fit for you.

"*Even though I feel challenged by my relationship with [name],*

I believe in the goodness in both of us.

Even though it's hard to trust that the changes I want will happen,

I choose to have compassion for myself and for [name].

The relationship can be so challenging.

Sometimes I feel very frustrated.

I want this relationship to thrive.

But I'm not sure how to make it get better.

Sometimes I overreact.

Sometimes I shut down.

When I think about the problems in the relationship, I feel tension in [name body part].

I can tap to reduce that tension.

I can start to relax.

I want to be more compassionate.

I don't want my fear or resentment to control me.

Am I afraid of getting hurt?

Am I afraid of being controlled?

Sometimes it's hard to stay calm and listen well.

What would it be like if I listen more deeply?

I choose to be open to a more complete understanding.

I appreciate the effort I'm putting into this relationship.

I also want to honor [name's] perspective.

I want to be respectful.

I choose to have deep compassion for [name's] struggles.

I look forward to the next step.

I'm inspired by the possibilities.

I can tap through any resistance or barriers that come up in me.

I may already be sensing new hope and understanding."

After going through this sequence two or three times, you will probably find that you are already feeling more empowered about the relationship. Gauge this with another SUD rating on the amount of distress you feel when you think about your desire for the relationship to improve. You have also prepared yourself to take it further by next applying the guidance in this chapter.

MAKING YOUR RELATIONSHIPS MORE FULFILLING: THE INNER JOURNEY

In this chapter we will share some of what we've learned and how you can use acupoint tapping to better move through challenges that, for us, were so often snares into struggle and despair. While our focus will largely be on committed partnerships, the chapter is designed for anyone, whether or not you are currently in a long-term relationship. Rather than a manual for couples, as was *The Energies of Love*, this chapter focuses almost exclusively on the *inner* journey of being in a relationship. It may apply to the way you relate to a current partner or it may prepare you for a future partner. While same-sex or trans relationships involve many dynamics and considerations that differ from those of heterosexual partnerships, the challenges we address here apply to all. We have grouped them into seven broad themes:

1. Moving through emotional intensity without escalating.

2. Shifting the way you respond to behaviors in your partner that had been triggers for anger, hurt, or resentment.

3. Tracing emotional challenges—that play themselves out again and again in your relationships—to formative childhood experiences.

4. Healing these lingering emotional wounds.

5. Transforming the *patterns* that grew out of these early wounds.

6. Completing other "unfinished business" in your emotional life, including "baggage" from earlier relationships or an earlier time in your current relationship.

7. Establishing a vision of the relationship you desire and rewiring your brain to support that vision.

We invite you on a journey that will explore each of these topics. Although the focus is on the inner work required for sustaining a gratifying long-term intimate partnership, many of the principles apply to any relationship that matters to you, from friendships to parent-child dynamics to coworkers.

1. Moving Through Emotional Intensity Without Escalating

Whether or not you are in a close relationship, life presents ample opportunities for encountering situations that may provoke strong emotional reactions. We are wired for the fight-flight-freeze response, and it may be activated by a disrespectful coworker, an aggressive driver, or a spouse in a cranky mood. It's not that emotions are wrong. They guide us in our decisions, large and small. They become problematic when their intensity escalates to the extent that the emotional centers of your brain "hijack" the reasoning centers so you are unable to think clearly or act effectively.[6] Because human survival depended on staying together with a small clan, we evolved to be hypersensitive to emotional disruptions with those closest to us. We are most likely to experience hair-trigger outbursts with the ones we love.

The High Road and the Low Road. In *Parenting from the Inside Out*, the neuropsychiatrist Daniel Siegel and early childhood expert Mary Hartzell identify two fundamental types of responses to emotionally difficult situations: the "high road" and the "low road."[7] The high road is driven by advanced brain structures that emerged later in evolution. They are located "higher" in the cerebral cortex, toward the top of the head. The low road is dominated by subcortical brain structures, such as the amygdala, which regulate automatic behaviors, notably the fight-or-flight response. When taking the high road, your responses are well considered, adaptable, and situationally appropriate. When overly stressed or otherwise in a situation that triggers low-road reactions, you may be overcome by intense emotions such as fear, sadness, or rage, resulting in "reactions rather than thoughtful responses."[8] Low-road behaviors are familiar to all of us from both sides. We've received them and we've delivered them. Unresolved childhood issues make us more susceptible to these storms of tumultuous feelings and inappropriate behavior.

Using Energy Methods to Stay on the High Road. You've already seen throughout this book that energy techniques can send deactivating signals to the threat centers of your brain. But is it possible to use them in the middle of a heated exchange when your instincts are to fight or retreat? If you follow your raw impulses when your front brain is being pushed offline by your limbic system, it doesn't always work out so well. But how do you stop a freight train so you can work with your energies during an escalating encounter?

Havening. Well, you could say, "Give me a moment," take a deep breath, and shift your attention away from the interaction so you are fully engaged with noticing what is happening in your body. Then place each hand on its opposite shoulder and smooth them down to your elbows. Do this three or four times, continuing to breathe deeply while focusing inwardly. Known as "Havening,"[9] the movement crosses your energies from each side of your body to the other and calms Triple Warmer (the energy system involved with the fight-or-flight response). It also generates delta waves, which have a sedating effect on regions of your brain that are involved in processing emotionally charged experiences.

Take a Moment to Tap. This may be all you need to get back on the high road. If not, you might say something like, "I want to be fully present for you right now, but I'm distracted by [report the feelings or sensations you noticed without in any way returning to the disagreement]. I'm going to take another moment to stimulate some energy release points." From here, you could do any of the methods presented in the Appendix on steps you can take if the program becomes unsettling. "Tapping on the Reaction You Are Having" (p. 359) would be a good choice. Just go through the 12 acupoint tapping points once or twice. Words aren't needed since you are already in an emotionally charged state. Then turn inward and report to the person any changes in your emotions or sensations. This brings the other person into your process in a manner that is likely to increase empathy and align your energies so the conversation can continue with greater attunement (or it might cause the other person to judge you as being crazy, but at least you get some sympathy).

Tap While You Talk, Tap While You Listen. Another technique people who are close to one another can use is a "Tap While You Talk, Tap While You Listen" technique. Dawson Church explains,

> The moment you feel a rise in emotional intensity with someone you love, immediately start tapping. [This] tells your body that there's no need to go into the fight-flight-freeze response, that the current situation is not a threat to your physical survival, and that you're not traveling along the same dysfunctional neurological highway you've constructed in the past.[10]

Make a Pact. If the other person is your partner, colleague, or friend, you might explain in advance that you keep these approaches for retrieving your equanimity in your back pocket. That way it is already understood so you don't have to explain it while using it. It can be a pre-agreed ritual for defusing the tension that may emerge in any close relationship. In fact, in our *Energies of Love* book and workshops, we have couples make an ironclad "pact" that whenever either of them is starting to get triggered, they immediately stop the conversation and turn to energy exercises before proceeding.

All of these techniques build on the principle that a simple energy intervention can lead you away from primitive brain responses that escalate tension and toward front-brain control where your capacities for reasoning, patience, and empathy are more available to you.

The test driver we will feature in this chapter is Sasha, a 53-year-old accomplished singer who had trained in energy medicine but was relatively new to energy psychology.

Sasha's Work with an Intense Reaction

From her journal:

Some years ago, my husband began to collaborate with a new business partner. They began spending a lot of time together. Most of it was at our house. (We have a business that doesn't need an outside office, so much of our work when I'm not on the road is at our home.) The new partner was a woman. I have had many recurring trust issues in my life with other women and the men that I am in relationship with.

During this period, my husband and I started going through a very difficult time. We had two teenage children. We faced a great deal of financial stress, work stress, and living stress. I was traveling a lot for my work, which took me to different time zones. It was hard to link up or to talk and connect, and it seemed like communication with my husband just went completely down the drain.

When I had met with his new business partner, she had often expressed how lonely she was being a single woman and that she was really wishing to have a deep connection with someone and start a family. From the strain of our situation and the time I had to spend away from home, a new bond was formed between my husband and this woman that was deeper than I was comfortable with. But when I expressed my concern to him, he just brushed it off, as if it were part of my imagination and everything was fine. After one extremely long and faraway trip, I decided that I was going to take a break from traveling and focus my attention on healing my home life and relationship. This threw off what the woman—let's call her Sue—had become accustomed to.

One day Sue came to our house complaining that now that I was home, it was making it difficult for them to work late to plan, schedule projects, and grow the business. At first I was very calm and expressed honestly that there were a lot of things that my husband and I needed to work on. I was actively changing my work life in order to put things back in place, and I was sure the business would be fine if they adjusted their work hours to not cut into our evenings.

At this suggestion, Sue flew off the handle and began saying that she was my husband's best friend and how dare I try to impede on their success. It suddenly spiraled out of control. Of course, from the words she was saying and my previous trust issues, I felt the trigger go off in me, and I began to fight back. It turned into an ugly violent argument outside on our lawn. At that point, she stormed back to her car and drove off. I blamed the whole situation on my husband.

We fought for weeks about this, and some of the arguments and things that were said still haunt me to this day, even though Sue is no longer in our lives and the situation eventually got "resolved." I have dreams about it where I think I will react differently, and it still unfolds out of control and makes me feel sick to my stomach. I have often ruminated on how I might have been able to control my emotions and not let Sue get the best of me.

After doing the tapping routine on this (I did it about five times, with some energy work and rest in between), something shifted. I could deeply understand the situation that unfolded among the three of us. I felt an element of emotional learning that I had not experienced during the real-life situation. Now, as the tapping helped move

the emotions and stuck energies, I feel as if I can listen in to the emotions I'm feeling during the scenario, as well as to have more compassion for Sue in the hurt and anger she was experiencing. The tapping has also brought me to a place where I have been able to discuss the incident with my husband in an honest and open way, as opposed to turning him into the "enemy" because of my inability to process my own emotions.

Your Turn

Describe in your journal a situation where, in your judgment, you responded in a way that was extreme and unhelpful. It may have been with your current partner, a past partner, or any other relationship that matters to you. If a situation doesn't come to you, imagine one that might occur. Use the Basic Tapping Protocol as presented in Chapter 2 to reach the point that you can imagine being in the situation without overreacting. You can apply this to as many situations as you wish. It gives you practice for moving through emotional intensity without getting stuck on the low road.

2. Shifting the Way You Respond to Behaviors in Your Partner That Had Been Triggers for Anger, Hurt, or Resentment

In addition to being able to process emotional overreactions from your past, you can use energy techniques to make you less likely to overreact in the first place. One approach is mental rehearsal, which was featured in the previous chapter and is also basically what you were just doing with the previous instruction. If you know you are vulnerable to getting hooked by a certain person or topic, you can imagine a scenario in which you are likely to overreact and tap down the intensity of your emotional response. As the intensity decreases, you can also create a scenario where your response is just what you would like it to be and tap it in to secure the ideal response.

Doing this for a number of imagined provocative situations has an inoculating effect so you are more likely to meet the real-life situations with greater peace and composure. While we suggest you do this, we are also aware that you have been learning how to use the Basic Tapping Protocol to defuse emotional overreactions throughout the book. Here, instead of taking you through that process once more, we are going to go into deeper dynamics that will make you less vulnerable to triggers with your intimates.

Attachment Style. A concept that has become popular in professional circles and self-help literature is *attachment style*.[11] Your attachment style reflects the way you interact with others, particularly in your intimate relationships. It involves basic questions such as "Am I worthy of love?" and "Can I rely on others to meet my most basic needs?" Your attachment style was formed early in life—typically between your earliest months and two years—based on interactions with your parents or other primary caregivers. It is one of the most primary of your guiding models, and it can be broadly characterized as *secure* or *insecure*.

Secure attachment during childhood paves the way for greater ease with intimacy in adulthood. Individuals with a secure attachment style are generally optimistic regarding their primary relationship. They have a strong sense of self-worth; they expect closeness, warmth, and comfort in their relationships and tend to find it. They communicate their needs and emotions effectively, and they accurately interpret and respond to the emotional cues of their partner. They are able to emotionally soothe themselves as well as others, and they can move easily between intimacy and independence, resulting in the emotional and behavioral *interdependence* necessary for a successful relationship.

Insecure attachment in childhood lays the groundwork for later difficulties with intimacy. Children with insecure attachment did not receive the imprinting from their caregivers that would help them learn to establish secure bonds or regulate their own nervous systems, leaving them vulnerable to emotional problems throughout their lives. Insecure attachment behavior in intimate relationships may fall into either of two polar extremes: anxious clinging or emotional avoidance.

The potential for developing a secure attachment style can be found in your genes. It is what nature intended. For many people, their style of relating is relatively secure. But there's nothing like being in a long-term intimate partnership to discover the gaps. While a book isn't going to make anyone's attachment style leap from extremely insecure to unwaveringly secure, we can guide you in developing skills that will increase your ease and security with intimacy.

Self-Soothing. A fundamental skill that supports secure attachment is the ability to soothe yourself when you are feeling emotionally vulnerable. Because infants lack the ability to calm themselves when they are distressed, they must rely on their caregivers to provide comfort. They learn coping strategies for soothing distressing emotions or difficult experiences, for better or for worse, from the responses they receive.

Ideally, the ability to self-soothe was acquired during early interactions with your parents or other caregivers. You were upset. Your parent offered comforting words and got you playing with your favorite stuffy. You felt better and began to learn that shifting your attention to a pleasant activity allows an emotional upset to settle naturally. If, as an adult, you depend exclusively on your partner to soothe your upsets, your relationship will suffer under this excessive burden. Adults who have not developed adequate

self-soothing skills become overly reliant on their partner for emotional comfort and resentful when it is not provided.

Fortunately, skills for improving your mood and bringing calm, nurturing, and pleasure to your life can be learned at any age. They generally rely on your senses. Donna enjoys relaxing in a hot bath. We both enjoy going for walks in beautiful natural settings. Energy techniques for self-soothing, like those presented throughout the book and in the Appendix in particular, are always in our toolbox. Other popular forms of self-soothing include music, dance, art, sports, and meditation. These are simple, readily available, and generally free or almost free.

However, for those who did not learn in their formative years that they could make themselves feel better, calmer, or more relaxed, times of distress can result in an internal panic. This may lead to clutching toward others or escape into drugs, junk food, or other addictions. It may not occur to them, when feeling distraught, that they can take simple, healthy steps to improve their mood and outlook.

Whether or not self-soothing comes easily to you, it is an ability that can be further developed. One approach is to identify a calming technique you can count on and stimulate energy points to create a mental association between feeling needy and the technique, so it becomes a reflex. Phrases can be in the format of Choices Statements: *"When I feel lonely, I choose to sit on the porch and listen to Enya."* *"In dark times, I choose to do my favorite*

Pilates routine." "When Bob isn't there for me, I choose to savor Fido's undying love." If any objections to your plan emerge, you can then use the Basic Tapping Protocol to address these Psychological Reversals.

Putting Resources in Your Emotional Bank Account. In addition to creating a default self-soothing routine, you can invest in four commonsense ways to "put money in the bank" so your reserves are already stronger in the face of events that might be upsetting. They involve simple physical or interpersonal actions that are in your control: enough sleep, enough exercise, enough physical touch (even if you don't have a partner who can provide this, you can give hugs or trade massages with a friend), and enough emotional contact (which may take some creativity, but it is available from many sources). Paradoxically, as you become more adept at self-soothing, the easier it becomes for a partner to provide comforting support.

While emotional overreactions to your partner may be addressed in any number of ways using tapping, strengthening your ability to calm your "low road" reactions is one of the most powerful, and it is our focus right now. Here is how Sasha approached it.

Sasha's Default Calming Technique and How She Built More Emotional Reserve

From Sasha's journal:

One thing I do in dark times is to get in my car and put on my favorite music and sing at the top of my lungs in order to feel connected with my true happy self again. Another is to pull out picture albums of my childhood and go down memory lane thinking of childhood adventures that rekindle a love I have for my journey here in this life.

For establishing emotional reserves, I focused on getting more sleep. For the Choices Statement, I used *"Even though I often do not get enough sleep, I choose right here and now to change that habit."* Tapping on the Reminder Phrase *"Not getting enough sleep"* helped alleviate the pressure I feel to "get to bed at the right time" and shifted it to a feeling of "getting to bed to rest is something I'm doing *for* me."

Your Turn

Describe a calming technique that you find reliable or can imagine being dependable (see earlier examples involving Enya, Pilates, and Fido, as well as Sasha's). Create a Choices Statement that pairs this technique with circumstances that might make you feel needy or vulnerable. Say it out loud three times, rubbing your chest sore spots with the first phrase and placing your hands over your Heart Chakra with the second. You can repeat this several days in a row until you feel the connection has been made. If internal objections arise, address them using the Basic Tapping Protocol.

Finally, take an inventory of the four ways of establishing emotional reserves: sleep, exercise, physical touch, and emotional contact. Consider whether you would like to increase your reserves in any of these areas and, if so, create an Acceptance Statement (Sasha's was *"Even though I don't get enough sleep, I deeply and completely accept myself"*) that evolves into a Choices Statement (e.g., *"Even though I don't get enough sleep, I choose right here and now to change this habit"*). Tapping on the Reminder Phrase (e.g., *"Not getting enough sleep"*) will reduce the charge on the issue, and the Choices Statement will open a pathway to changing the habit. You can also turn to the techniques in Chapter 6 for establishing desirable habits.

3. Tracing Emotional Challenges to Formative Childhood Experiences That Play Themselves Out Again and Again in Your Relationships

Jeremy was 36 when he married Melissa.[12] He was eager to help raise her seven- and nine-year-old sons. He had gotten to know them quite well during the year prior to the marriage; he had brought them to baseball games, zoos, parks, and other local attractions; and he had participated in their hobbies. The boys liked their stepdad and the attention he was giving them, and the new family was blossoming within an atmosphere of affection and promise. Melissa's ex-husband, Steve, the boys' biological father, had not been particularly eager to spend time with his sons during the marriage, but he also loved them. Because of a job change after the divorce, he had moved to another town several hours away, but he had been reliable in taking the boys for the afternoon every other Sunday.

During his courtship with Melissa, Jeremy had never met Steve. But now that Jeremy had moved in with the family, the twice-monthly visits became a fixture in his life. He was civil enough toward his new wife's ex, but he avoided having much contact with him when the boys were being picked up or dropped off. During the first Christmas vacation after the marriage, Steve arranged to take the boys for a week, and the three of them flew to Orlando for a Disney marathon. The boys were so excited about it that they seemed to talk of little else for the week prior to and for weeks after the trip.

When Steve came for the next Sunday visitation, Jeremy could hardly look at him. He began to criticize Steve's parenting style to Melissa, point out his culpability in the divorce, and generally paint an ugly picture of the man who had fathered her children. At first Melissa acknowledged the truth in some of the observations, but over time Jeremy became increasingly vehement in his criticisms. This grew into a loaded theme in their interactions on the weekends when Steve would be arriving, and Jeremy began questioning the boys about their visits with their father, as if looking for more fodder for his rants. He was eventually unable to hide his disdain toward their father from the boys.

Jeremy's jealousy toward Steve continued to escalate, and the acrimony was seeping into other areas of the family. As Steve's visits approached, tension would descend onto the household. The boys were confused. Melissa began to judge Jeremy harshly. She had more than once called him a "spoiled brat." This was the state of things when they scheduled a couples counseling session with David. Jeremy knew at some level that his reactions were not rational, but this knowledge did not hold a candle to the strength of his emotions. When Jeremy was triggered, Steve was an evil man sabotaging all of Jeremy's fine efforts with the boys and the family, and there was no other reality to consider.

After hearing both of their renditions of the problem, David spoke to the part of Jeremy that knew his reactions to Steve were extreme. David explained that when intense emotions are triggered, they are very real, whether rational or irrational. He suggested tapping to take the edge off the intensity of Jeremy's responses to Steve. Neither Jeremy nor Melissa had any experience with energy psychology, but the couple who referred them had worked with David and described the method, so they were game for whatever could help, however strange it might look. While Jeremy was not particularly open to considering that his assessment of Steve might be wrong, he was interested in feeling less consumed by his reactions.

They proceeded, following essentially the same steps you have been using throughout this book. The scene that Jeremy chose for his SUD rating was from the previous Sunday, watching as Steve's car pulled into the driveway. It was a 10 on the 0-to-10 SUD scale. After four tapping cycles, it had gone down to a 7, but even after further tapping it seemed to be stuck there. David asked, "How do you know it is a 7?" Jeremy said that he felt pressure in his chest and a tightness in his throat. David asked him to explore the feelings in his throat. Jeremy said it is almost as if he were trying to hold back tears. David asked if he could recall one of the first times he had that feeling. Jeremy immediately recalled a memory from age 10 when his parents brought a foster boy into the family. It was just a temporary favor for a relative of the boy until a permanent placement could be found, but it changed everything for Jeremy.

As an only child, Jeremy had enjoyed his parents' full attention and affection. Suddenly that was history. The foster boy had many problems. Both of Jeremy's parents held full-time jobs, and their limited time and resources shifted from Jeremy to the new boy. Jeremy, at 10, did not have words or concepts that could help him come to grips with the loss. He felt emotionally abandoned by both of his parents. He could not fathom why they had brought this troublesome person into their home, and he hated the foster boy. He began starting fights and creating acrimony wherever he could. This strategy seemed to eventually work. After about a year, the agency found a permanent placement for the boy, and Jeremy never saw him again. All of this was buried in the recesses of Jeremy's psyche. He hadn't thought about it for years, and no other circumstance in his adult life had triggered his unprocessed feelings around that chapter from his childhood. He had never thought to mention it to Melissa, but the parallels between the foster boy and the situation with Steve became immediately obvious to all three of us. We'll return to Jeremy and Melissa in the following section.

Early Experiences That Created a Blueprint for Current Events. Being able to calm overreactions and soothe emotional upset, the skills we've focused upon so far, may go a long way toward emotional self-management. But if unresolved trauma or unmet emotional needs from your past are interfering with your current relationship or a future one,

more is needed. Managing the intense emotions that can be evoked when interacting with your intimate may require a focus on unresolved issues from the past. Admittedly this can be a lifelong project.

Many people find the "spiral theory" of personal development mentioned earlier to be encouraging. Rather than repeating the same lessons, we return to old issues from a higher level of personal evolution. The more effectively you deal with an issue during the current round of the spiral, the more the issue becomes a source of experience and wisdom rather than a limitation when an analogous situation appears.

Your Emotional Reactions to Your Partner. More than 100 human emotions have been identified, and most of them are combinations of a few basic emotions shared by people of all cultures, such as anger, fear, sadness, disgust, surprise, anticipation, trust, and joy.[13] The way these emotions are expressed is then shaped by the culture. The word *emotion* comes from the Old French *esmovoir*, which means "to excite." While psychologists define this fundamental concept in a variety of ways, all agree that emotions involve arousal ("to excite") and that they influence how we process our thoughts and experiences.

At the most basic level, in the life of an infant, an internal event (such as hunger, pain, warmth, or cold) or an external event (such as a loud sound or a warm blanket) results in simple appraisals: "This is good" or "This is bad." While this is the prototype for the more nuanced emotions that will come later, this basic assessment of good or bad, explains the psychiatrist Daniel Siegel, "prepares the brain and the rest of the body for action."[14]

The neural pathways that help a child learn to regulate their nervous system are laid down by the parents' responses to the infant's expressions of positively or negatively toned arousal. Through those early interactions, you learned how to manage your inner states. If your parents' reactions to you were attuned to your internal experiences, you were more likely to develop a solid foundation for navigating life with confidence in the validity of your feelings and thoughts.

On the other hand, if your early caregivers failed to validate your internal experiences in their moment-to-moment interactions with you, your foundation for trusting your feelings and thoughts as valid guides became shaky. Children are wired to incorporate emotional responses and behaviors that mimic those of their caregivers through mirror neurons. As mentioned in the previous chapter, mirror neurons are brain cells that are activated when a behavior is witnessed, establishing neural pathways for repeating the behavior. If the lack of attunement is severe, as in cases of abusive, emotionally disturbed, or severely neglectful parents, children are launched on their journey through life with a fundamentally flawed compass. They may find themselves regularly suppressing, distorting, or becoming overwhelmed by their emotions and experiences.

Early caregivers not only validate or fail to validate the child's internal experiences but they also model how to respond when others express their emotions. A girl may take it upon herself to provide a fearful mother with the support the girl actually needs from her mother, or she may try to disappear in the presence of an angry father. Even when they no longer fit, such patterns often carry over into our adult relationships. A parent whose internal state is dominated by fear or anger reinforces the child's fears or anger.

Connecting Your Emotional Reactions to Earlier Experiences. Your ability to manage your emotional reactions to current relationships has its foundations in your early interpersonal experiences. When low-road reactions occur, and particularly when they repeat themselves, notice what triggers them. Even if you can't identify the triggers, your partner probably can. Just as Jeremy's responses to Steve became a springboard for his long-forgotten yet formative year with the foster boy, you will be invited to recall a memory that is a precursor of current difficulties.

This exploration will make the memories accessible for healing using the tapping protocols you have been learning. In the following scenario, you will be using the Affect Bridge (p. 109) to identify an early incident that still impacts your relationships. Sasha began with the feelings that still lingered about the woman who had grown so attached to her husband.

Sasha's Memory and Reflections about It

From Sasha's journal:

The Affect Bridge technique brought me back to a scene I had witnessed many times as a child. My parents were in an argument. My mother was hurt, comparing herself negatively with other women my father found attractive. My father was discounting whatever she said, calling it hysteria. My mother began to scream, as people do when they are being gaslighted (not a phrase I knew when I was growing up—but my father did it constantly, telling my mother that her thoughts/feelings/opinions didn't make sense). People being gaslighted *need* to be heard, witnessed, and understood. Soon they were in a screaming match.

As a little girl watching this, I felt heartbrokenly sad but helpless to do anything about it. So I got accustomed to it. My mother screamed all the time. I thought everyone's household was as loud as mine. When I moved out into the world on my own, my boyfriends would say, "What are you yelling at?" I'd say, "This isn't yelling, this was normal talking in my household," as if it were a badge of honor.

With super-traumatic childhoods of their own, and as children of World War II, my parents were running on empty and easily triggered. Their relationship was turbulent from the beginning. My mother got pregnant unplanned. She was not thinking of having another child. She was divorced from her first husband, with whom she had two children. My father had been a wild child who loved seducing women. He had no roots in the ground.

I don't have any proof that my father ever "cheated" on my mother, but she certainly made it seem like he had. Throughout their relationship, this tug of war continually existed. In any case, my father was a big flirt. He could not go to a party with my mother without them coming home in a fierce argument about who he had flirted with, how he had dishonored my mom, and on and on. Many nights were filled with drunken screaming matches followed by days filled with awkward silences.

Tiptoeing around the house during the silent spells was a skill I perfected. I had learned how to navigate a battlefield. When entering my own relationships, this was my framework. Jealousy, suspicion, and mistrust were some of the earliest tools I developed to try to protect myself. I have learned through therapy that jealousy is my personal fallback. Therapy has taught me to try to be curious about it, to dissect it, analyze it, embrace it, and integrate it. *Much* easier said than done. There has been a stream of women in and out of my intimate partnerships, and I have had to battle inner demons about them.

I never know quite what is suspicion, madness, or reality. Are they *really* trying to get between me and my husband or is this just the distorted lens of how I see relationships? To make it worse, my mother presented other women to me with judgment and distrust. So I have had difficulty forming long-term relationships with women due to this inherent suspicion, even without a man and romantic relationship being involved.

Your Turn

Identify a pattern in your relationships that seems to interfere with the intimacy and satisfaction you desire with your partner or loved ones. It may be as simple as not speaking up in a situation where, for instance, your partner is keen to see a particular movie but you would prefer a different one. Or it might be that you become irritated with very little provocation. Or you simply don't make time for the relationship. Or it might involve extreme jealousy or violent outbursts. Bring to mind a specific incident in which that pattern was playing out. Notice a dominant feeling or sensation as you focus on it. Use the Affect Bridge to ride it back in time to an earlier experience characterized by a parallel feeling or sensation. Describe and reflect on it in your journal. You will be processing it in the following section.

4. Healing These Lingering Emotional Wounds

Returning now to Jeremy and Melissa, after having discovered the hidden roots of Jeremy's irrational jealousy toward Steve, we tapped on every aspect of the memory we could identify, staying with each until it was down to a 0: Jeremy's loss of his parents' attention; his frequently having to hold back his tears when he felt lonely and abandoned; his confusion and puzzlement about what he had done wrong to deserve having so much attention withdrawn from him; the invasion into his family; his hatred for the new boy; the fights he had with the new boy; his being punished for starting the fights and feeling like a bad boy after 10 years of being a good boy; and even his confusion when the new boy suddenly disappeared.

Fortunately, since a round of tapping takes only about a minute, all of this was accomplished within that first two-hour session, David's standard for initial sessions with couples. Jeremy was by then able to talk lucidly and calmly about the foster boy's invasion into his young life. And he could reflect on how Steve's visits with the boys were bringing up feelings that traced back to his experiences with the foster boy. He was entertaining the possibility that his sense that Steve was purposefully trying to destroy the family Jeremy was building had something to do with this earlier scenario. Focusing again on watching Steve's car pulling into the driveway, Jeremy gave it an SUD rating of 3. A couple more tapping cycles and it was down to a 0.

We chose this case because so much was accomplished in a single session, making it easier to convey the steps that were taken. Healing deep emotional wounds may require multiple sessions, tapping on numerous incidents from your past. If you are discovering old wounds that seem to be calling for attention, be patient with yourself. While it may require some time and effort to clear unresolved experiences that are interfering with your current relationships, the benefits can be substantial and long-lasting.

How Sasha Brought Healing to Her Formative Childhood Experiences

Sasha obviously had many painful memories tied to witnessing the hostility between her parents. While she had described some of them in previous therapies over the years, they hadn't been emotionally resolved, and they were at the base of guiding models that hindered her relationships: "Intimacy is measured by the intensity of the fights and drama in the relationship." "Men will hurt me; women will help them do it." "Trust is for fools."

Sasha first tapped on the memory of her parents having returned from a party one night. She guessed she was about 12. She had been awakened by their screaming. The initial SUD was a 10. She applied the Basic Tapping Protocol and got the amount of distress she felt in bringing the memory to mind down to 6. She identified a Psychological Reversal that she put into this Choices Statement: *"Even though relationships are always either angry or silent, I choose to recognize that my parents aren't the only available models."* This gave some relief, and the SUD about the memory went down to 4. Several aspects then came to her mind, including *"It's my fault that I can't get them to be nice to each other," "This is what I have to look forward to in my own marriage," "A feeling of breathlessness in my chest."*

She gave each aspect an SUD and tapped the amount of bodily distress it caused down to 0. As the intensity of the original memory diminished, she began to see some of the ironies in the distorted type of intimacy her parents' marriage presented to her. She worded a new Acceptance Statement, this time with some humor: *"Even though my parents had the emotional intelligence of a couple of snails, I love and deeply accept myself."* She battled her SUD about the memory of being awakened by her parents' screaming down to a 0. She did this with several other memories of her parents' fights. Each became easier to fully resolve than the one before it since they shared many of the same aspects. Once an aspect had been resolved, it didn't usually carry over to the next memory.

A surprising insight emerged when Sasha reflected on her need to argue. It involved the early patterning that held "fighting is a measure of intimacy." She wrote in her journal:

It seemed to stem from my ancestors. Ancestral patterns along my feminine line involved keeping their mouths shut, not being honored, feeling pain, and experiencing repression. I started to realize that the fighting that my mother would instigate was connected to her mother and grandmother and on and on. It wasn't just anger about my father's flirting. It felt connected to generations I wasn't even aware of. I started tapping on imprints that seemed encoded in my DNA. What memories were alive in me that were carrying my female ancestors' lives of guilt, shame, suppression, fear, and repressed anger? Many tears flowed that sometimes felt like mine while other times had a texture of "timelessness."

Your Turn

Returning to the scene you entered using the Affect Bridge, use any of the tools in Chapters 2 and 3 to reduce the emotional charge on that experience and to work with any aspects or Psychological Reversals that arise. This may lead you on a long and complex journey, but even if you limit your focus to reducing the impact of a single unresolved formative experience, it is likely to play out as a positive change for your current or future relationships.

5. Transforming the *Patterns* That Grew Out of These Early Wounds

Even after healing or resolving earlier experiences, patterns that have been established around these wounds may continue to persist. While you may find many benefits to having accomplished deep transformative change, the surrounding structure of your life may still need to catch up. The steps for the outer changes will be patterned after the inner changes. We'll share two examples here: one from Jeremy and the other from Gwen, another of David's clients.

For Jeremy, while the tapping was quick and very effective in healing the residue from the disorienting change in his life when the foster boy came into his home, the uproar he had created in his marriage still needed repair. We were able to address this toward the end of the initial session by bringing the focus to Melissa. She had just seen and been moved by the transformative work Jeremy had done, yet she was still reeling from her dismay about the rapid decline of her new marriage and her sense of betrayal. Jeremy had gone from an apparently ideal stepfather to an angry, jealous, irrational force in their home. Witnessing Jeremy's work had already put all of this into a welcome new light, but her hurt and distrust lingered. We began by tapping on her sense of bewilderment and betrayal. By the end of the session, she was able to revisit the strange course of her young marriage with relief rather than horror.

On a follow-up meeting two weeks later, Jeremy described what he had done with the boys and with Steve. He had asked the boys if they had ever felt jealous about each other. He helped each of them recognize times this had happened and got them to talk about how it felt to be on each side of jealousy. He used this as a jumping-off point to explain how he had become jealous of their father and to reassure them that this was now in the past, providing glimpses of his process. Upon Steve's next visit, Jeremy went out to the driveway to greet him before he came into the house. Jeremy began, "I have a story to tell you, Steve," and he recounted the highlights of the counseling session, with apologies and expressions of appreciation for the ways Steve was stepping up and playing a positive role in the boys' lives.

In the second example, Gwen was the youngest of five children. She had been unplanned. Her parents were already overwhelmed by the needs of their first three children when the fourth, Gwen's closest older brother, was diagnosed with cerebral palsy at age two. Gwen showed up a year later. By the time she was four, she had established her role in the family as "Mommy's little helper." She would assist in the preparation of school lunch bags each evening. She would comfort her older siblings when they were upset. As she got older, she was alert for their needs and would figure out innovative ways to help meet them. She had learned to keep her own needs in the background so that she didn't add to her parents' overpowering burdens.

Gwen grew up to be a model citizen and then wife and mother. She was active in community groups and would uncomplainingly do the tasks no one else wanted. She never said no to a request. In her neighborhood, she was the one who would bring food to anyone who was ill or grieving. In her marriage, her husband would have his underwear folded and his meals meticulously prepared. Her children were accustomed to the creative ways their mother would dote on them. When Gwen entered therapy, at age 35, she was overwhelmed with her life and soul-deep exhausted. As she and David explored her formative experiences and the guiding model that emerged from them, they named the theme "The Helping Hand Strikes Again!" She began tapping on the many aspects of this model and the experiences that shaped it. She had adapted to her needy family by minimizing her own needs and attending to those of everyone else. Her sense of self-worth was tied to this role, and when her pain that she was not valued in any other way revealed itself, it was intense. Tapping allowed her to defuse these memories so they no longer had her reliving the compulsion to help.

As Gwen addressed the emotional pain she had carried but repressed her entire life, new insights began to flood her. After watching a television program about people who had been displaced by warfare, Gwen had a series of dreams in which she was trapped in a refugee camp and had to use her wits to get free. Freedom from the oppressive grip of her unrelenting impulse to offer herself up whenever someone had a need or desire became the theme of her therapy. As she made strides in liberating herself from this deeply embedded pattern, however, her world did not applaud her progress. Everyone was accustomed to benefiting from what she was now trying to eradicate from her life. The final stages of the therapy involved a form of assertiveness training where she became practiced in saying no and stating, while tapping, the simple fact that she isn't available. This shifted everyone's expectations quite effectively, despite their initial disappointment and the adjustments it required of them.

Patterns Sasha Decided to Change

Sasha reflected in her journal:

My pattern of so readily going into "fight" mode grew out of the early life situations I've been exploring. This led me to fight with childhood friends, cutting off relationships prematurely, sometimes without any explanation. Numerous friendships have been victims to my deep-seated trust issues.

Looking back, I don't really know if I might have been able to trust the person, but I instead allowed the triggers to lead the way. Even if I did try to trust them, a lack of learning true intimacy and relationship skills was more of the driving factor to cutting off friendships and relationships.

Tapping helped me reduce the anxiety during "build-ups" of feeling that a fight is coming on. It was able to at least stall the instinct so I could walk metaphorically 360 degrees around the situation and analyze the driving forces. All of this cemented in for me two insights that seem to come from opposite directions, one about fighting and one about quiet:

1. I used to gauge how intense and true my relationships were by how many fights we could have and then resolve. It was as if the fight was a necessary component for the quality and depth of intimacy. In discussing this insight with my husband, we identified all the other ways available to us for intimacy that beat the daylights out of having to fight so we could make up.

2. Learning a pattern of "The Silent Treatment" after fights taught me to not really go into the depths and resolve the issue but rather to hold back my truths, bite my tongue, and swallow my thoughts, as if there was shame associated with them, probably from being *ashamed* because I usually instigated the fight in the first place. This insight led to me asking my husband to gently call me on it if I revert to "The Silent Treatment." It's a pattern I'm committed to changing.

Your Turn

Reflect on whether a current pattern in your life corresponds with outdated learnings that grew out of the early experiences you have been exploring. If you can identify such a pattern in your life, are you interested in changing it? If so, what steps would be required? Consider the examples provided by Jeremy, Gwen, and Sasha and put the changes that fit for you into motion. Use the Basic Tapping Protocol as needed to support you in taking those steps.

6. Completing Other "Unfinished Business" in Your Emotional Life, Including "Baggage" from Earlier Relationships or an Earlier Time in Your Current Relationship

Charlotte and Silas had been married for 28 years when they came in for couples counseling. Their youngest daughter had just moved away for college, and they were looking forward to a new phase in their lives. They had arranged for an educational tour in Greece and were thinking of another in Tibet the following year. But just as the empty-nest possibilities for greater intimacy were opening, Charlotte found herself pulling away from the relationship. She couldn't explain why, but she was aware that she had become increasingly critical of Silas, often angrily, and she had lost interest in sex.

In the eighth year of their marriage, Silas had a brief affair with a coworker while Charlotte was consumed with the care of their two young daughters. When Charlotte learned of the betrayal, she was enraged and devastated. She and the girls moved in with her parents. Silas was consumed with guilt and terrified that he had irreparably wrecked his family. He abruptly ended the affair and begged for forgiveness.

Charlotte wasn't interested. As she initiated divorce proceedings, they began working with a mediator to negotiate finances and visiting arrangements. In the process, they began talking to each other with a level of honesty that had become unfamiliar for them. They realized how much they had grown apart in the past couple of years. The mediator sensed an emerging ambivalence in Charlotte about the divorce and suggested that she see a therapist to explore her complex feelings about taking this critical step. The therapy was empowering for her. After working through her pain about the affair, she set terms for Silas to earn his way back into the family. She was reassured when he met those terms with gratitude.

In couples counseling with David nearly two decades later, Charlotte discovered that her newly emerging anger and withdrawal traced back to Silas' affair. When she took Silas back into the family after he acquiesced to her terms, she felt renewed passion for him and believed she had fully processed her hurt, anger, and sense of betrayal in her therapy sessions at the time. But this was also in the context that there was a great deal of incentive to continue her life with the father of her children. With the departure of their youngest, that incentive was no longer there, and her psyche was doing a new reckoning of the situation, largely outside of Charlotte's awareness.

As this became obvious, the counseling revisited every aspect of the affair, Charlotte's reactions to it at the time, and Silas' current perspective about it. The principle of the "spiral" was at play: that issues that seemed resolved at one point in our lives reemerge, letting us come to terms with them from new levels of experience and maturity. Tapping on the lingering hurt and anger around the affair, which Charlotte thought had been put to bed long before, resolved them at a deeper level.

Another layer in Charlotte's restlessness was that she had developed a sense of independence and self-sufficiency she didn't have 20 years earlier. For Silas, he had no ambivalence about wanting to be with Charlotte for the rest of his life. This was reassuring for Charlotte, but not enough. The counseling included tapping on ways that her newfound sense of independence could be expressed within the marriage by changing patterns in which Silas had been the de facto decision-maker.

Sasha's "Unfinished Business"

Of several incidents that came to her mind, Sasha focused on one from early in her marriage:

The beginning of my marriage had a lot of turmoil brought on by aggressive and turbulent outbursts from my husband's ex-wife that were directed at me. They were hurtful and exhausting. My husband and his ex have a son together, and the interactions between her and me were always darkened by her demeaning statements and passive-aggressive comments.

There are elements that I didn't think could ever get resolved because my husband didn't want to intercede and become involved in the arguments. I felt that no one had my back.

From my vantage point, I was doing everything I could to create a caring and loving atmosphere for their son during the times he was in our household. I abided by all the "rules" his ex had laid out on how the visits were to go. On top of all this, she would write odd and strange emails or letters to my husband with slightly intimate statements, which I found inappropriate. All this was consistently swept under the rug under the guise of me "being insecure" and "letting her get the best of me."

From childhood I have had to fend for myself due to the volatile nature of my parents' relationship. In therapy I had discovered that I held resentment that in all the mental abuse and narcissism my mother afforded me, my father never stepped in. He would just stay in the bedroom, hide away from the madness, and then apologize to me the next day.

But the damage had been done. I do not feel like I had a positive masculine force in my childhood providing protection or nurturing. I didn't receive this from my mother either. Now I have a defense mechanism that goes up when I am in a new situation where I feel a woman is looking to take advantage of my husband, or even tries to get close to him. Immediately I am reminiscing about past situations that mirror the nature of my own childhood home, like when my husband's ex was so toxic.

My SUD rating reflecting on this started at a 10. After using the bridge technique to go back into the first times I felt these emotions as a child and then to tap through those, it dropped to a 7. Then it took me quite a while to do more tapping on the specific conversations I began to remember and the demeaning statements his ex had said to me, all along tapping through the emotions. After about eight tapping cycles, the SUD was at a 1. I'm not completely unattached to the memories, but they are not charging me emotionally.

7. Establishing a Vision of the Relationship You Desire and Rewiring Your Brain to Support That Vision

In the previous chapter on peak performance, we focused on ways that tapping on Power Phrases and visualizations can bring about neurological shifts that alter your automatic thoughts and behaviors. Remember that tapping embeds them more deeply into your nervous system. Once the Psychological Reversals attached to them have been removed, this becomes an extraordinarily powerful way to change old guiding models.

When applying this approach to your relationships, you are likely to have the most creative and compelling visions after you have had some success with the six topics covered above. By untethering your relationships from knee-jerk responses and baggage from your past, you free your psyche to wander into the land of possibility. That is why we saved establishing a vision for last.

Linda and Lynne (Lynne's given name was also Linda, but when their relationship was becoming a "thing," she changed it to help preserve everyone's sanity) had done a great deal of deep psychological work on their partnership. Lynne was inclined to be accommodating—for example, having volunteered to give up her name—and her accommodations were giving Linda power in setting the terms for the relationship that Lynne didn't really want and secretly resented. This tendency inhibited their intimacy. In jointly envisioning the couple they wanted to become, they both imagined an easy give-and-take between them in making decisions small and large, from what to have for dinner to whether they would move to a more hospitable setting as climate change was making their current location less desirable. For this technique, being as specific as possible is helpful. So, it wasn't just a vague vision of an idyllic relationship that they cultivated. They made a difficult decision they were already facing and imagined navigating it in just the way they hoped.

At the time, relatives of Linda had just tragically died in a car accident, and Lynne and Linda were faced with the difficult decision of whether to adopt the family's three-year-old son. In envisioning their deliberations as easy and positive and in a good flow, they went through the steps you learned in the previous chapter until both found the vision quite believable (SUB of 8 and 10, respectively). When they returned to the actual discussion, Lynne held her own as they came to a mutually agreeable decision, which in this instance was to not adopt. If you are in a partnership, crafting the vision together can be bonding and instructive. If you are not in a partnership, focusing the vision around a friend, boss, employee, family member, or even an imagined future partner can be powerful.

Once you have made reasonable progress on the six issues addressed above, you have opened the energy to take your relationship into new dimensions. Your imagination can be a bridge for getting there.

Sasha's Positive Visions

Sasha created two visions: one for her marriage and one for her friendships. For her marriage, she envisioned having a husband who is invested in couple's therapy as a way to deepen understanding, dive into collaboration about where the relationship is headed, and come up with common life goals. "I often feel as if both of us are headed in different directions, and he has resistance to getting a third party—a therapist—involved to help us navigate into a deepened relationship. As I first created the vision of

my husband agreeing to go to therapy, the believability was a 2. After three tapping cycles, imagining myself being increasingly persuasive with him to seek marriage counseling and to enter it with optimism and a positive attitude, it was up to 8. I still don't know if he will agree, but I do know that I will present my hopes more effectively."

Focusing on her friendships, Sasha reflected, "I have had the most difficult time creating friendships. I long for meaningful conversations, sharing information and ideas, experiences, caring, and support. I created a vision of meeting people with common interests, who are equally curious about my life as I am about theirs and forming friendships with them. As I tapped on starting to develop such a friendship with a new neighbor, the believability was 0. None! In fact, the tapping brought up feelings of abandonment and loneliness. It was quite difficult, even painful. Truthfully, I will have to return to this because I feel it is tethered to messages and experiences with my mother that have still not been resolved. This is one that will be continued."

Your Turn

Choose a person you feel close to—whether a life partner, family member, friend, or colleague—but would like to feel still closer. Envision what you desire for the relationship. Think about what gets in the way of your taking the next step toward greater intimacy. Select a scene that epitomizes this issue, whether one that actually occurred or one that may occur. It might or might not touch on the challenges so far addressed in this chapter. Be specific. Where are you in this vision? What are you wearing? What is it that has come up? Imagine that you are able to move through the situation in a manner that you consider ideal. Rate its believability (SUB rating, where 10 is completely believable). Follow the steps on pages 123–124 for using tapping methods to increase the believability of a desired scene. Repeat as often as needed, visiting aspects as they emerge, until the rating is up to at least an 8.

SOME WAYS ENERGY METHODS HAVE AND HAVEN'T WORKED FOR US

We have personally used every technique in this book as well as all of the techniques in *The Energies of Love*. Along with crafting them for our clients, we frequently used them ourselves to deal with our relationship crisis of the week during the difficult early years of our time together. While we feel blessed and grateful for the ways we now love and enjoy each other, we wish we could say it was always easy. It wasn't. We'll give you one example. It involved the EFT "Tap While You Talk, Tap While You Listen" technique (p. 283).

In introducing this method, Dawson Church explains that for many couples, well-traveled pathways in the brain are so deeply established that the couple gets "sucked into the same old lose-lose situation,"[15] even when they know they are going to crash if they travel along that path. Since tapping intervenes at the level of your brain chemistry, it slows emotional reactivity, signals safety to your limbic system, allows you to take a breath and, in that moment, look at your partner through fresh eyes and actively listen rather than just react in old ways. The first time we tried this, it worked beautifully. We had been looking for an opportunity to experiment with it before we wrote about it.

Donna was in a situation where, due to unforeseen circumstances, she had to change some plans without consulting with David. She knew this would cause some inconvenience for him, and she was already on edge when they talked about what had occurred. One of her most deeply entrenched life patterns is to cause no "trouble." When she did cause trouble, she expected the other person to be hurt, angry, or upset. Besides this anticipation already having a built-in self-fulfilling quality, it was so rare that Donna inconvenienced the people closest to her that they tended to feel surprised and hurt if she didn't meet their expectations. So, as she began the conversation with David, she already felt upset that he was (presumably) irritated, as if there could never be any room for her to make her own (possibly inconvenient) decisions. This of course has the effect of bringing out a defensive emotional response in the partner.

Hearing the tone in Donna's voice, David said, "Whoa! This is the moment we've been waiting for! I'm going to start tapping, and I hope you will too." David was indeed a bit put out by the abrupt change in plans, but (tap, tap, tap) he hadn't gone into the reaction Donna was anticipating. When she essentially accused him of having gone there, it did not hook him. He of course doesn't know what would have happened if he weren't tapping, but he later reflected that listening while tapping seemed to help him receive Donna's emotional charge without taking it personally. As Donna tapped while explaining the circumstances, as well as when listening to David's response, she recognized that he was taking her in deeply and understood what occurred, and (voila!) we were both quickly done with it.

However, the next time we were in an emotionally charged situation and used this "Tap While You Talk, Tap While You Listen" technique, it made things much worse. An effect of tapping while telling a story is that it helps you go more deeply into the story, uncovering emotions to which you did not have conscious access. If the incident you are tapping on touches into a theme that has a great deal of unresolved emotion, you may simply escalate the situation, uncovering layer after layer without resolving a thing before the next unresolved emotion or memory has surfaced. If you find that continuing the conversation while tapping is escalating the negative emotions or starting to spin out of control, it is time to change strategies—immediately! You can, for instance, use any of the techniques in the Appendix or shift the tapping from the conversation to the emotions being unleashed.

While energy techniques, adjusted moment by moment as you've been learning to do from one SUD rating to the next, usually achieve the desired effect, given the complexity of a relationship, you should certainly use any technique with discernment. We'll close this chapter with an episode from our marriage when we had to use everything we knew to turn things around. Based on our three decades at the time of teaching "The Relationship Rollercoaster" and then "Energies of Love" seminars, we were asked to write *The Energies of Love*. As we convey in that book,[16] we found it an exciting invitation, but we had a somewhat superstitious hesitation. We have known several couples over the years who have written books on couples work whose marriages dissolved shortly after their book was published. We did not want to tempt the relationship gods. Along with the personal catastrophe and awkward embarrassment that would be involved, we were wary about the arrogance of holding ourselves out as a couple who had somehow "figured out" the sweet and not-so-sweet mysteries of love.

Sure enough, as soon as we were earnestly discussing the book with the publisher, our relationship took a serious downhill turn. Our organization happened to be growing exponentially at the time. We were both under tremendous pressure. Not surprisingly, given the chasms between the ways each of us approaches the world, we weren't seeing eye to eye on many of the critical decisions we were making that would shape the future of our organization and our life's work.

The differences in our ways of understanding the world when we are under stress were becoming so exaggerated that misunderstandings were amassing. In situations like this, Donna becomes highly expressive emotionally, while David wants to crawl into his interior cave and regroup. So, Donna would feel unmet and discounted, and this would escalate her sense of distress. Feeling pressed not to retreat, David tried to center himself for each hot topic we would encounter, but he began to respond in a way that he could "hardly believe was me."

With unrelenting tension between us, and both of us locked into our threat-response styles, David would be pushed over the edge of his calm defenses. He would begin to scream at Donna, swear at her, and generally exacerbate a situation that was already too escalated. While your stress style is a way of processing information that has built-in strengths, when you are pushed far enough, your reasoning abilities can regress to roughly the equivalent of a four-year-old during a tantrum. That your partner can send you down the rabbit hole into another encounter with your unresolved wounds seems part of nature's grand scheme to help you evolve. After each incident, David would commit himself to not getting triggered the next time.

He would use all the techniques he knew. He could bring to mind the last fight and use tapping to decrease his emotional response while recalling it, and that seemed to help. He would then enter the next encounter centered, clear, and confident, but within five minutes, he'd find himself screaming again and slamming doors. What ominous portents for writing our magnum opus on relationships! One day after it had happened for about the 15th time in three months, he went out to the hot tub of the condominium where we were staying. Conveniently, no one else was there. David decided to try a mindfulness practice to go deeper into his understanding of what was happening. Here is his account of what occurred:

I set my intention on noticing the texture of my experience at the time of these explosions and right before them. With that in place, I simply followed my breathing and noticed what emerged. At first, there was a lot of inner chatter, self-justifications, self-judgments, anger at Donna, seeing Donna's sweet countenance having turned fierce in frustration and anger, fear of being discovered to be a fraud, images of the headline in our energy e-letter announcing the divorce of the self-proclaimed relationship virtuosos. I just noticed each and let it go. Back to the breath. Then a very vague image emerged. But I was able to place it. It was the bus stop where I was left off every day after school during first grade. Another boy and I were the only two left off there.

Unfortunately for me, he was the class bully, a wiry but very strong boy who for some reason was called Pudgy. I recall that his father was a police officer and that he was the toughest kid and the best fighter in our class. I, on the other hand, was tall, skinny, highly uncoordinated, painfully shy, and socially awkward—the perfect target for bullies of far less stature than Pudgy. So it wasn't a big rush for him to beat me up, and I usually got away with just a punch to the stomach

or jaw, just enough to make me cry. Once he was satisfied that he had done enough damage to reaffirm his dominance, he would turn away and walk home.

But on the day that came up in my vision, something ominous had happened in school. The teacher was angry at the class for being particularly unruly. She kept us in instead of letting us go as usual to the playground for recess. But she had to deal with us needing a bathroom break, so she had all the boys line up in one line, all the girls in another, and marched us to the lavatories. But first she gave a warning that if one of us spoke, the entire class would have to put their heads down for 30 minutes afterward, a most unwelcome punishment for children with growing, restless bodies. If we retained perfect silence during the bathroom break, she would instead read us a story we were all eager to hear.

After I finished at the urinal, I walked up to the sink to wash my hands and another boy walked up to it at the same time. I stepped back and invited him to go first. At that unfortunate moment, the teacher happened to glance into the boys' bathroom, saw my mouth moving, and that was that. The whole class spent the next interminable half hour with our collective little heads on our folded little arms on our uncomfortable little desks. The teacher did not announce the name of the culprit, but she said it was someone she never would have suspected. Of course, by the end of the school day, everyone knew it was me. I could not have been more humiliated or felt more ostracized.

It also gave occasion for Pudgy to give me an extra-vigorous beating that day. And that was the scene that emerged out of the initial vague image of the bus stop. I was surprised it came up right then, in part because I had decades earlier dealt with my relationship with Pudgy ad nauseam in psychodynamic talk therapy. I felt done with it, processed, complete. I didn't, at first, see any relationship between this memory and my arguments with Donna. But even as I kept bringing my awareness back to my breath, I had opened a portal that kept presenting different aspects of the memory and then connections to my current problem.

While no one would ever see Donna as a bully, with the pressures on us, the complex demands of the organization, and the curse of having agreed to hold up our relationship up as a model, we became about as acrimonious as we'd ever been in our 33 years together at that point. I felt I was giving my

heart and soul to the organization, and Donna's disagreement and judgment of my best efforts felt as unfair as becoming the class villain for politely indicating that the other boy could use the sink first.

The sense of unfairness and injustice was the invisible link between what I was playing out with Donna and what was still unhealed in my psyche. My sense of feeling bullied became the psychological context of our interchanges. I would be in discussion with Donna about a sensitive issue and suddenly and uncharacteristically find myself screaming at her as if my life depended on it. I was desperate as not only was each unresolved encounter damaging our relationship but the unsolved problems were also hurting our organization in ways that were making our lives more difficult.

By tapping on the memory and other aspects of the theme of being bullied, the triggers lost their power, and my reactions to more recent altercations could also be neutralized. I've not been hooked in one of those discussions since. This had a positive domino effect. Now Donna could express her frustrations and be heard rather than fought, allowing genuine problem-solving to occur, and we were soon back on track with each other.

The steps David took when life had thrust him beyond his usual coping strategies began with identifying a childhood experience that was at the root of the current difficulty. This is where many transformational approaches—from Freud's psychoanalysis onward—begin. The difficulties we run into with our partners often have an analog in our past. What is *new* is a deepened appreciation of the role of the body in matters of the mind. A powerful new order of psychological healing is emerging with somatic psychotherapies that work with the body as well as the psyche, and acupoint tapping is one of the most powerful and direct methods. May tapping smile on your relationships.

CHAPTER 9

When Disaster Strikes

Energy psychology is rapidly proving itself to be among the most
powerful psychological interventions available to disaster relief workers
for helping the survivors as well as the workers themselves.[1]

—**Charles Figley, PhD**
Chair of the Veterans Administration
committee that first named PTSD

THE NEED TO TREAT the emotional fallout following the rapidly proliferating disasters in today's world is vital, and accumulating evidence demonstrates that acupoint tapping can provide immediate, effective relief and help people start rebuilding their lives more quickly after catastrophic events.[2] Even for those of us who only witness the aftermath of disaster, whether in person or through the media, seeing multitudes suffering is overwhelming. Mind-numbing compassion fatigue has become widespread. We may want to do something—anything—to help, but what? As this chapter will show, energy psychology makes it possible to marshal a strong positive response to address the most terrible events that can happen to a human being. However, we want to open the chapter with a word of caution that if you have experienced a traumatic event that is still raw in your psyche, whether

recent or from decades ago, this chapter may be upsetting. But it also may be empowering. Please be discerning in the way you approach it.

IN A COMMUNITY WITH RECURRING DISASTERS

To give an example of the power of energy psychology following horrific events, we'll start with wildfires. Each warm season brings countless fires to California, with many escalating into giant conflagrations that have destroyed entire communities and taken many lives. Kristin Miller, a clinical psychologist and a resident of Northern California, has been bringing energy psychology to those impacted by the devastating fires that have raged through her community year after year. Dr. Miller has found utility and efficiency in acupoint tapping with what she describes as its "highly portable set of nonverbal, self-administered skills for managing stress and trauma." She began engaging her community by "showing up at every possible place where people gathered to listen to their stories and share skills." She further reflected:

The stunning realization following wave after wave of outreach in my community was that no one had the skills to calm their survival system and to process the trauma. This was true whether I was working with the firefighters, other first responders, hospital staff, county mental health providers, trained counselors, school staff, or the Red Cross shelters. But as these skills are becoming more embedded in our community, the road to recovery becomes more clear.

When the exhausted medical personnel, county workers, and firefighters came off our blackened, treeless hills, we met them to process their post-event distress. Many had worked 70 and 80 days straight, trying to control the wildfires. Some had seen much death, having to drive past dead bodies to get people out of towns that were on fire. Others had circled their trucks around people to keep the flames at bay as people were grappling for their lives. All experienced feelings of powerlessness as the fires roared indiscriminately, dismantling all plans for an effective firefight, as when the whole town of Paradise burned down in less than two hours.

I came into a room of men in a Red Cross shelter just hours after they had escaped from the November 2018 Camp Fire (which caused 86 deaths) with only their lives. One man was in fight mode, angrily screaming into his cell phone. Another was rocking back and forth, trying to regulate himself. Another was checked out totally, frozen in a vacant stare. Another man seemed more open for engagement. He recounted gruesome collective stories about what the men in the room had experienced. I had him do some regulating breathing with me. Soon, one by one, each man joined in. We were then able to add some tapping. They all settled, and their nervous systems were regulated in about 20 minutes. Not long after, this team came out of their "cave" and began serving everyone else. While they had been as traumatized as all the others, they became a calming force within the shelter.

Additional examples and case studies are, sadly, burgeoning as the frequency of catastrophic events worldwide accelerates. The number of major recorded natural disasters from 2010 to 2019 nearly doubled (from 4,212 to 7,348) compared with the decade before. From hurricanes and floods to tsunamis, wildfires, and tornadoes, extreme weather events are now dominating this century's disaster landscape.[3]

In addition to this influx of natural disasters, industrialized countries in the twentieth century have experienced an exponential growth in human-made disasters.[4] Mass shootings, terrorism, genocide, warfare, and violent conflicts impacting civilian populations—combined with an increased frequency of industrial accidents—are tragically contributing to this escalation. As a result, more and more people and communities are in need of post-disaster psychological treatment.

PSYCHOLOGICAL IMPACT

Whether natural or human-made, disasters lead to serious disturbances and disruptions not only in the lives of individuals but also in the functioning of a society. An estimated one in five disaster survivors are emotionally traumatized for long periods of their lives.[5] Even for those not directly affected, the number of heart-wrenching situations we are exposed to daily on TV or social media overwhelms our sensibilities.

Disaster response management teams have understandably focused on physical needs, while the mental health problems provoked by disasters have often been a "neglected area."[6] In addition to PTSD, psychological harm following catastrophic events may include anxiety, depression, shock, despair, grief, sadness, anger, denial, maladaptive behaviors, substance abuse, insecurity, sleep disturbances, mood swings, suspiciousness, paranoia, obsessions, loss of accustomed role in the community, and stress-related physical illness.

If you have survived a disaster, are still plagued with some of these symptoms, and have read this far in the chapter, we will remind you that the general approach presented in Chapters 2 and 3 can be applied to those symptoms. Meanwhile, Chapters 4 and 5 directly address the most common psychological symptoms following catastrophic events: anxiety, depression, and PTSD. In this chapter, we will look at ways energy psychology is being applied worldwide in the wake of disasters.

ENERGY PSYCHOLOGY IN THE TREATMENT OF DISASTER SURVIVORS

Energy psychology has been a powerful aid in recovery following natural and human-made disasters in more than 30 countries. The striking successes have been attributed to its ability to rapidly regulate the neurological aftermath of trauma. Several international humanitarian relief organizations have adopted energy psychology as a primary treatment in their post-disaster missions, and they are also developing ways to scale the approach.[7]

When we became interested in applying energy psychology in the aftermath of disasters some two decades ago, one of the pioneers in this area who helped orient us was Carl Johnson, a psychologist who had been a PTSD specialist with the US Department of Veterans Affairs. Toward the end of his career there, Dr. Johnson learned Thought Field Therapy. He found a tapping approach to be far more effective than the tools that had previously been at his disposal, and he regretted that he hadn't had them his entire career. In the decades following his retirement, he regularly traveled to sites of some of the world's most terrible atrocities and disasters to volunteer psychological support.

One of the more powerful examples he gave us took place about a year after NATO forces ended the systematic campaign of terror, murders, rapes, and arson in Kosovo in the late 1990s. Dr. Johnson found his way to a small village in Kosovo where the brutalities had been particularly severe. He met with Dr. Mustafe Shala, the village's only physician. Often in small villages, the local physician is the primary professional resource for mental health as well as physical difficulties. Dr. Shala's clinic had been bombed, and he was working from a trailer next to its remains. He had suffered the same traumas as everyone else in the village. Dr. Johnson provided him with a tapping session. Dr. Shala was amazed by how much relief he experienced. He offered to refer people in his village to Dr. Johnson.

Dr. Shala posted a sign that free treatments for war-related trauma were being offered on a particular afternoon. Many in the community were dealing with nightmares, insomnia, intrusive memories, and an inability to concentrate. Dr. Johnson described how a long line of people seeking treatment formed outside of the trailer. Everyone had positioned themselves as far away from one man as possible. Dr. Shala told Dr. Johnson, with some concern, that they were all afraid of this man. Dr. Johnson brought him in for the first treatment.

Dr. Johnson was seasoned in working with hardened war veterans after his career in the VA. He recalled that the man "had a vicious look. He felt dangerous." But he had come for help, so with Dr. Shala translating, Dr. Johnson asked the man to bring to mind his most difficult memory from the war. Everyone in the village was haunted by traumas of unspeakable proportions: torture, rape, witnessing the massacre of loved ones. As the man brought the trauma to mind, his face tensed and reddened, and his breathing quickened. Though he never put his memory into words, the treatment began. Within 15 minutes, according to Dr. Johnson, the man's demeanor had changed completely. His face had relaxed and his breathing normalized. He no longer looked vicious. In fact, he was openly expressing joy and relief. He initiated hugs with both Dr. Johnson and Dr. Shala. Then, still grinning, he abruptly ran outside, jumped into his car, and roared away as everyone watched, perplexed.

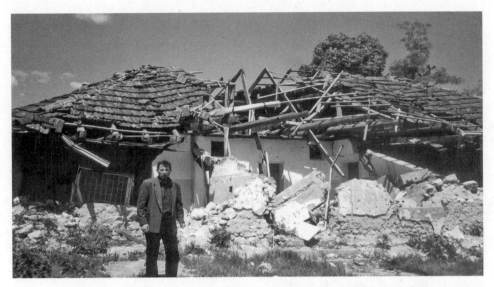

Figure 9.1. Dr. Mustafe Shala, the Kosovo physician, in front of his bombed-out clinic, next to the trailer in which the tapping treatments took place.

The man's wife was also in the group waiting for treatment, and Dr. Johnson brought her in next. In addition to the suffering she had faced during the war, she had become a victim of her husband's rage. The traumas she identified also responded rapidly to the tapping treatment. Just as her treatment was being completed, her husband's car roared back. He came in with bags of nuts and peaches from trees at his home and offered them as unsolicited payment for his treatment. He was enormously grateful, even gleeful, indicating that he felt something deep and toxic within him had been healed. He again hugged the doctors as well as his wife. Then, extraordinarily, he offered to escort Dr. Johnson into the hills to find soldiers who were still in hiding, too damaged to return to life in their villages. These were his own people—ethnic Albanians—as well as enemy Serbs who had inflicted so much suffering on his small village.

In Dr. Johnson's words, "That afternoon, before our very eyes, we saw this vicious man, filled with hate, become a loving man of peace and mercy." Dr. Johnson further reflected how often this would occur—that when these traumatized survivors could gain emotional resolution of experiences that had been haunting them, they became more loving and creative. While survivors, even after a breakthrough session like this, are still left with the formidable task of rebuilding their lives, the treatment disengages the intense limbic response from cues and memories tied to the disaster, freeing them to move forward more constructively.

When we asked Dr. Johnson how he determines if treatment for a traumatic event has been successful, he replied,

It has been successful when there is no suffering or anguish upon recalling the event. But at the same time, there is no reduction in sensitivity, distortion of values, or impairment in the ability to love. The memory is retained, but it is no longer in neon. There is still an awareness of the horror of the event, but it no longer has its grip on the person's soul. Where the memory had controlled the person, now the person has control of the memory.

OTHER REPORTS FROM THE FIELD

Dr. Johnson, himself a distinguished psychologist well versed in research methods, kept careful records of his work with 337 individuals following disasters in the four countries he visited in the years following his retirement. He reported that 334 of these traumatized individuals showed the above signs of having overcome their PTSD following their treatments. While this is an astounding claim given the degree of suffering he was working with, reports from dozens of countries where acupoint tapping has been used after disasters

corroborate one another in terms of rapid relief and long-term gains. The range of catastrophic events have included earthquakes, hurricanes, tornadoes, floods, wildfires, mass shootings, genocide, ethnic warfare, and industrial accidents. We will provide a brief sampling based on our many interviews with practitioners who have provided these services.

Sandy Hook Elementary School Shooting

This widely reported heartbreaking tragedy occurred on December 14, 2012, in Newtown, Connecticut. A 20-year-old former student of the elementary school shot and killed 28 people, including 20 children ages six and seven, six adult staff members, his mother, and himself. Nick Ortner, who happens to be a long-time resident of Newtown, is also the founder of one of the most influential organizations promoting an acupoint tapping approach to healing and personal development.[8] His mother, a school psychologist at a nearby elementary school, had worked closely with the school psychologist and principal who were killed at Sandy Hook.

Deeply touched on many levels, Ortner was determined to use his knowledge of energy psychology and EFT, as well as his local and global connections, to generate genuine healing for the traumatized community. On the day of the shootings, he contacted his colleague Lori Leyden, PhD, an internationally known trauma expert. She has introduced acupoint tapping and other disaster-relief methods following some of the world's worst recent disasters involving genocide and mass shootings.[9] Ortner asked Dr. Leyden's advice about providing an immediate response and facilitating long-lasting healing. That discussion turned into a collaboration. Three days later, Dr. Leyden arrived to begin organizing a long-term therapeutic and self-care initiative for the many people in Newtown affected by the shooting.

From the day Dr. Leyden arrived, she began conducting sessions with individuals as well as groups. Because the effects of long-term trauma are well known, and because of her success working with survivors of horrific violence, Dr. Leyden was able to immediately bring her experience to the task of establishing a community approach for Newtown that incorporated long-term, sustainable practices for relief. She made a commitment to the project and wound up living in Newtown for the next three years. Her goal was "to come in quietly, listening and observing, supporting local efforts, and providing the team an unobtrusive method for assessing needs while offering therapeutic and self-care assistance to those who needed it most." Sylvia Burwell, who was the US Secretary of Health and Human Services at the time, put those three years into perspective when she said in an interview, "While natural disasters capture headlines and national attention short-term, the work of recovery and rebuilding is long term."

Ortner sent out a request for volunteers to his 500,000-member mailing list. Ortner and Dr. Leyden then handpicked 35 volunteer tapping practitioners out of hundreds of responses to help create and build a long-term model for Newtown. Training in applying their facility with acupoint tapping to post-disaster situations began on January 5, 2013, 22 days after the shooting. The volunteers spent 35 to 60 hours in training, along with many more hours in supervision, to prepare for the immediate and long-term needs of those directly and indirectly affected by the tragedy. Dr. Leyden tells how at the start of the first day of the training, she asked who feels prepared to work with a parent whose six-year-old son or daughter was murdered. Eager to serve, everyone raised their hand. After a day of role-playing, she asked the same question again. Realizing that they didn't have the experience yet to take on this level of trauma, nobody raised their hand at the close of that first day of training.

Particular focus and outreach went to the parents and other family members of those killed, the children who survived the shooting, the school's teachers and other staff, and first responders, including police, firefighters, emergency medical technicians, medical examiners, and funeral directors. Rather than attempt to summarize the vast number of individual and group tapping sessions or related workshops and community events, we've collected a few representative comments by recipients or providers of the services:[10]

- **Scarlett Lewis, Mother of Six-Year-Old Jesse Lewis, Slain During the Shooting.** "In my attempt to heal from the tragedy of losing my son, an experience that has broken my heart and made me question going on with my own life, I sought many different types of help. Initially I sought traditional talk therapy that left me retraumatized and feeling worse. Nick Ortner introduced me to tapping, and I always finish these sessions with a deeper understanding of myself, feeling better, with a lightness of being and hope. Tapping makes me feel better when nothing else does."

- **Physician and First Responder, from the Office of the Medical Examiner.** "Dr. Leyden offered her services just days after the tragedy. She has been out to our office three times and has done multiple sessions each visit, spending several hours with technicians, doctors, investigators, and other staff directly involved with the Sandy Hook shootings. Her tapping and breathing exercises, as well as the group discussions, have been very helpful to me and my staff. I personally am sleeping better and functioning better."

- **Lynn Johnson, Director, Center for Serenity, Hartford, Connecticut.** "I have been so honored and moved to be a part of this project. Dr. Lori Leyden, Nick Ortner, Jondi Whitis, and the whole group have really inspired me. I have developed a program for young children, called the 'Feel Free Tap,' which is a version of EFT for grades K to 3. I loved sharing it with the group and can't wait to take it out to the wider community!"

- **Bonnie Skane, Volunteer.** "Being part of this volunteer team is such an honor and a blessing. In spite of this terrible tragedy, we have been seeing many little miracles happening every day. It's such a joy to help someone who is experiencing tremendous emotional pain, anxiety, and stress find relief with EFT! I truly believe that we change the world by changing ourselves, and EFT is simply an amazing tool that gives us the ability to release our negative emotions and choose positive ones instead."

- **Eric Leskowitz, Psychiatrist, Harvard Medical School.** Dr. Leskowitz provided this advice to the organizers: "Based on my clinical experience and reading of the research literature, EFT is the treatment of choice for rapid intervention in traumatic situations like Newtown that trigger overwhelming emotions in individuals and groups. Its use can prevent the future development of full-blown PTSD by empowering people to develop control over their own nervous systems."

A poignant "full-circle" story following the Sandy Hook tragedy involved a 12-year-old boy whose six-year-old brother was killed during the shooting. While the boy's mother had quickly embraced tapping, the boy was highly skeptical. He was understandably extremely angry about losing his brother and hadn't attended school since the tragedy two months earlier. Dr. Leyden had previously worked with orphaned genocide survivors in Rwanda, first for healing but then teaching them to become "heart-centered" leaders. The program was later formalized as Project LIGHT: Rwanda. Graduates of the program are referred to as "ambassadors," and a goal of the initiative is to connect traumatized young people around the world to support one another.

A Skype meeting was arranged between the 12-year-old boy in Newtown and two of the Rwanda ambassadors—young people like himself who had been through the worst of human tragedies. During the long call, they shared deeply, tapped together, and genuinely bonded. The boy in Newtown was so inspired that he returned to school the next day to make a speech to his classmates about why it is important to care about people who have experienced horrendous tragedies no matter where they live. Completing the full circle, he went on to create a nonprofit organization that raised money for some of the Rwanda ambassadors to attend university.

Hurricane Katrina

A hurricane can wreak horrific devastation in minutes. On August 29, 2005, Hurricane Katrina hit New Orleans and the surrounding areas, causing more than 1,800 fatalities and $125 billion in damage. A team of 12 Thought Field Therapy practitioners from eight states was invited by three medical and social service organizations in New Orleans to provide treatment and training to their staffs four months following the hurricane. The medical and social service personnel were inevitably victims of the disaster as well as helpers, and the strategy taken was to make their treatment part of their training. A total of 161 participants received treatment and training at six different sites.

Written evaluations were obtained from 87 of the tapping participants. Of these, 86 stated that they experienced positive changes and/or elimination of the problems they were experiencing at the time. The psychologist Caroline Sakai (who had also done the work in the Rwanda orphanage described in Chapter 4) compiled data on the 22 participants she treated. Their emotional issues included anger, anxiety, depression, eating to counter anxiety, frustration, guilt, survivor guilt, hurt, loss, loss of control, need for improved performance, overwhelm, panic, physical pain, resentment, sadness, shame, stress, traumatization, and worry. Each problem area was given a 0-to-10 SUD rating. Before treatment, the average score for the 51 problem areas described by the 22 clients was more than 8.

After treatment, usually consisting of a single individual session of under 15 minutes (which followed a half-hour group orientation), the average among the SUD ratings was less than 1.

In addition to the TFT team, EFT practitioners worked in the immediate aftermath of the hurricane and later with those who had been displaced. Sophia Cayer, who is highly experienced with tapping, described her work with a woman who had been traumatized not only by the hurricane but also by her subsequent time in a shelter after her home had been destroyed. A month after Katrina, this woman was so depressed that she was unable to function, spending much of her time crying uncontrollably. Cayer continued,

> When I sat down with her, she had one hand over her face, sobbing and unable to speak. I gently asked for permission to take her hand and see if I could help her relax. She agreed, and I began gently tapping on the energy points on her hand. Within a few moments, her tears began to subside. She was still unable to voice her experience, so I just kept tapping and talking with her. I used a specific EFT technique that offers relief without the person having to verbally describe the event.
>
> Among other issues, she was haunted by the screams and sounds of gunshots during the nights she spent in the shelter. While she was still, for the most part, unable to speak, I continued working with her, with her tears coming and going. After several minutes, her head was held high and she was able to speak. Then she smiled. Later that evening, I saw her at a gathering for survivors. Her friends, who had initially put me together with her, seemed amazed, reporting that she was her cheerful self again. I will always remember her smiles and hugs of gratitude.

Cayer reflected that with tapping, "even if it is only a single session, it doesn't leave the person stranded. It is not a matter of just soothing them and then letting them go. They are given powerful tools they can regularly use as they move through the crisis and beyond."

Refugee Camps

Becoming a refugee means enduring one crisis after another, and virtually all people who are forcibly displaced face substantial mental health challenges.[11] Enormous numbers—some 184 million people[12]—are currently refugees who were forced to flee their homes due to natural disasters, persecution, violence, or other threats. One in three of these individuals suffer from chronic depression, anxiety, or PTSD.[13]

The Moria refugee camp in Greece was Europe's largest camp when Gunilla

Hamne and Ulf Sandström, the cofounders of the Peaceful Heart Network (peacefulheart.se), were called there to assist with a disturbed eight-year-old boy who was "out of control." The Peaceful Heart Network has developed an acupoint tapping approach, called the Trauma Tapping Technique (TTT), that relies on a minimal use of words. Derived from TFT and EFT, this streamlined approach is particularly well suited for healing the immediate distress of trauma. It can readily be taught to disaster survivors and paraprofessionals or brought to large groups.

The boy in the Moria camp was acting out violently within his family and against others in the camp. He was described to Hamne and Sandström as "biting, throwing objects and stones, destroying tents, peeing everywhere, and tearing his clothes." The father was very caring and patient and tried his best to manage the boy. The mother had become numb and passive. The whole situation was creating chaos in the family; and with people so cramped, it had reached the point where the family was at risk of being forced to leave the camp with nowhere else to go. Hamne and Sandström describe their experience:

We went to one of the tents and did some drawing and acrobatic activities to connect. Suddenly the boy started to destroy everything in the tent, including the books and toys, fetching big stones and throwing them at everyone. He broke the metal legs of a table and demonstrated that he could use them as weapons. He demanded more pens, which he then broke into pieces. When the boy had calmed down, we demonstrated our exercises and techniques to the father and the other children of the family. The interpreter also participated. We had seen that the father could hold the boy and hug him, and therefore it should be possible for him to do the tapping with the boy.

When we had finished, we told the father that he should do the tapping as much as possible. Some days later, we saw the interpreter. He gleefully informed us, "I want to give you wonderful news. The father told me that he is using the tapping with the boy, and it is going extremely well! The father was super happy and the boy is super calm and lovely." The interpreter hugged us.

Along with their work with refugees, the Peaceful Heart Network has collaborated with local aid workers and groups in bringing TTT sessions and trainings to an estimated 250,000 individuals, addressing a wide range of post-disaster challenges in many countries. In Nepal, more than 900 tornado survivors received individual or group TTT sessions. In the most violent areas of Beni in the Democratic Republic of Congo, approximately 3,000 internally displaced persons, mainly youth and women, were served. Following Cyclone Idai in Zimbabwe, the Network reached approximately 100 people whose homes had been swept away. In the world's largest refugee camp, Bidi Bidi in Uganda, the Network has continuous engagement with refugees through a local pastor whose trainers have reached more than 2,000 people since 2018. In Colombia, they have been training social workers in a group that supports victims of trafficking. Seeing so much success around the world is inspiring, yet we know so much more is needed and possible.

Industrial Accidents

Pittsburgh's Critical Incident Stress Management (CISM) Team is composed of local professionals who volunteer their expertise following catastrophic events. Jim McAninch has used TFT as a CISM Team member following industrial accidents for more than three decades. Here is one of his accounts:

I was called to a site where an employee of a small company had been electrocuted. A worker had instructed his coworker to push a panel button, and the coworker was electrocuted on the spot. The survivor and six others watching had to deal with the horrible scene and their unsuccessful attempts to save the man's life. They were all traumatized by the horrific death. The intense odor of burning flesh remained vivid in each of their memories. For two of the witnesses, the death also caused past traumas to resurface.

One recalled the gruesome car-crash fatalities he'd witnessed as a tow truck operator for 20 years. The worker who had instructed that the button be pushed had years earlier found his wife dead in a snowbank. In the current disaster, after the electricity was no longer passing through his coworker's body, he had unsuccessfully tried to resuscitate the burned man, adding to his trauma and guilt. And, as a morbid reminder, he couldn't get rid of the smell or taste of the vomit that had come into his mouth during the resuscitation effort.

I treated him first as the group watched. Using TFT, I assisted him with his anger and guilt until the SUD was down to 0. I then had the others get into pairs and copy the treatment on themselves and on each other, until the trauma-related emotions were all down to 0. A week later, when I returned to do follow-up, each of the survivors was able to recall and talk about the tragedy without experiencing retraumatization.

McAninch described numerous situations where much of the emotional distress following terrible accidents was quickly resolved using TFT. While the speed and power seen in the above story is not unusual, in some cases McAinich needed to return to provide multiple sessions or make referrals for individuals who were severely affected. He noted that, as in the above case, past losses and traumas often resurfaced and became another focus for the sessions.

THE RESEARCH

While these accounts of the effectiveness of tapping protocols following disasters, and hundreds more like them, are dramatic and inspiring, they are not science. Putting on the skeptic's hat, we might ask if perhaps people who are called to work in disaster settings have an aptitude for providing effective support in crises, and the specific methods they use are only tangential. Would the same techniques be as effective in the hands of others who don't have these special qualities? Before tapping resources and recommendations are adopted by major disaster relief organizations, objective evaluations of outcomes must be produced.

This is challenging, however, because the unexpected nature, chaos, and pressing demands that suddenly emerge when a disaster strikes work against systematic assessments when trauma response teams arrive immediately after a catastrophic event. Existing research on tapping protocols in post-disaster situations was usually conducted months, years, or even decades after the disaster occurred, when established research

procedures were more feasible. Because the effects of trauma often persist for decades, however, this research is appropriate and necessary, and the outcomes after treating chronic PTSD with acupoint tapping in the years following a disaster have been impressive, as summarized in Chapter 4. A systematic review of six clinical trials investigating the use of tapping in treating PTSD found unusually strong outcomes.[14]

For instance, in a study of civilian survivors of systemic violence years earlier, 145 adult survivors of the 1994 genocide in Rwanda were randomly assigned to TFT treatment or a control group. The TFT group experienced significantly more improvement on PTSD symptom scales, and these were sustained at a two-year follow-up.[15]

In a clinical trial nearly two decades after the 1992–1995 wars in Bosnia, 18 adults were selected based on severe ongoing emotional distress tracing back to their horrific experiences during the wars, which included severe injuries, torture, beatings, rape, sexual humiliation, and watching others being assaulted or murdered.[16] Each of the participants received four 1-hour sessions over a two-week period using a tapping protocol. A standardized civilian PTSD symptom checklist was administered prior to the treatment, at the end of the treatment, and at a four-week follow-up. Again, reduction of symptoms reached a high degree of statistical significance, and the benefits were sustained on follow-up.

A 2010 earthquake in Haiti caused more than 200,000 deaths and $8 billion in damage. Seventy-seven of the survivors were assessed for PTSD on a standardized symptom inventory. Forty-eight scored in the clinical range. After two days of instruction in EFT, none of the participants showed a score in the clinical range. Post-test symptom and symptom severity scores decreased by an average of 72 percent.[17]

These are all impressive findings, but we also need to note that it is generally advocates of energy psychology who conducted these studies of the effectiveness of tapping protocols in treating the emotional wounds following traumatic events. Another series of studies, however, was conducted by researchers who did not particularly favor the approach. Numerous investigations have used advanced statistical methods to compare the outcomes of psychotherapies that have been applied following disasters or other forms of severe mental duress.[18] A broad array of therapies was assessed. Not surprisingly, the analyses revealed a wide range in their effectiveness for reducing trauma-based symptoms and improving functioning. Six of these comparison studies included an energy psychology protocol. The acupoint tapping therapies were among the most effective interventions. As discussed in Chapter 4, they demonstrated the strongest outcomes compared to 36 therapies in one study[19] and the strongest outcomes in relation to

17 therapies in another.[20] The evidence is mounting that acupoint tapping is among the most potent interventions available in post-disaster situations. Let's take a closer look at how they work.

THE FOUR TIERS OF ENERGY PSYCHOLOGY INTERVENTIONS FOLLOWING DISASTERS

Acupoint tapping protocols can be applied at any time following a catastrophic event, from minutes to years. After attending to physical needs, establishing safety, and fostering trust and rapport, a four-tier framework categorizes energy psychology interventions in post-disaster situations according to their purpose and the time elapsed since the event.

First Tier: Psychological First Aid

The first concern after physical safety has been established following a catastrophic event involves immediate emotional relief and stabilization. Much as a paramedic might instruct someone having an anxiety attack to perform a breath-control technique that is incompatible with hyperventilation, energy psychology uses interventions that interrupt the fight-or-flight response. In the midst of a disaster, the relief worker might demonstrate diaphragmatic breathing to a traumatized individual, saying, "Everyone feels overwhelmed now. How about we take a few slow deep breaths?" This could be followed by suggesting, "Now let's add to our breathing by tapping on some stress-release points. Just tap where I tap." The tapping sends deactivating signals to the amygdala that rapidly decrease elevated emotional responses in stressful situations. This simple procedure can be a potent intervention for providing psychological first aid in the immediate aftermath of disaster. Practitioners often start with the most comforting interventions available for fostering relief and stabilization, such as diaphragmatic breathing, self-hugs, gentle rocking, offering reminders that the person survived and is safe now, and introducing tapping as appropriate.

Second Tier: Reducing Limbic System Arousal Following Trauma Triggers

Beyond immediate relief, acupoint tapping can transform self-limiting stress-response patterns that can develop after a traumatic event. Fear, rage, or anguish may have become neurologically associated with a particular internal or external cue. For instance, someone who barely survived a flood accompanied by thunderstorms might now experience full-on terror whenever there is lightning and thunder. By bringing to mind vivid images of lightning and thunder while tapping, they can be freed from the involuntary threat response. Reducing hyperarousal in the parts of the brain involved with emotional processing, self-defeating emotions, thoughts, and behavioral patterns can counter flashbacks and nightmares. Uncoupling extreme stress responses from memories, chilling fantasies, or external triggers is a widely recognized key to the successful treatment of PTSD.[21]

Third Tier: Overcoming Complex Psychological Difficulties

When someone experiences a traumatic event, a variety of complex issues that had been operating beneath the surface may emerge. These may show up in the person's relationships, work, or health, and they often trace back to childhood difficulties that haven't been adequately processed. Such issues can be addressed using a tapping approach, particularly once adequate progress in the first two tiers has been accomplished. By combining tapping with carefully selected memories, emotions, or beliefs, energy psychology can address each element of a complex psychological issue. Whether it's resolving a traumatic memory that's tied to obstacles in overcoming more recent trauma or addressing beliefs developed in childhood that contribute to pessimism and hopelessness, untangling these various elements frequently becomes a focus of ongoing treatment. This type of comprehensive approach may be critical in post-disaster counseling if a complete healing is to occur.

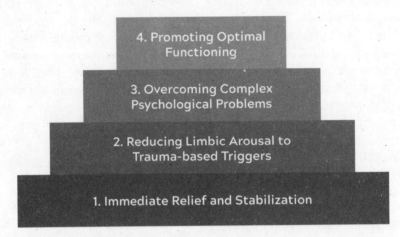

Figure 9.2. Themes for focusing energy psychology interventions at various timeframes following a disaster.

Fourth Tier: Promoting Optimal Functioning

Even after stabilizing emotional responses and addressing long-standing problems that a catastrophic event may have brought to the surface, the existential issues of life remain. In fact, a catastrophic experience may accentuate fundamental human questions about the meaning of life, uncertainty about the future, the reality of evil, and awareness of the inevitability of death. Yet people who have seen the worst of life can thrive emotionally and spiritually. Coming to terms with such issues reorients the person to living the rest of their life with an expanded consciousness and greater alignment with their deeper being. In fact, as the Russian author Leo Tolstoy is commonly attributed as saying, "There is something in the human spirit that will survive and prevail, there is a tiny and brilliant light burning in the heart of man that will not go out no matter how dark the world becomes." Many people have found a tragic event to mark a major advance in their lives.

The term *post-traumatic growth* describes "positive psychological changes that are experienced as a result of struggles with highly challenging life circumstances."[22] Previously unknown strengths and resilience are often discovered following a catastrophic event. Interviews with energy psychology practitioners suggest that an energy-attuned approach can help uncover and nourish that "tiny and brilliant light," fostering feelings of spiritual connectedness and promoting serenity, confidence, and courage.[23] Although these are ongoing issues and often involve intense psychological challenges, people can achieve greater personal stability and a higher level of functioning after traumatic experiences. Understanding this inspires hope in the aftermath of devastating experiences.

EFFICIENT DELIVERY

In Lori Leyden's previously mentioned work in Rwanda, the organization that arranged which villages and groups she would meet with had allotted six days for her to work with 100 orphans who were also heads of their households. They ranged in age from 19 to 25. At the time of the 1994 Rwanda genocide, when they were orphaned, they were only five to 11 years old, yet they were each left to care for two to six other orphans with no visible means of support for food, rent, education, or daily living expenses. With close to 100,000 orphans from the war and hundreds of thousands more children orphaned due to their parents dying of HIV/AIDS, the Rwandan government did not have the capacity to care for these orphans.

Since individual counseling with 100 people over six days wasn't going to go very far, Dr. Leyden decided to meet with the entire group on each of the six days. She could still have one-on-one sessions, but she could amplify their impact by conducting them in front of the large group. Using what is called "Borrowing the Benefits," everyone in the group would, before each one-on-one session, tune in to their own area of greatest concern, give it an SUD rating, and then bring their attention to tapping along with the person working with Dr. Leyden in the front of the room, using the wording that person used.

The first session focused on a young man, about 20 years of age, who had been caring for three other orphans since the genocide. He was still struggling with intrusive memories about the genocide 13 years earlier. He rated his distress as being "above 10" on the 0-to-10 SUD scale. He, Dr. Leyden, and the entire group tapped on these and similar statements, one at a time:

"My mind does not feel safe."

"My memories will never go away."

"I will be terrorized by these memories for the rest of my life."

"I'm afraid to sleep because of these memories."

After 25 minutes of tapping, he reported that he was at a 2 on the SUD scale. He commented, "My mind feels safe now. I know I am safe right now. I'm looking forward to sleeping tonight." Meanwhile, Dr. Leyden reported sensing a palpable shift in the room. She said, "There was a quiet sense of peacefulness that wasn't there before the session." As she checked in with the rest of the group, all 100 participants reported being at a 2 or below on their original issue. Specifically, one person after another reported feeling new levels of safety.

As the week progressed, the young man reported that his sense of calm persisted at home each evening. He was able to sleep peacefully. Others who had one-on-one sessions in front of the group addressed additional themes, including these, as the group tapped along with them:

"Helplessness of being an orphan."

"Hopelessness of not having a bright future to look forward to."

"Healing for the wounds of rape."

"Terror that the intrusive memories of my parents being murdered in front of me will keep returning."

"Pain of often going hungry."

"Anxiety of not being able to provide basic needs for the younger children I am caring for."

During the sessions, the participants reported how the new sense of safety helped them cope better with the challenges they faced daily. They also taught their "families" to tap at home, which made them feel more in control of their situation and better able to help others when they were feeling stressed or traumatized. Dr. Leyden commented that it was for her "another reminder of what I've seen hundreds of times: the power of the tapping to reregulate the physiological dysfunction that occurs when a person has been traumatized."

"Borrowing the Benefits" seems to work even with people who have little in common. But it can be extraordinarily powerful when they have all gone through the same catastrophic event or other hardships. Groups also have the power of "contagion" as people entrain with one another emotionally. As the person on the stage heals, a healing energy pervades the group. As the person on the stage is inspired, an energy of inspiration pervades the group. As the person on the stage feels hope, an energy of hope pervades the group.

In addition to working with large groups instead of relying on individual psychotherapy, energy psychology has been efficiently delivered through lay counselors, electronic media, and the strengthening of local resources. Mental health professionals in a community confronted with a disaster are being taught how to use tapping; survivors are teaching it to other survivors; politicians are being educated about the availability of rapid, efficient treatments; and communities are learning how to deliver them. While the experience of seeing those afflicted by catastrophic events will always be heartbreaking, we also find it exciting and gratifying to be part of this sea change in the ways humanity is able to bring about emotional recovery following agonizing disasters.

IMPLICATIONS

All this brings us to an obvious question: Why wait for disasters? Imagine a world where it is widely recognized, based on the growing evidence, that combining the stimulation of acupuncture points with the best practices psychology has to offer takes those best practices a quantum leap forward! Imagine a world where every therapist and paraprofessional possess these skills, no matter their theoretical orientation, so when disaster strikes, external response teams do not need to bring in acupoint tapping. Local therapists and their communities can already be prepared. This is doable. The basics of energy psychology aren't that hard for therapists to learn, regardless of their theoretical orientation. And it would be a viable response to the overwhelming size of the need as catastrophic events afflict increasing numbers worldwide.

CHAPTER 10

Bringing Energy Psychology
to a World in Distress

Energy psychology offers revolutionary tools for moving forward in healing ourselves and helping humanity deal with its current lineup of impending catastrophes.[1]

—Eric Leskowitz, MD
Department of Psychiatry, Harvard Medical School (ret.)

HEALING AND PERSONAL DEVELOPMENT aren't the only uses for energy psychology. The easy availability of acupoint tapping holds promising implications for our society. The collective consciousness of humanity impacts your life every day. At its extreme, the challenges that may well be pushing our species toward an excruciating extinction all trace to a crisis in consciousness. If we can't raise our awareness to see what is required and muster our collective will to change direction, we are rapidly heading toward a horrific point of no return.

At the personal level, energy psychology is all about shifting direction. It is strikingly effective in modifying the mental models that govern a person's life. But an energy approach can also be used for collective transformation. You may or may not choose to become active in influencing the direction of that transformation, but the experience you have had with this program positions you to involve yourself in ways that may not have previously been available to you. You will see in this chapter that energy psychology can be applied at a wider level to shift the social beliefs and practices that shape humanity's mutual activities. Before we dive into those possibilities, let's pause for a brief review.

WHAT YOU HAVE LEARNED SO FAR

Tapping has presented an energy psychology approach and offered instruction in ways of applying it. We have been referring to the essentials of the method as the "Basic Tapping Protocol."

The Basic Tapping Protocol

The set of techniques you learned in Part I provided you with the ability to transform self-defeating mental models and initiate two fundamental processes for coping and thriving:

- to send *calming* signals to parts of your brain that become overactive when you are upset or navigating a situation that is problematic for you, and

- to send *energizing* signals to "executive regions" of your brain so you can manage challenging situations more successfully.

If you "lift the hood," you will find that these are common denominators for all forms of effective psychotherapy. Energy psychology brings about these actions rapidly and in ways that are different from conventional psychology.[2] In a nutshell, it works like this:

1. When you tap on acupuncture points, the tapping immediately generates signals in the form of electricity, called piezoelectricity.

2. These signals are transported to your brain along a set of energy pathways that are embedded in your body's connective tissue.

3. Regions of your brain that are engaged when thinking of a problem or issue become like magnets, attracting the signals generated by the tapping.

4. This occurs nearly instantly and can be systematically applied to the issue and its many aspects, resulting in an easing of emotions such as fear, anger, or jealousy while energizing brain regions involved with problem-solving and stress management.

5. The benefits tend to be permanent.

Literally having at your fingertips the ability to send calming or energizing signals to pertinent brain areas at will is a game-changer in taking charge of your mental landscape.

Best Practices

In Part II we have explored the best practices psychology has to offer for challenges that most people face (e.g., worry, sadness, self-defeating habits) as well as for more extreme versions of these challenges (e.g., chronic anxiety, depression, addictions). We've also applied acupoint tapping protocols *within the framework* of these best practices. By combining established methods such as psychological exposure and cognitive restructuring with the stimulation of acupoints, you are bringing tapping to psychology's most reliable approaches for a wide range of emotional challenges. Meanwhile, psychotherapists using the book are able to integrate a tapping approach with what they already do well.

Moving Forward

If you have gotten this far using the book's procedures, we congratulate you and thank you for trusting us. Through repetition you have learned and internalized one of the most effective approaches psychology has developed for teaching people how to master their inner lives. You have also applied the procedure to several concerns that matter to you and—we have reason to believe, based on our work with hundreds of individuals as well as considerable research—you have most probably experienced benefits that matter to you.

We encourage you to continue to use the Basic Tapping Protocol. The next time a difficult feeling that seems tied to the past occurs . . . tap. The next time you notice a habit or pattern of behavior that isn't serving you . . . tap. The next time you face a challenge in your work, family, or love life that you don't know how to handle . . . tap. Tapping sessions around such issues will bring up aspects and unresolved issues that will appear less and less as you address them. The effects are cumulative. Your guiding models evolve. You will be attracting a better tomorrow as you break the chains, link by link, that keep you from being at your best today.

Gary Craig and Gabriëlle Rutten go so far as to encourage people to tap each evening on the "worst moment of my day."[3] Stressful events, even minor disturbances, accumulate. Regularly clearing them keeps you functioning at your best. In addition, issues that frequently recur reveal deeper patterns that get in your way and can be shifted by addressing them and their various aspects using acupoint tapping.

COMING TO TERMS WITH THE TERRORS OF MODERN LIFE

As we move into the broader applications of an energy approach, we'll start with your personal relationship with a world that is, by any measure, in perilous distress. The theme of this book is, in a sentence, that acupoint tapping protocols can, in positive ways, help you evolve the inner models that shape your feelings, choices, and ultimately your life. But what of the developments that are far beyond your personal story or your control? While tapping cannot change the outer world, it can help you navigate through it so your resilience is supported and your spirit stays strong.

Many people on the planet enjoy comforts and pleasures that royalty could not have imagined a few centuries ago. Most are not so fortunate. Everyone, however, lives in the shadow of fears that are difficult to contain. Many are living on the edge of a continual low-grade fight-or-flight response. While the fight-or-flight mechanism is one of nature's most dazzling achievements and helped our ancestors survive, it is being called up today to manage all forms of stress and challenges for which it was never designed, such as an argument with your spouse or child, a glitch in your computer, or gridlock traffic. The media is a huge source of stress, unceasingly broadcasting personal tragedies, worldwide unrest, mass shootings, deadly conflicts, and natural disasters that can exact a vicarious toll on you.

We will focus next on seven themes that have been helpful to us personally and to our students and clients. These topics include surrendering, not surrendering, divisiveness, suffering, chaos, overwhelm, and despair. Each has a counterpoint (e.g., despair/faith), and we will suggest a way to accept and embrace the inherent dilemmas and how to use tapping so that your guiding model about each dilemma becomes more grounded and effective. You can go through all seven—each of which our test drivers found to be useful—or select the ones that speak to you most directly.

1. Surrendering Meets Acceptance

You eventually have to face it. The universe is more powerful than you, and you can't control everything that is happening! It is ultimately empowering to not try to change what can't be changed. Any other stance is a formula for breaking your spirit.

For each of these seven topics, we are going to suggest an *"Even though . . . I choose to . . ."* Choices Statement as a starting point for tapping on the relevant issues. The technique acknowledges a fundamental conflict—even a paradox—and transforms it into an empowering guiding statement for moving forward.

A Choices Statement for Meeting Dilemmas Involving Surrender

"Even though I can't control my destiny or the destiny of humanity . . .

I choose to recognize, marvel at, and finally surrender to the fundamental uncertainty woven into existence."

Adjust or completely reword this while staying with the *surrendering* theme and proceed to the section on "Tapping Through the Dilemma." If you wish, just do Steps 1 and 2 in the "Tapping Through the Dilemma" instructions, or complete all the steps to take it deeper.

Tapping Through the Dilemma

1. Give a 0-to-10 SUD rating on the amount of distress you feel in your mind and/or body when tuning in to the first phrase.

2. Say your "Meeting the Dilemma" Statement three times, massaging your chest sore spots on the first phrase and holding your hands over your Heart Chakra on the second.

3. Do a tapping sequence through the 12 points, saying the first phrase of your statement at each point (without "Even though"). You are using the tapping to neutralize the negative in order to make room for the positive. Repeat until the SUD has gone down as far as you can get it—for instance, if it won't go down further after two subsequent rounds of tapping.

4. Do another tapping sequence, this time alternating between the first and second phrases.

5. Do the Integration Procedure (p. 62).

6. Do your final tapping sequences on the second phrase alone, expressing a choice (or an explicit statement of acceptance such as *"I love myself and accept my feelings"*).

7. Do another SUD rating for the first phrase. If you discover new aspects about the situation, Psychological Reversals, or Tail-Enders, note them and consider applying the Basic Tapping Protocol to them as well.

2. Not Surrendering Meets Courage

The reason for following *surrendering* with *not surrendering*, its opposite, falls into the sphere of the Serenity Prayer, which is a staple of spiritual and self-development literature: "God, grant me the serenity to accept the things I cannot change, the courage to change the things I can, and the wisdom to know the difference." Do not let the reasons for despair overshadow the fact that you have resources for making a real difference in your world and being a force for good, however you define it. Just as trying to change what can't be changed can break your spirit, if there is too much focus on what can't be changed, you lose sight of what is possible for you.

A Choices Statement for Meeting Dilemmas Involving Not Surrendering

"Even though the world's problems may seem hopeless . . .

I choose to discover ways I can influence my own destiny and the destinies of those I touch."

Adjust or completely reword this while staying with the theme of *not surrendering*. Return to the section on "Tapping Through the Dilemma," and complete at least the first two steps. Then move on to dealing with divisiveness.

3. Divisiveness Meets Inclusion

The social landscape teems with disagreement, discord, and dissension. Perceived hostility in "civic discourse" can be destabilizing to one's psyche. The great scholar of mythology Joseph Campbell observed that while all mythological systems direct the "expansive faculty of the heart" toward the in-group, they deliberately direct "every impulse toward violence" toward the out-group. He characterized this as an "archaic but dominating myth" that must be transformed "if humanity is to survive."[4] While we may feel pressure and see cause to villainize those who disagree with us, we can each do our part to embrace a higher perspective that transcends and transforms the "archaic myth" that Campbell believes can lead to our demise in today's world.

Our friend Jean Houston, who is a cultural historian, philosopher, and activist, teaches in her "Social Artistry" trainings that the word *politics* is derived from the Greek word, *politeia*, which implies an active engagement in which people empower each other to enhance their communities.[5]

A Choices Statement for Meeting Dilemmas Involving Divisiveness

"Even though the blistering divisions among people are deeply disturbing . . .

I choose to find ways to take loving actions that are rooted in our fundamental unity with each other and with life."

Adjust or completely reword this while staying with the *divisiveness* theme, return to the section on "Tapping Through the Dilemma," and complete at least the first two steps. Then move on to the following section, which addresses suffering.

4. Suffering Meets Compassion

Suffering and evil are the two realities that religions bank on to draw followers, yet no religion, philosophy, or scientific discipline has adequately explained either without faith that there is a higher purpose for each. Meanwhile, watching intense, undeserved suffering shakes most of us to the core. And now, with electronic communication being a large part of our mental diet, we see enormous amounts of suffering. Some people—such as doctors, other medical personnel, and psychotherapists—make it the driving force in their lives to alleviate suffering. Others close their hearts or even judge the victims, partly because the vicarious pain or sense of needing to help is too much to bear. How can we keep ourselves centered and not lose heart when witnessing great suffering?

A Choices Statement for Meeting Dilemmas Involving Suffering

"Even though my heart aches knowing so many people are suffering . . .

I choose to let this awareness strengthen my heart, expand my compassion, and help me find at least small ways to relieve suffering whenever an opportunity arises."

Adjust or completely reword this while staying with the *suffering* theme, return to the section on "Tapping Through the Dilemma," and complete at least the first two steps. Then move on to dealing with chaos.

5. Chaos Meets Hope

Social structures are breaking down all around us. But cultural chaos and threat are seeds for the emergence of new forms that have never before existed. These sit silently in the archetypal realms, ready to beckon the next step in humanity's evolution, waiting for the conditions that will allow them to manifest. They exceed the creativity of your imagination, wondrous though it is. In their *Future Humans Trilogy*, Jean Houston and Anneloes Smitsman explore ways the patterning for a more conscious and evolved humanity already resides deep in our psyches and even in our DNA.[6] The two of us find this understanding to offer great hope amid the social chaos that can be seen everywhere.

A Choices Statement for Meeting Dilemmas Involving Chaos

"Even though the social chaos all over the world terrifies me about humanity's future . . .

I choose to recognize that new hope-inspiring social forms are emerging and to align myself with them."

Adjust or completely reword this while staying with the *chaos* theme, return to the section on "Tapping Through the Dilemma," and complete at least the first two steps. Then move on to dealing with overwhelm.

6. Overwhelm Meets Peace

The sheer amount of information we receive and process daily exceeds what was required of any generation before us. Beyond that, the issues raised by what is reported in the news and other sources challenge our guiding models. Never before have we been given intimate glimpses into such a range of human dilemmas or witnessed such diverse and often discordant ways of dealing with them. So, we are always undergoing some sort of reorientation. This is not necessarily a bad thing. It makes us wiser quicker. But it can be overwhelming, becoming another source of despair and debilitation.

A Choices Statement for Meeting Dilemmas Involving Overwhelm

"Even though I'm overwhelmed by all that is unfolding today . . .

I choose to embrace the fact that this point in history is my time to be in this world."

Adjust or completely reword this while staying with the *overwhelm* theme, return to the section on "Tapping Through the Dilemma," and complete at least the first two steps. Then move on to dealing with despair.

7. Despair Meets Faith

When we said "no religion, philosophy, or scientific discipline has adequately explained suffering or evil without resorting to faith that there is a higher purpose for each," it may have sounded like we were dismissing faith as a desperate, irrational reach for comfort. The notion of a higher purpose is easy to espouse but harder to envision. An analogy used in theological seminaries is that our trying to understand God or the force that created the universe is like an amoeba looking back up the microscope and trying to understand the scientist. One needs only to gaze at the stars to sense the immensity of creation. We humans—slower and weaker than many predators who would like to eat us—have persisted through one impossible challenge after another. Will we survive the current planetary crisis? Only time will tell. But we do know that forces that are beyond our comprehension are at play and have already shepherded the unlikely evolutionary journey of *Homo sapiens*. Having faith that this larger intelligence doesn't want to squander all the evolutionary capital it has invested in creating such conscious beings is more likely to bring out your best than a pessimistic guiding model that we are all doomed and may as well give up.

We hope this has been useful for finding a more centered and empowering place within yourself for facing problems that go far beyond your sphere of responsibility. We do have one caveat. Just as healing the emotional wounds of a trauma doesn't change what occurred or how terrible it was, cultivating more empowering inner models for addressing terrible situations doesn't make them less terrible. But it does help you find your way through them more effectively and with greater peace and composure.

After going through this process, one of our test drivers commented that she was surprised by how much this focus on larger problems reduced her personal anxiety. She had been afraid it would do the opposite. Another wrote:

This section feels very important because it emphasizes that no matter what our belief systems, we all face these predicaments. Admitting my own uncertainties is a big step toward understanding what others are facing. We are all united in confronting these dilemmas, and addressing them personally and collectively would be a big step in helping move society forward.

If you complete any of these processes, you are building a more resilient guiding model for adapting to the issues affecting your world. And your efforts will be vastly repaid if the reward is that you gain greater peace about what you cannot change and a sharpened focus on where you can be most effective. You might want to repeat some of the statements out in nature so you can resonate with the energies of the Earth, plants, and trees that are the handiwork of the forces that put you here on the planet.

FROM INNER RECKONING TO HELPING CREATE A BETTER WORLD

Our brains evolved for the world of our distant ancestors, but the world we find ourselves in today is demanding a major transformation from a fight-or-flight, friend-or-foe mentality to neural pathways that are programmed for an increasingly interdependent world. Previous generations have had potent rituals for bringing individuals into harmony with their society's needs, norms, and beliefs. Systematic tools for empowering individuals to adjust in their own unique ways to a rapidly changing world are, however, a relatively new development.

In the West, they trace to the emergence of psychotherapy in the late 1800s. Now, with approaches such as energy psychology, you can efficiently initiate precisely targeted self-directed neurological change. Could similar principles be applied to advance the welfare of large groups or cultures?

The ability to deliberately and precisely send beneficial electrical signals to targeted brain regions can help transform ancient programming that has become destructive in individuals. But it can also help a culture understand how such shifts can be made and how to create educational approaches based on these principles. Cultural and political forces can be mobilized to make such advances the new normal. The concept of "neural plasticity"—the capacity of the nervous system to modify itself in response to experience—suggests that we don't need to wait for natural selection to advance evolution in individual brains. New insights and even neural changes can be brought to the collective in ways that are empowering. The application of energy psychology to help entire communities in the wake of catastrophic events is already taking shape, as seen in the previous chapter.

To envision the ways an understanding of the energies that impact human consciousness can be applied for fostering beneficial social change, we will explore the evidence that supports seven disparate but interrelated premises:

1. Energy can carry memory and exhibit intelligence.

2. Energy fields influence physical and biological processes.

3. Energy can exert effects over a distance.

4. Energy fields have an invisible impact on human relations.

5. Collective fear can be understood as an energy field.

6. Energy fields can be harnessed for social good.

7. Personal and cultural potentials are coded in energy fields.

1. ENERGIES THAT CARRY MEMORY AND EXHIBIT INTELLIGENCE

Energies believed to be capable of coding complex information and making intelligent choices have played a central role in the worldviews of many societies throughout history.[7] At least 97 cultures have been identified whose healing systems and spiritual traditions, often extending back thousands of years, refer to a "human energy field" that is subtle and imbued with the capacity for discernment.[8] Words for these energies include *prana* in Sanskrit, *qi* in Chinese (also spelled *chi*), *ki* in Japanese, *wakan* for the

Lakota Sioux, *orenda* for the Iroquois, *ruah* in Hebrew, *barakah* in Arabic, and *pneuma* in ancient Greece.

Although such terms have sometimes been translated as "energy" in the West, each depicts a larger construct than the electromagnetic energies usually understood when scientists use the term. The concept of *qi*, for instance, provides the main theoretical foundations for ancient Chinese medicine, philosophy, culture, and natural science. While the tradition recognizes the observable "characteristics of energy, such as the ability to work and to be accumulated, stored, discharged, and projected from the body," notes the health researcher Wayne Jonas, MD, "qi also has characteristics of intelligence and information."[9] Attuning to these energies seems to be a pathway into levels of consciousness that transcend conventional Western frameworks.

How does modern science view these claims? The Russian physicist Yury Kronn, in his book *The Science of Subtle Energy*, explores what scientists refer to as "dark matter"—the 96 percent of the universe's "mass-energies" that don't fall within the electromagnet spectrum and can't be measured by the instruments of modern physics.[10] He argues that this energy follows laws that are fundamentally different from those of the visible world, and that they are more consistent with explanations found in ancient healing systems. He believes that it is from this strata of the universe that energies that follow laws not known in conventional physics emerge.

This convergence of ancient and contemporary understanding opens new possibilities for harnessing the power of the ever-present energies that surround us.

While these energies may seem bizarre at times, it's possible to catch glimpses of their very real effects. The examples we'll be exploring range from mysteries following heart transplants to memories stored in chakras, to wound healing, plant germination, embryo development, and the genesis of illness. All reveal energy fields that are capable of orchestrating detailed and nuanced changes.

The Stunning Experiences of Heart Transplant Patients

To illustrate how energy operates in ways that defy conventional thinking, we will look at experiences that have been reported by heart transplant patients. Claire Sylvia, herself a heart transplant recipient, described in her book *A Change of Heart* the way many people who have had a heart transplant may suddenly become obsessed with thoughts, memories, dreams, tastes, desires, or values that they later learn correspond with those of the person whose heart now beats in their own chest.[11] The following is from the case files of one of the foremost investigators of such reports, the neuropsychologist Paul Pearsall, PhD:

The heart donor had died from a fall while reaching for a Power Rangers toy sitting on the cement ledge just outside a high hotel railing. The recipient was a 5-year-old boy with an uncorrectable septal defect and severe cardiomyopathy.

Donor's mother: When I met the recipient family and little Daryl (the recipient) at the transplant meeting where donor and recipient families meet, I broke into tears and—if my husband hadn't caught me—I would have fallen to the floor. I saw it right away. Daryl smiled at me exactly like Timmy (the donor) always did. He had a very crooked smile and sort of looked at me sideways as if he was teasing me. It was that exact slanted smile. We sat and talked with Daryl, and it was uncanny how I could feel in my own heart my son's heart seeming to call out to mine. Like our dog wags her tail when she recognizes us, my heart began to race with glee. I asked if I could put my head to Daryl's chest and listen, and I could have done that for hours. My son's heart and mine seemed to fall into sync, and Daryl loved it and kept showing the slanted smile the whole time. What Daryl (the recipient) told us left us in total awe.

Heart recipient: I gave the little boy who gave me his heart a name. I called him Timmy, and I could tell he was just a little kid younger than me. I could feel that he had been hurt real bad by falling a long way. I can sometimes still feel the thump that killed him. He liked Power Rangers a lot like I used to, but he was probably too little to know what they really are. Sometimes at night I get woken up by my whole body jumping, and I can feel Timmy's heart like it felt when he fell—like a heavy thump. I wonder what happened to my old heart. It was broken but it did its best to take care of me, and I feel sorry for it sometimes and I cry.

Recipient's father: We never really knew until today how old Daryl's donor was. We knew he had fallen, but that's all. I guess Daryl got Timmy's age right by a lucky guess, and they needed a small child-sized heart for the transplant. I'll never know how he got his donor's name right. Maybe it's just chance because Daryl used to watch Tim the Tool Man Taylor on the television show *Home Improvement*. I do have to say that the crooked smile Daryl started having after his transplant always did bother me a little and now I can see where he might have gotten it from the donor. I don't know how, but I'm sure he did because he never smiled that way before.

Recipient's mother: Are you going to tell them the real "Twilight Zone" thing? Daryl used to love collecting and playing with his Power Rangers. When we brought him some after his transplant, he threw all of them in a box and said he never wanted to see them again. He hasn't looked at them again.[12]

While only a small percentage of heart transplant recipients attribute any unusual experiences to their donor, Daryl's account is common enough that many cardiac surgeons counsel families about this possibility prior to a heart transplant. Dr. Pearsall's investigations included many such dramatic cases. In another, a psychiatrist described one of her patients, an eight-year-old girl who received the heart of a murdered 10-year-old girl:

> Her mother brought her to me when she started screaming at night about her dreams of the man who had murdered her donor. She said her daughter knew who it was. After several sessions, I just could not deny the reality of what this child was telling me. Her mother and I finally decided to call the police and, using the description from the little girl, they found the murderer. He was easily convicted with evidence my patient provided. The time, the weapon, the place, the clothes he wore, what the little girl he killed had said to him . . . everything the little heart transplant recipient reported was completely accurate.[13]

Reports like these, which can't be explained by conventional science, shatter old ways of thinking and move human knowledge forward.[14] No explanation for these accounts (beyond that the many well-documented cases have been fabricated) makes more sense than the following:

- The heart has its own energy field. This is well known. In fact, the electromagnetic field of the heart is about 60 times greater in amplitude than that of the brain and up to 5,000 times stronger.[15]

- This energy field carries information that is highly detailed, and that can be registered in a person's awareness or reflected in their mannerisms. That is the part that busts the paradigm. Conventional science can't explain Daryl's crooked smile or sudden aversion to Power Rangers or the eight-year-old heart recipient's having precise knowledge about her donor's murderer.

Memories Stored in Chakras

A practical understanding of energy fields that carry highly nuanced information is part of the experiences of many energy healers. For instance, early in her career, Donna was focusing on the Heart Chakra of a depressed 36-year-old woman. Donna, who is highly sensitive to the energies in an organ, informed the woman that Donna was feeling like a girl of about seven who just lost someone she adored. It wasn't a parent but someone very important. Donna felt deeply the client's sorrow, like her grief was too much to bear and her heart was closing down. The woman replied in tears that Robert, her older brother, was unintentionally shot by a neighbor boy who was playing with his father's rifle. Robert died two days later. Donna was able to see and sense this information in the energy of the woman's Heart Chakra. After Donna applied energy-based interventions to heal the long-buried unresolved grief held in the woman's Heart Chakra—not unlike the procedures you have been using throughout this book—the woman began to reckon with having never again been able to love as fully as she loved her brother, which was followed by a large increase in her ability for intimacy within her marriage. Imagine how if health-care practitioners were this attuned to the information carried by specific organs—it would change their entire approach to healing.

Seed Germination Experiment Illustrating How Energy Can Carry Information During a Tapping Treatment

An inventive experiment investigating the effects of an acupoint tapping session for treating depression built upon earlier well-designed studies showing that when a cheerful person does a "laying on of hands" over the water used to irrigate a plant, the subsequent plant growth is more robust than when a depressed person treated the water.[16] The larger concept, known as the "green thumb" effect, has been demonstrated in a wide range of experiments.[17]

In the energy psychology experiment, okra seeds were surreptitiously attached to the back of a clipboard given to a 42-year-old woman diagnosed with a major depressive disorder while taking a standardized depression checklist.[18] The proportion of seeds that germinated and the amount of root growth 72 hours later was significantly less than for a control group of seeds that had not been in her presence. The woman was then given a two-hour treatment session using an energy psychology protocol to focus on her depression. Then she was again given the depression inventory, with another batch of okra seeds attached to the clipboard. The growth of these seeds was significantly greater than for the seeds that had been in her presence before the treatment or for the control seeds. Meanwhile, her depression score dropped from 20 (indicating moderate depression) to 3 (negligible depression) after the single session.

Just as the heart seems to carry information that can be transferred from the heart donor to the recipient, the woman's energy field appears to have carried *information* that was transferred to the okra seeds. That information seems to have had an entirely different effect prior to the treatment than it had after the treatment. The treatment presumably changed the woman's energy field, the information it carried, and the effects it brought about.

2. ENERGY FIELDS THAT INFLUENCE BIOLOGICAL PROCESSES

The seed germination experiment raises an important question for understanding the unexpected power of acupoint tapping. Did the information in the woman's energy field that transferred to the okra seeds also affect her general well-being? It is relatively easy to understand how tapping on selected acupoints sends signals to brain areas involved with a mental health issue, influencing the neural circuits in ways that help resolve previously identified symptoms. But broader improvements beyond overcoming the symptoms that are the target of the treatment have also been widely reported following tapping sessions.[19] Documented underlying physiological changes include improved cardiovascular functioning, boosts in immunity, decreased cortisol production, enhanced expression of genes involved with problem-solving and stress management, and optimized brain wave patterns.[20] The person is not only no longer suffering from depression or anxiety but also thinking more clearly, relating better to other people, healing from physical challenges, and navigating the circumstances life presents with greater ease.

To understand how shifts in the person's energy field may produce benefits beyond the reasons the person was using the tapping, we need to examine the nature of energy fields. We take you on this more scientific segue because it is an invisible but vital dimension of the work you have been doing throughout the book. We'll look at energy fields in wound healing, embryo development, and illness.

First, what are fields? In physics, a field is simply a region of space on which a force acts. You are familiar with how a magnet's field can organize iron filings, as illustrated in Figure 10.1. In biology, fields that influence bodily processes are known as "biofields."[21] They surround you and interpenetrate each of your organs. These are key concepts in medicine. The electrical activity of the heart is measured with an electrocardiogram (EKG). An electroencephalogram (EEG) measures the electrical activity of the brain. Biofields can be found at each level of the body that functions as a unit, from cells to organs to the entire organism, and they can also be spontaneously generated.

Wound Healing

The reason energy fields are so important for understanding tapping is that the body's electromagnetic fields influence the action of its cells, including its neurons. An everyday example involves wound healing. After a wound is sustained, an electromagnetic field develops and organizes cellular activity in the healing process, stimulating growth and repair.[22] The energy medicine researcher James Oschman, PhD, explains that the electrical field created at the site of a wound persists until the repair is complete, attracting mobile skin cells, fibroblasts, and white blood cells that close and heal the wounds. Finally, as the tissue heals, the current changes and "feeds back information on the progress of repair to surrounding tissues."[23] The influence of specific frequencies on cell generation and repair has been documented in more than 175 papers published in the scientific literature.[24]

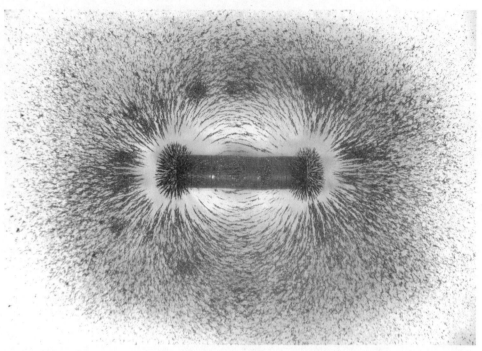

Figure 10.1. Biofields impact biological processes just as a magnet can organize bits of iron.

Embryo Development

The concept of a biological "field" first arose in embryology in the early 1900s as an underlying template for explaining the developmental process.[25] Just like the way an energy field coordinates cell activity in the healing of a wound, energy fields have been shown to direct physiological growth in the fetus and developing organism. This was vividly demonstrated in the 1930s by Harold Burr, PhD, a neuroanatomist at the Yale School of Medicine.[26]

When Dr. Burr measured the electrical field around an unfertilized salamander egg, he discovered that it was shaped like a mature salamander. It was as if the blueprint for the adult was already within the egg's energy field! The unfertilized egg already possessed the electrical axis that would later be aligned with the brain and spinal cord.

The Genesis of Illness

Dr. Burr went on to discover energy fields around various organisms, including molds, plants, frogs, and humans, and he was able to describe electrical patterns that differentiated healthy states from disease states. He discovered, for example, that when cancer-associated electromagnetic patterns were observed in mice, even ones that showed no physiological symptoms of malignancy, they eventually developed cancer. Dr. Burr found not only correlations between specific pathologies and the electrical characteristics of corresponding organs but also that physical illness is *preceded* by changes in an organism's energy field, and he demonstrated this in hospital studies with humans.[27]

After a recent analysis of Dr. Burr's work, the science writer Sally Adee wrote that Burr "was prescient: everything he theorized about bioelectricity has been validated in the 50 years since he said it."[28] For instance, the Tufts University developmental biologist Dany Spencer Adams put dyes that are sensitive to changes in voltage patterns on a frog embryo, making it possible to observe changing electrical patterns as the embryo develops. At one point in Adams' experiments, apparently random bright patterns that had appeared on the featureless embryo began to resemble eyes and a mouth. Subsequently the embryo's mouth and eyeballs developed precisely where the electric glow had foreshadowed them.[29] This parallels what Dr. Burr found with his salamanders. The blueprint for the developing organism was evident in the energy field before the anatomical structures developed. Since the genetic code doesn't contain any "instruction for anatomy,"[30] the most reasonable interpretation of Burr's and Adams' findings is that the embryo grows in response to direction from the surrounding energy field.

Since we were trying to establish energy medicine as a scientifically informed pursuit, we were thrilled to learn of Dr. Burr's experiments, conducted at a top-rated medical school some half a century before our careers even began. We often find ourselves pointing to his discoveries because they are vital for understanding how energy healing modalities that change the body's energies can *prevent* illness. Summarizing the implications of Burr's findings, Dawson Church noted that "cancer was showing up in the *fields of energy* before it showed up in the *of cells of matter*. . . . Energy fields form the templates around which matter condenses. Change the field and you change matter."[31]

3. ENERGY FIELDS THAT PRODUCE EFFECTS FROM A DISTANCE

Notice that in all the above examples—from heart transplants, to memories stored in chakras, to wound healing, plant germination, embryo development, and the genesis of illness—an energy field appears to be managing elaborate biological or psychological changes. Beyond these demonstrations that energy can carry nuanced information and exhibit intelligent behavior, another property that is critical for applying an understanding of energy for bringing about collective change is its ability to act across distances.

Among the most mind-bending properties of quantum physics is "quantum entanglement."[32] This involves the way two subatomic particles that have interacted continue to influence one another even when they have been separated. Albert Einstein famously referred to this as "spooky action at a distance."[33] Experiments have demonstrated that the effect holds at increasingly large distances, from centimeters to meters to miles, even across the distance from Earth to satellites in space.[34]

Do the principles of the subatomic world apply to the world we see with our senses? It has been tempting for science-fiction writers, new age philosophers, spiritual advisors, and alternative health practitioners to confound these quantum principles of the microworld by applying them to the everyday world. Such commentators have been roundly criticized as being dilettantes who don't at all understand the nature of the quantum world.[35] Quantum entanglement between humans has also been dismissed as belonging to the much-maligned domain of parapsychology, yet the evidence of its existence keeps accumulating and scientists are beginning to understand more about it.[36]

Vlatko Vedral, PhD, a physicist at Oxford University, asserted in the prestigious journal *Nature* that quantum entanglement "can exist in arbitrarily large systems involving not just two photons or electrons," but during events we can experience and observe.[37] We will give four examples: diagnoses from a different location than the patient, altering properties of matter from a distance, killing cancer cells thousands of miles away, and acupoint tapping from afar.

Diagnosing and Healing from Different Locations

Several studies using EEG equipment have shown that some individuals can influence the brain waves of others from a distance.[38] The healing effects of prayer have been documented even when the sick person is in a different location.[39] Individuals known as "medical intuitives" have diagnosed health conditions with no physical proximity. To systematically study such reports, the neurosurgeon Norman Shealy provided medical intuitive Caroline Myss the names and birthdates of patients he had diagnosed. Myss had no contact with or other information about the patients. Myss' clairvoyant diagnoses matched Shealy's medical diagnoses in 93 percent of the cases. Her statements were specific, such as "left testicle malignant, spread to left kidney"; "venereal herpes"; and "schizophrenia."[40]

Changing Properties of Matter from a Distance

Medical qigong, an ancient Chinese practice that involves controlling and directing energy for healing purposes, has been shown to be able to, from a distance, affect cell growth and increase survival time of tumor-embedded animals.[41]

One of China's most widely respected physicians, Yan Xin, MD, became famous for curing "incurable" diseases by using qigong to project chi energies to his patients to bring about healing. As his reputation grew, a group of physicists decided to investigate what might be happening. In one of their experiments, they had him direct chi energies toward a radioactive element to see if he could change the rate of radioactive decay.

According to physics, the radioactive decay rate of an element is one of nature's constants. Yet Dr. Xin was able, at will, to increase or decrease it by up to 12 percent, and he could do it from close up or thousands of miles away. More than 60 scientific papers have been published reporting on the remarkable phenomena observed in Dr. Xin's experiments, conducted under the auspices of the Institute of High Energy Physics of the Chinese Academy of Sciences and Tsinghua University in Beijing.[42] The radioactive decay experiment has now been informally replicated using meditative techniques.[43] In the way that people with highly refined abilities to mobilize energies can use those skills to impact matter with no physical contact, those of us with no such gifts can still tap on points on our skin that generate electrical signals that can shift the neural pathways controlling our thoughts and behavior.

Killing Cancer Cells from Thousands of Miles Away

Another qigong master, Jixing Li, was able to selectively kill human cancer cells kept in a laboratory that was 3,000 miles away. While in California, Li concentrated on the cells, which were placed in a growth medium in an incubator at Pennsylvania State University. The cells that were the object of Li's focused intention died. Another set of cancer cells, just inches away from the targeted ones, were not affected and continued to proliferate quickly.[44]

Newtonian science has no explanation for medical intuitives who can accurately diagnose patients despite no physical contact or healers who can destroy cancer cells on the other side of a country. Some form of subtle energy that eludes conventional scientific instruments must be involved. Commenting on the way that even the strongest electrical or magnetic fields can't influence the decay rate of radioactive elements, Dr. Kronn, the Russian physicist, speculated that "chi interacts with the particles that make protons and neutrons, quarks, or the even tinier particles, subquarks, which make up quarks. It means that subtle energy . . . belongs to and acts in the subatomic world."[45]

Tapping from Afar

For energy psychology, growing evidence suggests that acupoint tapping exerts a clinically beneficial influence even from a distance. From the earliest days of energy psychology, practitioners have been telling stories about treatments that were administered to someone at a different location. When David first heard of these reports, referred to as "surrogate tapping," he was annoyed. It was hard enough to try to convince his psychologist colleagues that tapping on the skin can send deactivating signals to the limbic system, let alone that it can be done from a distance. But as the reports continued to come in, he decided to find out what he could.

Based on a literature search and a request to the energy psychology community via e-letters and e-lists for case descriptions of surrogate tapping, David reported in a peer-reviewed journal that 193 unique cases of surrogate tapping had been identified.[46] Exactly 100 of them met the following criteria:

1. A "sender" had applied an energy psychology protocol to him/herself (self-tapping) intending to be helpful to a "receiver."

2. The sender did not physically tap on the receiver but may have been in the same room (as is often the case with infants or animals), or the two may have been isolated by distance. While the influence when the "sender" and "receiver" were in close proximity might be explained by visual cues, mirror neurons, or other factors, in more than a third of the cases, the two were in different locations.

3. The receiver did not apply the Protocol to him/herself.

4. The positive outcome was attributed by both the sender and the receiver to the surrogate tapping.

All 100 cases resulted in perceived benefits within these criteria. While controlled clinical trials would be necessary to establish a cause-effect relationship between the surrogate tapping and the improvements, the findings are at least provocative. More intriguing is the implication that energy psychology interventions may influence the therapist-client in-person relationship in ways that have not yet been discovered. Are broader outcomes also possible?

4. THE INVISIBLE IMPACT OF ENERGY FIELDS ON HUMAN RELATIONS

We want to bring into your imagination ways a mastery of energies that operate beyond those recognized by conventional science can help "humanity deal with its current lineup of impending catastrophes," as Dr. Leskowitz put it in this chapter's opening quote. Whether you feel helpless about these impending catastrophes or determined to work toward preventing them, engaging the energies interlaced with these societal conditions is within your means. Everyone on the planet has a vested interest in these outcomes.

The mission of the HeartMath Institute, a nonprofit in California, is to provide "heart-based, science-proven tools for raising humanity's consciousness from separation and discord to compassionate care and cooperation" (heartmath.org). Based on EKG and EEG readings, their research has shown that an individual's brain waves can entrain themselves with another person's heartbeat nearby.[47] We influence one another not only with our words, behavior, and status but also in ways we've never imagined.

The observation that an individual's heart rhythm influences a nearby person's brain waves, like guitar strings resonating with one another, is easy enough to comprehend. Many people report knowing before they walk in the door that their spouse is upset. Likewise, the way that an energy field orchestrates the phases of wound healing can also be observed in everyday experience. The energy field that appears around the wound emits instructions like a remote control changes the channels on your TV. Understanding that energy fields can influence events that aren't in proximity opens new possibilities for instigating social change.

This teases the imagination. Can energies that operate from a distance be applied to influence the outlook and behavior of groups or even communities? And even if they can, powerful tools may be used in good ways or ill. Even at the personal level, a corporation might use energy psychology to make its sales force operate with greater integrity or to make it more comfortable about deviating from the truth. The military could use it to increase a soldier's aptitude for teamwork or to decrease sensitivity about taking another person's life. These Orwellian possibilities may unfold for better or for worse, but unfold they will.

5. COLLECTIVE FEAR AS AN ENERGY FIELD

Al Gore, the former US vice president, coined the term "amygdala politics" to describe political decisions based on fear rather than on facts. He described the intentional manipulation of citizens to support more militaristic policies through "vicarious traumatization."[48] His book *Assault on Reason* begins by noting, "Fear is the most powerful enemy of reason. . . . Fear frequently shuts down reason."[49]

Acupoint tapping generates signals that rapidly *shut down* unrealistic fear. This changes the energy in the brain. But the energy of fear also resonates with others in a primal manner. Mass hysteria is an energy that can sweep a group. Those who are sensitive to subtle energies recognize this. Is it possible to reduce collective fear that clouds good judgment and, ultimately, social policy?

What if, prior to making decisions to counter perceived threats, politicians were to, as a group, tap on selected acupuncture points while imagining the worst plausible outcomes? This would not diminish their ability to make rational decisions about the situation. Eliminating exaggerated fear doesn't dull perceptions of an actual threat. The decisions following such an unlikely though conceivable practice would be *more* rational rather than less.

This possibility does not need to be limited to politicians (who would probably be the last to use it anyway). Town hall meetings, community focus groups, school boards, company boards of directors, management teams—any gathering that influences collective choices—could use the "Borrowing the Benefits" technique (p. 327). Tapping could routinely be applied to counter irrational fears about the issue on the table and validate legitimate threats before decisions are finalized.

6. ENERGY FIELDS CAN BE HARNESSED FOR SOCIAL GOOD

Devices that interact with human intention were developed in the 1990s at the physicist William Tiller's lab in the Stanford Department of Materials Science and Engineering.[50] The Princeton Engineering Anomalies Research (PEAR) program, which operated for nearly three decades under the aegis of Princeton University's School of Engineering and Applied Science, studied the interaction of human consciousness and sensitive physical devices.[51] In hundreds of experiments, the investigators demonstrated that when a group of people, such as a crowd at a football game, is focused on the same event—particularly when strong emotions are activated, such as at the moment of a touchdown—mechanical devices such as random number generators are affected.

While these effects are very small, they are statistically significant. The devices generate patterns that aren't random. Even more striking is the fact that such devices have responded to events happening hundreds of miles away.

As these devices demonstrate, and as we have attempted to show in this chapter, energy carries nuanced information, acts intelligently, influences physical and biological processes, and can act from a distance. How might such properties of energy be harnessed for the collective good? Some real-world examples follow.

The HeartMath Institute has put some of these principles into practice for improving worldwide conditions with its Global Coherence Initiative (heartmath .org/gci/). The first large experiment of this nature was conducted in 1973.[52] It led to the mind-boggling conclusion that the energy being put out by a group of meditators reduced crime rates. Crime in Washington, DC, had increased steadily over the first five months of 1973. At that point, a crime prevention project brought thousands of transcendental meditation practitioners into the city for a two-month experiment between June 7 and July 30.

The organizers publicly predicted that crime would be reduced by 20 percent. This prediction was ridiculed by the chief of police, who asserted that the only thing that would decrease crime that much that summer would be "20 inches of snow." A week after the study's start, violent crime, as measured by FBI Uniform Crime Reporting statistics, began decreasing and continued to drop until it had been reduced by 23.3 percent by the experiment's end. After the meditators went home, crime began to increase again. While this result may have been a coincidence, similar studies have led to comparable findings.[53] A worldview that includes an understanding of subtle energies and organizing fields fills in gaps so that these apparently implausible anomalies become plausible.

A playful investigation into this phenomenon was conducted by Dr. Leskowitz. Interested in the widely recognized "home field advantage" dynamic, Dr. Leskowitz interviewed players on the Boston Red Sox baseball team. A star outfielder noted that the players "regularly discuss the impact that the energy of the Red Sox fans has on our performance and ultimately the outcome of the game."[54] This takes "field" in home *field* advantage into new dimensions.

At a more far-reaching level, the researcher and social activist Lynne McTaggart has been working with teams of scientists and volunteers from over 100 countries to create the first "global laboratory," conducting controlled experiments on the effects of mass intention.[55] Her online groups send a specific thought to create an outcome that the team of scientists then evaluates. Significant measurable changes have been produced in various experiments, from making seedlings grow faster to lowering violence in ghettos or war-torn areas to healing individuals with PTSD.

7. PERSONAL AND CULTURAL POTENTIALS ARE CODED IN ENERGY FIELDS

Perhaps the most important quality of the energies we have been discussing, in terms of personal and cultural evolution, is that they seem to activate inherent potentials. The term *entelechy*, introduced by Aristotle, refers to the internally guided journey toward completion and possibility. At the purely biological level, the electrical field surrounding Harold Burr's salamander eggs held the entelechy for the adult. It encoded the development of the mature salamander. For humans, entelechy is the deep organizing pull toward the individual's psychological and biological potentials.[56]

The reason this is important for personal growth is that the best therapists are able to evoke a client's highest possibilities, and entelechy explains the energetic dynamic by which potential becomes manifest. A guiding model that we, the authors, hold is that deep patterns for health, self-actualization, and happiness are natural. They exist as the entelechy within each person, and in ways that are more difficult to map, they exist in cultures and humanity as a whole. At the individual level, the job of the healer, therapist, or educator is to perceive them and go about helping the person activate them. At the cultural level, it is a shared journey to perceive the best in human nature and cultivate it. We are reminded of the comment attributed to Michelangelo—that he "saw the angel in the marble and carved until I set him free."[57] Fostering your own entelechy is perhaps the most consequential tool offered by energy psychology.

To the extent that you apply a constructive energy-informed approach to your personal challenges, you become a happier and more effective individual. To the extent you incorporate these understandings into your community activities, you become a more constructive and empowered citizen.

Conclusion

AS WE CLOSE THIS volume, we are reflecting on our first book on acupoint tapping. Published in 2005, it was called *The Promise of Energy Psychology*. The publisher suggested we call it "The Power of Energy Psychology." Even though we had by that point been witnessing and were often dazzled by the power of the method, we didn't feel the research evidence was in yet to justify that title to the professional community. By the time of this writing, however, nearly two decades and more than 150 scientific studies later, it is clear that the approach is effective with a wide range of conditions, outcomes are achieved with surprising speed, and benefits are lasting.

We are confident asserting that energy psychology protocols could empower most people on issues ranging from being nervous before a talk, bringing up their kids more capably, dealing with a traumatic event, and finding greater balance in a topsy-turvy world. The approach has appeared at a time in the culture's development when individuals are psychologically stretched in unprecedented ways, and the need for *unprecedented* types of support to help all of us operate at our best is urgent.

It is on this stage that we believe energy psychology is emerging as a major player. We close by renewing our invitation that you take advantage of this empowering innovation and make it a major player in your own life. Blessings!

Appendix

If the Program Becomes Unsettling

Clients often think they've gone crazy or "lost it" when shifts in consciousness happen. . . . It's our task to help define these events as positive, transformative incidents that are a natural part of self-discovery. [1]

—Dorothea Hover-Kramer, RN, EdD

Cofounder, Association for Comprehensive Energy Psychology

A CHALLENGE IN PRESENTING the potent techniques in this book is that any tool that is useful for psychological exploration can bring up strong emotions and painful memories or unleash dormant psychological problems. We have made every effort to present the program so you can adjust it to your own needs, pace, and sensitivities. If you are coming to this section out of a felt need instead of simply to see what it contains, a variety of tools are available here for getting yourself back on track.

Distress while working through difficult issues is inevitable, yet working through unprocessed feelings and experiences is a necessary part of personal evolution. A caveat, however: if the distress becomes extreme and persists even after applying the techniques in this Appendix, please enlist the support of a resourceful friend or mental health professional before continuing with the program.

TAPPING ON THE REACTION YOU ARE HAVING

Dawson Church was doing a demonstration with a woman who wanted help regarding bouts of extreme shyness and a tendency to go silent in certain social situations. Just standing in front of the large group attending the demonstration, her shoulders slumped, as if trying to make herself take up less space, and her voice became tiny. With the tapping treatment, her SUD rating went from an initial 8 down to 6, but it stayed at 6 for the next two rounds. At this point, a terrifying childhood memory surfaced. She and her mother had walked into their home while a burglary was in progress. Her mother started to scream, and the intruder began to viciously beat her mother. The girl ran and hid behind some curtains. She was sure the burglar was searching for her and managed to silence her own tears and screams of terror.

Now with the memory rushing back in vivid detail, she went through the same kinds of physiological reactions, presumably, as when the incident occurred: shaking heavily, face blanched, heart pounding, hardly breathing. Of course, at this point Dr. Church saw the symptoms but did not yet know the story. He offered reassuring words while unwaveringly instructing her to continue tapping. By the second trip through the tapping sequence, her breathing had returned to normal, and she had stopped shaking. A couple more rounds of tapping (no Acceptance Statement, no Integration Procedure, just the emotional first aid of stimulating the acupoints while she was experiencing the stress response) and she was able to describe what had occurred. Then her work was able to proceed by focusing on various aspects of the memory, neutralizing them one by one.

She had totally repressed her memory of this incident, but whenever she felt any stress in front of other people, she had to fight against herself to be able to speak. Asked to test the degree to which she had overcome her shyness following the tapping, she described her experience to the large group in full-bodied posture and voice.

As in this case, activating a past trauma may make you feel like the problem is getting worse. Shifting your focus to the reaction you are having in your body and emotions while you continue to tap is the default procedure when this occurs. If, however, the sense of overwhelm is intolerable or makes it too hard to continue thinking about the situation, energy *medicine* techniques that are specifically designed to counter overwhelm and panic are the next step.

A SIMPLE CALMING TECHNIQUE YOU CAN USE ANYTIME ANYWHERE

Assuming you have already tried tapping on the reaction you are having, which will usually be enough to bring you back to center and into a sense of renewed balance, the immediate need is to calm your nervous system. Fortunately, simple energy techniques can override the biochemistry of anxiety and panic. We'll start with one that is very basic and can be used anywhere, anytime.

The Calming Hug/Heart Hold

1. Sit or stand comfortably with your arms crossed, right hand wrapped around the left side of your body about four to six inches below the start of your armpit.

2. Place your left hand above the elbow of your right arm (see Figure A.1).

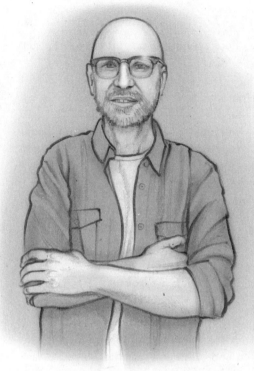

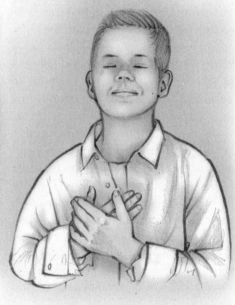

Figure A.1. The first step of the Calming Hug/ Heart Hold, an anywhere, anytime technique.

Figure A.2. The second step. The Heart Hold can also be done independently.

3. Rock from side to side if that is comforting, or simply stay still.

4. As you begin to feel calmer, place your hands over your Heart Chakra at the center of your chest (see Figure A.2).

5. Breathe in slowly through your nose and out through your mouth, taking deep breaths, with the exhalations being much longer than the inhalations. If it helps to pace yourself, you could breathe in while slowly counting to six and breathe out while counting to 12. Notice how your shoulders relax.

This may seem too simple when you are extremely upset, but it does a great deal. The Calming Hug eases Triple Warmer, the energy system that activates the fight-or-flight response. It also connects Triple Warmer's energies with the energies of Spleen Meridian, which responds to stress and distress in a more tranquil and grounded manner. Meanwhile, crossing your arms stimulates communication between your left and right brain hemispheres, facilitating a more balanced response to the distress.

As you are bringing gentle pressure to your chest during the Heart Hold, your parasympathetic nervous system is being activated, which relaxes your entire body. You are also bringing energy to your Heart Chakra, which is associated with balance, calmness, and serenity.

Finally, breathing deeply into your nose and out of your mouth connects two of the most important meridians for staying calm and grounded: Central and Governing. This type of conscious breathing shifts you from the sympathetic nervous system's fight-or-flight activity into the parasympathetic nervous system's rest-and-recover mode. It also engages your vagus nerve, reducing fear and anxiety while modulating your mood. You may be surprised by how effective deep breathing

along with these postures can be for generating genuine calm from within.

The Calming Hug/Heart Hold is a simple, powerful technique you can use anytime you are beginning to feel overwhelmed, off-center, or emotionally triggered. If you practice it a few times when you don't need it, you will have it memorized and available for when you do need it.

MORE ENERGY TECHNIQUES FOR CALMING YOUR NERVOUS SYSTEM

Additional techniques that are particularly potent for countering distress and calming your nervous system include the Hand-on-Chest Tap, the Blow-Out, and the Stress Hold.

The Hand-on-Chest Tap

Place one hand on your chest. With the fingers of your other hand, tap on the ridge below the "V" where your little finger and ring finger meet (see Figure A.3). These points are used in the Basic Tapping Protocol, but tapping on them at any time can have a powerful effect. They are on the Triple Warmer Meridian and ease the fight-flight-freeze response.

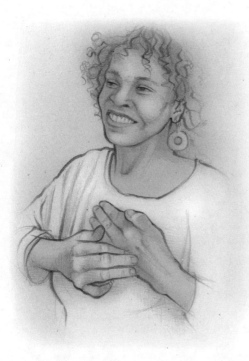

Figure A.3. The Hand-on-Chest Tap is a simple technique that helps turn off the threat response.

The Blow-Out

The Blow-Out is a brief, active technique to do if you are storing a great deal of frustration, distress, or anger. Simply "blow out" the energetic residue of your accumulated feelings by doing the following:

1. make fists as you bring your hands and arms in front of you,

2. swing your arms down and then around behind you,

3. lift them above your head, and

4. rapidly, and with some force, send your fists down to your sides, letting these pent-up emotions out with a sound.

Purse your lips as you blow out the feelings. Open your hands when they have come all the way down (see Figure A.4). Repeat this several times. End by doing the movement once more, but this time slowly and deliberately. Now with some of the energies cleared, do the Stress Hold.

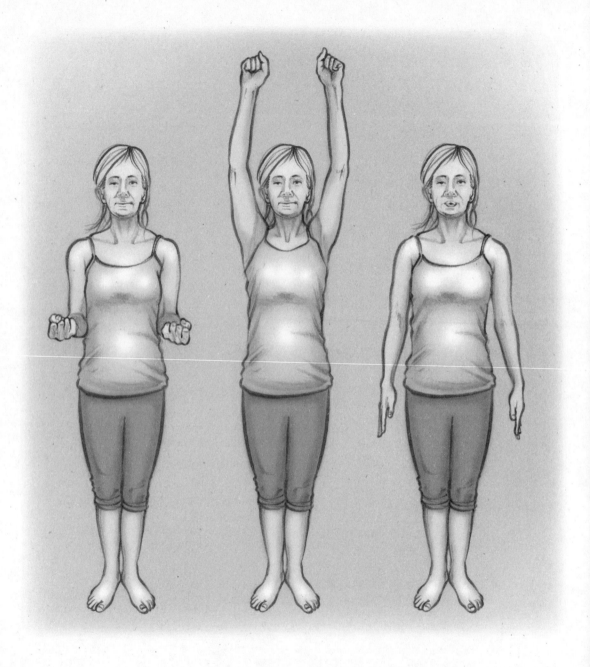

Figure A.4. When distress, frustration, or anger build, the Blow-Out is a simple physical technique for sending their energies out of your body.

The Stress Hold

When your body becomes stressed, blood is redirected from your brain to your arms, legs, chest, and other areas to support the fight-or-flight response. The Stress Hold neutralizes this response by sending blood back to your brain. It can be powerfully relaxing for your body and mind, and it is very easy to do. It can be done standing, sitting, or lying down. Place the palm of one hand over your forehead and the palm of your other hand over the back of your head, just above your neckline (see Figure A.5). Hold comfortably for a couple of minutes while inhaling through your nose and exhaling through your mouth.

The Calming Hug/Heart Hold, the Hand-on-Chest Tap, the Blow-Out, and the Stress Hold are powerful, and each can be done in a moment. The Daily Energy Routine is a more comprehensive energy practice that can have many benefits for your body, mind, and spirit, particularly if done on a daily basis. It takes only a few minutes.

THE DAILY ENERGY ROUTINE

Energy imbalances are a first place to look if your SUD won't go down, and the Daily Energy Routine (DER) is a simple, straightforward correction for energy imbalances! We want to share its origins with you, so you realize it is more than just a bunch of techniques we simply threw together.

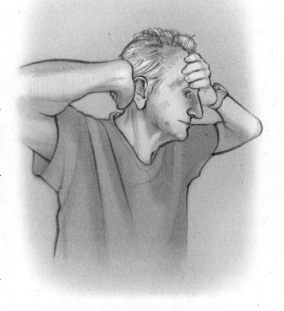

Figure A.5. The Stress Hold—a gentle physical technique for calming the energies of your nervous system.

It was 1997, and we were writing Donna's first book, *Energy Medicine*. As the manuscript was developing, it was becoming more and more detailed and comprehensive. It had been two years in the making, and these leaps in its evolution were feeling like giant accomplishments.

But suddenly we realized that with so many techniques for working with the body's numerous energy systems, we were concerned that all the information and procedures would overwhelm people. Plus, everyone seems to be incredibly busy. So we set out a challenge for ourselves. What could we teach people that they can do every day in just a few minutes to get their energies strong and flowing and keep them that way?

Over the previous two decades, Donna had treated more than 10,000 people in individual 90-minute sessions. She almost always gave her clients techniques to use at home so that what was achieved during the session would be reinforced. David asked her to make a list of the techniques she might assign as homework. From these, he asked her which ones seemed to be the most powerful. Then, from that list, he asked her to identify the ones that are the most universal. What works for just about everyone? He next asked her to select from that smaller list the ones that, as a set, would really keep people's energies humming and that they could do in five or six minutes.

Thus was born the Daily Energy Routine. Our DER videos have been viewed by more than two million people, and we know from our practitioners that thousands of individuals around the world are regularly using the method. Based on the appreciative feedback our practitioners consistently receive, we have abundant anecdotal evidence that this simple set of procedures yields strong benefits for body, mind, and spirit. It is particularly handy to use as a kind of first aid measure if a tapping session seems stuck.

You can follow Donna in doing the DER at der.energytapping.com. You will find two versions there: one with explanations (12 minutes) and one without explanations (five minutes), which people use after viewing the longer video. Of course after going through it a few times, you will have internalized it and won't need the video to lead you.

The DER is proving itself to be a wonderfully effective practice that can keep all your energy systems in a good flow. Countless health practitioners encourage their clients to do the routine every day because they know that it is one of the easiest ways for people to optimize their health and mental well-being. Over the years, we have received hundreds of emails describing how the DER has helped people overcome persistent ailments that medical interventions couldn't correct. Here is just one of them. Marie Long, who started doing the DER in her 80s, wrote:

I feel younger and more supple than ever in my life. I recently visited my son in Japan and was riding with him on his motorbike! I thoroughly enjoyed it. Me, who never even wanted or has ridden even a pedal bike, is now experiencing a great new adventure at 87. It has been 26 months since I started doing Donna's Daily Energy Routine, and I will continue to do it for the rest of my life. I have reversed my diagnosed osteoporosis, displaced vertebrae, collapsed lung, and so much, much more! The "piddling little exercises," as my granddaughter calls them, take only about five minutes a day with benefits beyond my belief. Coming from allowing myself to sink into the poor-me-redundant-granny-nobody-needs-me victim role, I am now a geriatric delinquent biker, and my son and granddaughter are very proud of me! The Daily Energy Routine is certainly my "keep young" secret.

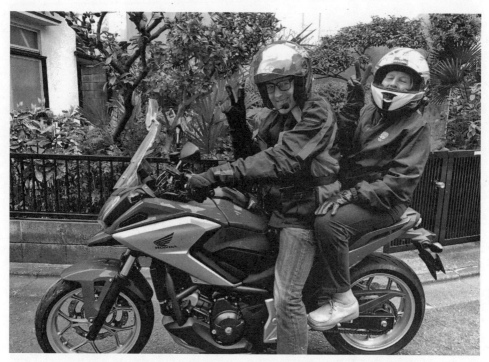

Figure A.6. Marie Long (in back), at age 87, with her son at the handlebars attributes the DER to her having reversed her medically diagnosed osteoporosis, displaced vertebrae, and collapsed lung.

You will find that this routine is as simple as it is powerful. It consists of just eight easy steps. The entire routine usually takes only five to seven minutes. We hope you will try it. If it feels as good to you as it does to most people, continue to do it daily. Again, you can follow Donna in doing the DER at der.energytapping.com.

ACEP'S TOOLS FOR RESILIENCE

We were proud to have been consulted when the Association for Comprehensive Energy Psychology (ACEP) was creating a web resource that presents their "Tools for Resilience" (energypsych.org/page /ResilienceTools). It provides a wealth of additional resources for difficult times.

OTHER PRACTICAL STEPS YOU CAN TAKE DURING A PERIOD OF DISTRESS

Beyond your tapping sessions and the quick energy first-aid techniques just presented, additional activities that support your sense of calm and well-being can build greater personal peace and resilience for trying times. Here are a few suggestions:

Tool 1: Breathe Deeply

The easiest and most direct activity you can do when you're feeling triggered is to take a few deep breaths, even without the Calming Hug/Heart Hold. Your breath is the only autonomic process over which you can take conscious control. When you are in fight-or-flight mode, your blood pressure rises, your pulse rate increases, your breathing quickens, and your breath becomes more shallow. Breathe in through your nose, letting your belly fill with air. Breathe out very slowly through your mouth. By taking control of your breathing, making it slower and deeper, your blood pressure and pulse rate go down as your emotions are soothed. Doing this whenever you are triggered trains your body that it doesn't need to escalate its threat responses.

> Your breath is the only autonomic process over which you can take conscious control.

Tool 2: Breathe In Peace, Breathe Out Stress

Take four long, slow breaths, inhaling through your nose and exhaling through your mouth. With the inhale, imagine that peace, joy, and wisdom are filling your body. With the exhale, imagine that a gray cloud of stress, worries, or troubles is leaving your body.[2]

Tool 3: Cultivate Calm

Find ways to fully rest and relax your body, mind, and spirit. What activities help you feel peaceful? This could be as easy as taking a quick nap or a relaxing bath, listening to serene music, walking in nature, having a comforting cup of tea, or getting a massage. Some people meditate, do yoga poses, practice stretching exercises, or use progressive relaxation techniques. Any of these activities is relaxing. Doing them on a regular basis builds a reservoir of peace and a habit of greater calm. For more than a quick fix, you might arrange for a vacation or a weekend stay at a bed and breakfast and leave your daily responsibilities and the pull of social media behind. Sometimes a simple change of context can go a long way toward fostering deep relaxation and restoration, even when your distress is over the top.

Tool 4: Find Support from Another Person

Reach out to a friend who cares about you. Invite this person to be a sounding board and source of support as you sort through your thoughts and feelings. Life coaches, spiritual advisors, and psychotherapists can also be powerful resources in troubled times.

Tool 5: Play with an Animal

Pet your cat, run with your dog, babysit your neighbor's pet, visit a petting zoo. Being in communion with animals lowers anxiety, depression, and stress levels; provides companionship; and improves immune-system functioning, among other benefits.[3]

Tool 6: Hang Out in Beauty

Beautiful, peaceful locations can do wonders for the soul. If possible, visit a physical space that brings you pleasure. This could be immersing yourself in a secluded area surrounded by trees; walking on the shore of a river, lake, or ocean; taking in a field of wildflowers; or preparing a quiet nook in your home where you feel safe and protected. Make a conscious effort to remember what you see and feel during your time in this space so you can call it up in your mind anytime you need an extra dose of tranquility.

Tool 7: Use Your Imagination

Even if you can't get to an inspiring setting, you can vividly imagine being in a special sacred space, by a mountain stream, lying under a towering oak, watching a sunset at the ocean. Or perhaps recall a cherished childhood hideaway. Giving such imagery your attention while breathing deeply will cause your nervous system to respond in much the same way it would respond in the actual setting.

Tool 8: Get Active

Stimulating your body with a fun, uplifting physical activity such as swimming, dancing, or jumping on a trampoline can help to discharge trapped energies. Simply taking a walk is mentally and physically refreshing as well as readily available. The benefits of regular physical exercise for your brain, emotions, and health are well established.[4]

Tool 9: Seek Inspiration

We are naturally drawn to creative works that have the power to transport us beyond the realm of the ordinary. They allow us to glimpse the innate beauty, creativity, and courage that are an essential part of the human spirit. Such attunement is one of the most effective ways to rise above the trials and tribulations of everyday life. Find books, movies, music, poetry, other art forms, or sacred ceremonies and rituals that inspire, motivate, and uplift you.

Tool 10: Eat for Peace and Health

While people respond to foods differently (one reason for the plethora of dietary books and advice), make it a priority to find the kinds of nourishment that will support your well-being and resist foods that heighten your anxiety or dampen your mood.

Tool 11: Be Patient with Yourself

Consciously participating in your own evolution involves releasing familiar but outdated ways of thinking and behaving, as you have been doing in this program. While this is a good thing, it can also be destabilizing for your psyche. Opening your heart and mind to new perspectives may be as challenging as it is desirable. You are faced with the paradox that you are wired both to evolve and to keep things the way they are. You want your life to be better, but part of you also fears change. Progressive and conservative forces battle it out not only in societies but within each of us. What you *can do* is to embrace the paradox. Foster your efforts for personal evolution while accepting yourself just as you are. You can use tapping to cultivate patience, acceptance, creativity, and even humor about the paradox: *"Even though I get into this same mess over and over again, I'm getting lots of practice working my way out of it!"*

Tool 12: Reach to Your Inner Guidance

Archetypes are elements of your psyche that can connect you to powerful, positive energies that are far beyond your conscious mind. A potent way of accessing a helpful archetype is to go within and visualize yourself talking to an inner guide or inner wise person who can nurture and advise you. Your inner wisdom figure could be someone you know, a person you know of, or someone who exists only in your imagination. Most people doing this visualize a spiritual or religious figure, a mentor they admire, or someone they looked up to as a child. Once you see this archetypal figure in your mind's eye, ask a question or simply ask for guidance and listen carefully for the response. Our final suggestion is that you cultivate an active relationship with your inner guidance by asking for help and advice whenever you are needing an extra dose of insight.

Downloads and Other Resources

IF YOU WISH TO find an energy psychology practitioner, course, or training program, we keep a list of resources at resources.energytapping.com. The various links to articles and videos mentioned throughout the book follow:

energytapping.com. David and Donna's Energy Psychology website.

cancercase1.energytapping.com (pp. 8, 29). Video excerpts showing use of energy psychology in treating a cancer patient.

models.energytapping.com (p. 26). Expands the discussion in Chapter 1.

phobiacase1.energytapping.com (p. 29). Video excerpts showing the use of energy psychology in the treatment of a phobia.

resources.energytapping .com (pp. 49, 378). Listings of energy psychology practitioner organizations, training programs, and other resources.

der.energytapping.com (multiple mentions, beginning p. 84). Access videos of Donna doing the Daily Energy Routine with and without explanations.

dreams.energytapping.com (p. 124). A primer for using tapping with dreams.

tapping-words.energytapping .com (p. 125). Journal article: "Words to Tap By."

800surveys.energytapping.com (p. 125). Journal article on reflections from 800 practitioners and clients.

vetcases.energytapping.com (p. 158). Excerpts from energy psychology treatments from four combat veterans with PTSD.

adversechildhoodexperiences .energytapping.com (p. 380). Journal article: "How Energy Psychology Remediates Emotional Wounds Rooted in Childhood Trauma: Preliminary Clinical Recommendations."

how-it-works.energytapping
.com (p. 388). Journal article: "Six
Empirically-Supported Premises
about Energy Psychology."

rwanda.energytapping.com
(p. 376). Video of Caroline Sakai,
PhD, describing her work with the
PTSD of an orphaned adolescent
in Rwanda.

energypsych.org/page/
resiliencetools (p. 365). The "Tools
for Resilience" page on the ACEP
website.

energypaper.energytapping
.com (p. 372). Journal article: "The
Energy of Energy Psychology."

disaster-relief.energytapping
.com (p. 386). Journal article: "Uses
of Energy Psychology Following
Catastrophic Events."

Notes

INTRODUCTION

1 Roger Callahan, "Roger Callahan on His Discovery of Tapping Therapy | TFT," Thought Field Therapy, November 7, 2013, YouTube video, 3:51, youtube.com/watch?v=dcmi6kWeKXs.

2 David Feinstein, "Integrating the Manual Stimulation of Acupuncture Points into Psychotherapy: A Systematic Review with Clinical Recommendations," *Journal of Psychotherapy Integration* 33, no. 1 (2023): 47–67, doi.org/10.1037/int0000283.

3 Eric Leskowitz, "Integrative Medicine for PTSD and TBI: Two Innovative Approaches," *Medical Acupuncture* 28, no. 4 (August 2016): 181–83, doi.org/10.1089/acu.2016.1168.

4 Dawson Church et al., "Clinical EFT as an Evidence-Based Practice for the Treatment of Psychological and Physiological Conditions: A Systematic Review," *Frontiers in Psychology* 13 (November 2022): 951451, doi.org/10.3389/fpsyg.2022.951451.

5 To see portions of the treatments, a 34-minute excerpt from the first three tapping sessions, at which point the cancer was clearly receding (as indicated by the CT scans), can be viewed at cancercase1.energytapping.com.

6 Dawson Church, *Mind to Matter: The Astonishing Science of How Your Brain Creates Material Reality* (Carlsbad, CA: Hay House, 2019).

7 Peta Stapleton, *The Science Behind Tapping: A Proven Stress Management Technique for the Mind and Body* (Carlsbad, CA: Hay House, 2019), xix.

8 Feinstein, "Integrating the Manual Stimulation," 47–67.

9 Donna Bach et al., "Clinical EFT (Emotional Freedom Techniques) Improves Multiple Physiological Markers of Health," *Journal of Evidence-Based Integrative Medicine* 24 (2019): 2515690X18823691, doi.org/10.1177/2515690X18823691.

10 Dawson Church et al., "Empirically Supported Psychological Treatments: The Challenge of Evaluating Clinical Innovations," *Journal of Nervous and Mental Disease* 202, no. 10 (October 2014): 699–709, doi.org/10.1097/NMD.0000000000000188.

11 Dawson Church, Peta Stapleton, and Debbie Sabot, "App-Based Delivery of Clinical Emotional Freedom

Techniques: Cross-Sectional Study of App User Self-Ratings," *JMIR mHealth & uHealth* 8, no. 10 (October 2020): e18545, doi.org/10.2196/18545.

12 The smartphone app is available as "The Tapping Solution" or see thetappingsolution.com.

13 David Feinstein, "Six Empirically-Supported Premises about Energy Psychology: Mounting Evidence for a Controversial Therapy," *Advances in Mind-Body Medicine* 35, no. 2 (2021): 17–32, how-it-works.energypsychology.com.

14 Leskowitz, "Integrative Medicine," 181–83.

15 Sally Adee, *We Are Electric: Inside the 200-Year Hunt for Our Body's Bioelectric Code, and What the Future Holds* (New York: Hachette, 2023), 8–9.

16 Adee, *We Are Electric*, 5.

17 Adee, 130.

18 Adee, 3.

19 Adee, 3.

20 David Feinstein, "Six Empirically-Supported Premises," 17–32.

21 David Feinstein, "The *Energy* of Energy Psychology," *OBM Integrative and Complementary Medicine* 7, no. 2 (2022): 15, doi.org/10.21926/obm.icm.2202015.

22 John White and Stanley Krippner, *Future Science: Life Energies and the Physics of Paranormal Phenomena* (New York: Anchor, 1977).

23 James Oschman, *Energy Medicine: The Scientific Basis*, 2nd ed. (New York: Elsevier, 2015), 41.

24 Dawson Church, *Bliss Brain: The Neuroscience of Remodeling Your Brain for Resilience, Creativity, and Joy* (Carlsbad, CA: Hay House, 2022).

25 Feinstein, "Six Empirically-Supported Premises," 17–32.

CHAPTER 1: THE GUIDING MODELS THAT MOVE YOU FORWARD OR HOLD YOU BACK

1 Adapted from David Gruder, "A Framework for Addressing Six Questions Self-Developers Have," DrGruder.com/6qsd, accessed August 2, 2023; paraphrased by Dr. Gruder.

2 Elizabeth Winkler, *Shakespeare Was a Woman and Other Heresies: How Doubting the Bard Became the Biggest Taboo in Literature* (New York: Simon and Schuster, 2023).

3 Norman Doidge, *The Brain That Changes Itself: Stories of Personal Triumph from the Frontiers of Brain Science* (New York: Penguin Life, 2007).

4 Christopher Hitchens, *The Portable Atheist: Essential Readings for the Nonbeliever* (Boston: Da Capo Press, 2007), xvi.

5 Gabor Maté, *Scattered Minds: The Origins and Healing of Attention Deficit Disorder* (New York: Penguin Random House, 1999), 238.

6   Natalie Jones et al., "Mental Models: An Interdisciplinary Synthesis of Theory and Methods," *Ecology and Society* 16, no. 1 (2011): 46, ecologyandsociety.org/vol16/iss1/art46/.

7   Jones et al., "Mental Models," 46.

8   Stuart Lightbody, *The 361 Classical Acupuncture Points: Names, Functions, Descriptions, and Locations* (Hackensack, NJ: World Scientific, 2020).

9   Juan Li et al., "Biophysical Characteristics of Meridians and Acupoints: A Systematic Review," *Evidence-Based Complementary and Alternative Medicine* (2012): 793841, doi.org/10.1155/2012/793841.

10 Helene M. Langevin and Jason A. Yandow, "Relationship of Acupuncture Points and Meridians to Connective Tissue Planes," *Anatomical Record* 269, no. 6 (December 2002): 257–65, doi.org/10.1002/ar.10185.

11 Dawson Church, *The EFT Manual*, 4th ed. (Santa Rosa, CA: Energy Psychology Press, 2018).

12 David Feinstein, "The Energy of Energy Psychology," *OBM Integrative and Complementary Medicine* 7, no. 2 (2022): 15, doi.org/10.21926/obm.icm.2202015.

13 Introduced by Gary Craig as the "Constricted Breathing Technique." Variations of the procedure are used as demonstrations in many introductory acupoint tapping classes. See "The EFT Constricted Breathing Technique," Gary Craig Official EFT Training Centers website, accessed March 21, 2023, emofree.com/fr/eft-tutorial/tapping-basics/breathing.html.

14 Developed by the psychologist John Diepold; described in John H. Diepold, Victoria Britt, and Sheila S. Bender, *Evolving Thought Field Therapy: The Clinician's Handbook of Diagnoses, Treatment, and Theory* (New York: W. W. Norton, 2004).

15 Leah R. Dickens, "Using Gratitude to Promote Positive Change: A Series of Meta-Analyses Investigating the Effectiveness of Gratitude Interventions," *Basic and Applied Social Psychology* 39, no. 4 (2017): 193–208, doi.org/10.1080/01973533.2017.1323638.

16 David Feinstein, "Six Empirically-Supported Premises about Energy Psychology: Mounting Evidence for a Controversial Therapy," *Advances in Mind-Body Medicine* 35, no. 2 (2021): 17–32, how-it-works.energypsychology.com.

17 Andrew C. Ahn et al., "Electrical Properties of Acupuncture Points and Meridians: A Systematic Review," *Bioelectromagnetics* 29, no. 4 (May 2008): 245–56, doi.org/10.1002/bem.20403.

18 Zhang-Jin Zhang, Xiao-Min Wang, and Grainne M. McAlonan, "Neural Acupuncture Unit: A New

Concept for Interpreting Effects and Mechanisms of Acupuncture," *Evidence-Based Complementary and Alternative Medicine* 2012 (2012): 429412, doi.org/10.1155/2012/429412.

19 Sviatoslav N. Bagriantsev, Elena O. Gracheva, and Patrick G. Gallagher, "Piezo Proteins: Regulators of Mechanosensation and Other Cellular Processes," *Journal of Biological Chemistry* 289, no. 46 (2014): 31673–81, doi.org/10.1074/jbc .R114.612697.

20 Langevin and Yandow, "Relationship of Acupuncture Points and Meridians," 257–65.

21 James Oschman, *Energy Medicine in Therapeutics and Human Performance* (New York: Elsevier, 2003).

22 Franck Di Rienzo et al., "Neuropsychological Correlates of an Energy Psychology Intervention on Flight Phobia: A MEG Single-Case Study," PsyArXiv Preprints, created November 17, 2019, doi.org/10.31234 /osf.io/s3hce.

23 Yuan Xu et al., "A New Theory for Acupuncture: Promoting Robust Regulation," *Journal of Acupuncture and Meridian Studies* 11, no. 1 (February 2018): 39–43, doi.org/10 .1016/j.jams.2017.11.004.

24 Beth Kearns, "All About the Tapping Points w/ Beth Kearns," August 3, 2016, in *Tapping Q&A*, hosted by Gene Monterastelli, podcast, MP3 audio, 42:14, tappingqanda.com/232.

CHAPTER 2: A BASIC TAPPING PROTOCOL

1 Dawson Church, marketing email for EFT Universe, October 27, 2020.

2 Roger J. Callahan, *Tapping the Healer Within* (Chicago: Contemporary Books, 2001), 7–10.

3 Peta Stapleton, *The Science Behind Tapping: A Proven Stress Management Technique for the Mind and Body* (Carlsbad, CA: Hay House, 2019), xxv.

4 Steve Wells and David Lake, *Enjoy Emotional Freedom: Simple Techniques for Living Life to the Full* (Woolombi, Australia: Exisle, 2010), 25.

5 Dawson Church, *The EFT Manual*, 4th ed. (Santa Rosa, CA: Energy Psychology Press, 2018), 367–70.

6 David Feinstein, Donna Eden, and Gary Craig, *The Promise of Energy Psychology: Revolutionary Tools for Dramatic Personal Change* (New York: Tarcher/Penguin, 2005).

7 Dawson Church, Peta Stapleton, and Debbie Sabot, "App-Based Delivery of Clinical Emotional Freedom Techniques: Cross-Sectional Study of App User Self-Ratings," *JMIR mHealth & uHealth* 8, no. 10 (October 2020): e18545, doi.org/10 .2196/18545.

8 David Feinstein, "How Energy Psychology Changes Deep Emotional Learnings," *Neuropsychologist* 10 (2015): 38–49.

9   Dawson Church, "Clinical EFT as an Evidence-Based Practice for the Treatment of Psychological and Physiological Conditions," *Psychology* 4, no. 8 (August 2013): 645–54, doi.org/10.4236/psych.2013.48092.

10 Carl Rogers, *On Becoming a Person: A Therapist's View of Psychotherapy* (New York: Houghton Mifflin, 1961), 17.

11 Donna Eden, *Energy Medicine: Balancing Your Body's Energies for Optimal Health, Joy, and Vitality*, rev. ed. (New York: Tarcher/Perigree, 2008), 109–46.

12 Church, *The EFT Manual*, 106.

CHAPTER 3: THE DETECTIVE WORK

1   Gary Craig, "Finding aspects within the EFT Tapping Process," The Gary Craig Official EFT Training Centers (website), accessed April 27, 2023, emofree.com/eft-tutorial/tapping-roots/aspects.html.

2   Daniel David, Ioana Cristea, and Stefan G. Hofmann, "Why Cognitive Behavioral Therapy Is the Current Gold Standard of Psychotherapy," *Frontiers in Psychiatry* 9 (January 2018): 4, doi.org/10.3389/fpsyt.2018.00004.

3   David Burns, *Feeling Great: The Revolutionary New Treatment for Depression and Anxiety* (Eau Claire, WI: PESI Publishing & Media, 2020), 452.

4   The Association for Comprehensive Energy Psychology maintains a regularly updated database of published studies worldwide: energypsych.org.

5   Summarized in David Feinstein, "Six Empirically-Supported Premises about Energy Psychology: Mounting Evidence for a Controversial Therapy," *Advances in Mind-Body Medicine* 35, no. 2 (2021): 17–32, advances-journal.com/wp-content/uploads/2021/05/Feinstein.pdf.

6   David Burns, *Feeling Good: The New Mood Therapy* (New York: HarperCollins, 1999).

7   Burns, *Feeling Great*, xiv.

8   Burns, xv.

9   Carl R. Rogers, *On Becoming a Person: A Therapist's View of Psychotherapy* (New York: Houghton Mifflin, 1961), 17.

10 Patricia Carrington, "Introducing the EFT Choices Method," patcarrington.com, April 19, 2019, patcarrington.com/introducing-the-choices-method/.

11 David Burns, "When Helping Doesn't Help: Why Some Clients May Not Want to Change," *Psychotherapy Networker*, March/April 2017, 19, psychotherapynetworker.org/article/when-helping-doesnt-help.

12 Burns, "When Helping Doesn't Help."

13 Burns, *Feeling Great*, 97.

14 Burns, 15–26.

15 Burns, 26–34.

16 Mary T. Sise and Sheila Sidney Bender, *The Energy of Belief* (York, PA: Capucia, 2022), 189–90.

17 Ann Adams and Karin Davidson, *EFT Level 2 Comprehensive Training Resource* (Fulton, CA: Energy Psychology Press, 2011), 92.

18 John G. Watkins, "The Affect Bridge: A Hypnoanalytic Technique," *International Journal of Clinical and Experimental Hypnosis* 19, no. 1 (1971): 21–27, doi.org/10.1080/00207147108407148.

19 Burns, *Feeling Great*, xv.

20 Burns, 480.

21 Maggie Adkins, "Inner Dialogues with EFT," in *EFT and Beyond: Cutting Edge Techniques for Personal Transformation*, ed. Pamela Bruner and John Bullough (Essex, England: Energy Publications, 2009), 78.

22 Church, *EFT Manual*, 241.

23 Steven Ungerleider, *Mental Training for Peak Performance: Top Athletes Reveal the Mind Exercises They Use to Excel*, rev. ed. (Emmaus, PA: Rodale, 2005), 24.

24 Robert Hoss and Lynne Hoss, *Dream to Freedom: A Handbook for Integrating Dreamwork and Energy Psychology* (Santa Rosa, CA: Energy Psychology Press, 2013).

CHAPTER 4: WORRY, ANXIETY, AND PTSD

1 Nick Ortner, *The Tapping Solution: A Revolutionary System for Stress-Free Living* (Carlsbad, CA: Hay House, 2013), 7.

2 Karen Hughes et al., "The Effect of Multiple Adverse Childhood Experiences on Health: A Systematic Review and Meta-Analysis," *Lancet Public Health* 2, no. 8 (2017): e356–66, doi.org/10.1016/S2468-2667(17)30118-4.

3 Caroline E. Sakai, Suzanne M. Connolly, and Paul Oas, "Treatment of PTSD in Rwandan Genocide Survivors Using Thought Field Therapy," *International Journal of Emergency Mental Health* 12, no. 1 (2010): 41–50.

4 An eight-minute video clip of Dr. Sakai describing this case can be accessed at rwanda.energytapping.com.

5 David Feinstein, "Uses of Energy Psychology Following Catastrophic Events," *Frontiers in Psychology* 13 (April 2022): 856209, doi.org/10.3389/fpsyg.2022.856209.

6 Gunilla Hamne, Ulf Sandström, and Peta Stapleton, "Evaluation of a Brief Trauma Tapping Training and Single Session Application," *International Journal of Healing and Caring* 23, no. 3 (September 2023): 22–28. doi.org/10.78717/ijhc.202323322.

7 William James, *Habit* (Ann Arbor, MI: University of Michigan Library, 1890), 31.

8 Ralph Adolphs, "The Biology of Fear," *Current Biology* 23, no. 2 (January 2013): PR79–R93, doi.org/10.1016/j.cub.2012.11.055.

9 Amanda Heidt, "Brain Circuitry for Fear and Anxiety Is the Same on fMRI," *The Scientist*, September 21, 2020, jneurosci.org/content/40/41/7949.

10 David S. Goldstein, "Adrenal Responses to Stress," *Cellular and Molecular Neurobiology* 30, no. 8 (2010): 1433–40, doi.org/10.1007/s10571-010-9606-9.

11 Brain imaging studies showing that tapping activates specific brain areas related to psychological symptoms and deactivates others are summarized in Chapter 9.

12 The phrases in the six "Quick Fix" boxes throughout the book were formulated in collaboration with Carol Look, whom we consider to be a master in bringing the benefits of tapping to large groups: carollook.com.

13 Amrisha Vaish, Tobias Grossmann, and Amanda Woodward, "Not All Emotions Are Created Equal: The Negativity Bias in Social-Emotional Development," *Psychological Bulletin* 134, no. 3 (2008): 383–403, doi.org/10.1037/0033-2909.134.3.383.

14 Rick Hanson, *Buddha's Brain* (Oakland, CA: New Harbinger, 2009), 41.

15 William Pearse, "The Anxiety Epidemic," *Inomics*, May 31, 2021, inomics.com/blog/the-anxiety-epidemic-1377345.

16 Tom C. Russ et al., "Association Between Psychological Distress and Mortality: Individual Participant Pooled Analysis of 10 Prospective Cohort Studies," *BMJ* 345 (2012): e4933, doi.org/10.1136/bmj.e4933.

17 Morgan Clond, "Emotional Freedom Techniques for Anxiety: A Systematic Review with Meta-Analysis," *Journal of Nervous and Mental Disease* 204, no. 5 (May 2016): 388–95, doi.org/10.1097/NMD.0000000000000483.

18 You will see that sometimes we refer to the "fight-flight-freeze response" and other times just to the "fight-or-flight" response. Fight, flight, and freeze are the three responses to threat that have evolved over eons. Fight and flight are initiated by the amygdala. Freeze is initiated by the vagus nerve. When we use "fight-or-flight," we are referring to responses initiated by the amygdala.

19 Peta Stapleton et al., "Reexamining the Effect of Emotional Freedom Techniques on Stress Biochemistry: A Randomized Controlled Trial," *Psychological Trauma: Theory, Research, Practice, and Policy* 12, no. 8 (2020): 869–77, doi.org/10.1037/tra0000563.

20 Marjorie E. Maharaj, "Differential Gene Expression after Emotional Freedom Techniques (EFT) Treatment: A Novel Pilot Protocol for Salivary mRNA Assessment," *Energy Psychology: Theory, Research, and*

Treatment 8, no. 1 (2016): 17–32, doi
.org/10.9769/EPJ.2016.8.1.MM.

21 Donna Bach et al., "Clinical EFT
(Emotional Freedom Techniques)
Improves Multiple Physiological
Markers of Health," *Journal
of Evidence-Based Integrative
Medicine* 24 (2019): 2515690X18823691,
doi.org/10.1177/2515690X18823691.

22 See directory at resources
.energytapping.com.

23 See "How to Tell the Difference
Between a Panic Attack and a Heart
Attack," Cleveland Clinic, April 2,
2021, health.clevelandclinic.org/the
-difference-between-panic-attacks
-and-heart-attacks/.

24 The National Institute for the Clinical
Application of Behavioral Medicine
(NICABM) offers a series of online
courses taught by some of the world's
top psychologists, psychiatrists, and
other trauma experts, with Bessel van
der Kolk, MD, being a major presenter.
These courses have been a primary
source for identifying the best
practices that the mental health field
has developed for treating PTSD and
related conditions (nicabm.com).

25 Bessel van der Kolk, *The Body Keeps
the Score: Brain, Mind, and Body in
the Healing of Trauma* (New York:
Penguin Random House, 2015).

26 Abram Kardiner, *The Traumatic
Neuroses of War* (New York:
Hoeber, 1941).

27 David Frausto Peña et al., "Vagus
Nerve Stimulation Enhances

Extinction of Conditioned Fear and
Modulates Plasticity in the Pathway
from the Ventromedial Prefrontal
Cortex to the Amygdala," *Frontiers
in Behavioral Neuroscience* 8 (2014):
327, doi.org/10.3389/fnbeh.2014.00327.

28 Stephen W. Porges, *The Polyvagal
Theory: Neurophysiological
Foundations of Emotions, Attachment,
Communication, and Self-Regulation*
(New York: Norton, 2011).

29 Robert Schwarz, "Energy Psychology,
Polyvagal Theory, and the Treatment
of Trauma," in *Clinical Applications
of the Polyvagal Theory: The
Emergence of Polyvagal-Informed
Therapies*, ed. Stephen W. Porges
and Deb Dana (New York: Norton,
2018), 270–84.

30 American Psychological Association,
*Clinical Practice Guideline for the
Treatment of Posttraumatic Stress
Disorder (PTSD) in Adults*, February
2017, apa.org/ptsd-guideline/ptsd.pdf.

31 Maria M. Steenkamp et al.,
"Psychotherapy for Military-Related
PTSD: A Review of Randomized
Clinical Trials," *JAMA* 314, no. 5 (2015):
489–500, doi.org/10.1001/jama.2015.8370.

32 Lisa M. Najavits, "The Problem of
Dropout from 'Gold Standard' PTSD
Therapies," *F1000 Prime Reports* 7
(2015): 43, doi.org/10.12703/P7-43.

33 Dawson Church et al., "Psychological
Trauma in Veterans Using EFT
(Emotional Freedom Techniques):
A Randomized Controlled Trial,"
Journal of Nervous and Mental

Disease 201, no. 2 (2013): 153–60, doi .org/10.1097/NMD.0b013e31827f6351.

34 Linda Geronilla et al., "EFT (Emotional Freedom Techniques) Remediates PTSD and Psychological Symptoms in Veterans: A Randomized Controlled Replication Trial," *Energy Psychology: Theory, Research, and Treatment* 8, no. 2 (2016): 29–41, doi.org/10.9769/EPJ.2016 .8.2.LG.

35 Peta Stapleton et al., "Emotional Freedom Techniques for Treating Post Traumatic Stress Disorder: An Updated Systematic Review and Meta-Analysis," *Frontiers in Psychology* 14, (2023): 1195286, doi.org /10.3389/fpsyg.2023.1195286.

36 Brenda Sebastian and Jerrod Nelms, "The Effectiveness of Emotional Freedom Techniques in the Treatment of Posttraumatic Stress Disorder: A Meta-Analysis," *Explore: The Journal of Science and Healing* 13, no. 1 (2017): 16–25, doi.org/10.1016/j .explore.2016.10.001.

37 Thanos Karatzias et al., "A Controlled Comparison of the Effectiveness and Efficiency of Two Psychological Therapies for Posttraumatic Stress Disorder: Eye Movement Desensitization and Reprocessing vs. Emotional Freedom Techniques," *Journal of Nervous and Mental Disease* 199, no. 6 (June 2011): 372–78, doi.org/10.1097/NMD .0b013e31821cd262.

38 Dawson Church and Audrey J. Brooks, "CAM and Energy Psychology Techniques Remediate PTSD Symptoms in Veterans and Spouses," *Explore: The Journal of Science and Healing* 10, no. 1 (January–February 2014): 24–33, doi .org/10.1016/j.explore.2013.10.006.

39 R. C. Brown et al., "Psychosocial Interventions for Children and Adolescents after Man-Made and Natural Disasters: A Meta-Analysis and Systematic Review," *Psychological Medicine* 47, no. 11 (April 2017): 1893–1905, doi.org/10.1017 /s0033291717000496.

40 Ifigeneia Mavranezouli et al., "Psychological and Psychosocial Treatments for Children and Young People with Post-Traumatic Stress Disorder: A Network Meta-Analysis," *Journal of Child Psychology and Psychiatry* 61, no. 1 (January 2020): 18–29, doi.org/10.1111/jcpp.13094.

41 You will see in the video that Gary Craig begins to tap on one of the veterans who has gone into extreme distress. Tapping on another person can be as effective as tapping on oneself, but self-tapping is generally preferred because it is empowering to know you brought about the relief, and it also teaches you how to use the method whenever needed.

42 Church et al., "Psychological Trauma in Veterans."

43 Dawson Church, *The EFT Manual*, 4th ed. (Santa Rosa, CA: Energy Psychology Press, 2018).

44 EFT founder Gary Craig wrote *EFT for PTSD* in 2009 (Santa Rosa, CA: Energy Psychology Press) with invited sections by several other prominent practitioners. A few of the Acceptance or Choices Statements in this section are taken or modified from that book. This one was presented by Ingrid Dinter.

45 Quoted in "Core Issues of Abuse: Forgiveness," Into the Light, accessed April 30, 2023, intothelight .org.uk/core-issues-abuse -forgiveness/.

46 Xiaoli Wu et al., "The Prevalence of Moderate-to-High Posttraumatic Growth: A Systematic Review and Meta-Analysis," *Journal of Affective Disorders* 243 (January 2019): 408–15, doi.org/10.1016/j.jad.2018.09.023.

47 Peter A. Levine, *Waking the Tiger: Healing Trauma* (Berkeley, CA: North Atlantic Books, 1997), 12.

CHAPTER 5: SADNESS AND DEPRESSION

1 Adapted from *Tools for Transforming Trauma* by Robert Schwarz (New York: Routledge, 2002), paraphrased by Dr. Schwarz.

2 Atticus, *Love Her Wild: Poems* (New York: Atria, 2017), 195.

3 Lowry A. Kirkby et al., "An Amygdala-Hippocampus Subnetwork That Encodes Variation in Human Mood," *Cell* 175, no. 6 (2018): 1688–1700.e14, doi.org/10.1016/j.cell.2018.10.005.

4 Martha Manning, "A Journey Through Fire: Surviving When Your Self Is in Ashes," *Psychotherapy Networker*, July/August 2018, psychotherapynetworker.org/article /journey-through-fire.

5 "Depressive Disorder (Depression)," World Health Organization, March 31, 2023, who.int/news-room/fact -sheets/detail/depression.

6 "Major Depression," US National Institute of Mental Health, last updated January 2022, nimh.nih.gov /health/statistics/major-depression.

7 American Psychiatric Association, *Diagnostic and Statistical Manual of Mental Disorders*, 5th ed. (Washington, DC: American Psychiatric Association Publishing, 2013).

8 Jason D. Boardman, Kari B. Alexander, and Michael C. Stallings, "Stressful Life Events and Depression among Adolescent Twin Pairs," *Biodemography and Social Biology* 57, no. 1 (2011): 53–66, doi.org/10.1080 /19485565.2011.574565.

9 Naomi R. Wray et al., "Genome-Wide Association Analyses Identify 44 Risk Variants and Refine the Genetic Architecture of Major Depression," *Nature Genetics* 50, no. 5 (May 2018): 668–81, doi.org/10.1038/s41588-018 -0090-3.

10 David Feinstein, "Using Energy Psychology to Remediate Emotional Wounds Rooted in Childhood Trauma: Preliminary Clinical Guidelines," *Frontiers in Psychology* 14 (October 18, 2023), doi.org/10.3389/fpsyg.2023.1277555.

11 Mekonnen Tsehay, Mogesie Necho, and Werkua Mekonnen, "The Role of Adverse Childhood Experience on Depression Symptom, Prevalence, and Severity among School Going Adolescents," *Depression Research and Treatment* (2020): 5951792, doi.org/10.1155/2020/5951792.

12 Fei-Fei Zhang et al., "Brain Structure Alterations in Depression: Psychoradiological Evidence," *CNS Neuroscience & Therapeutics* 24, no. 11 (November 2018): 994–1003. doi.org/10.1111/cns.12835.

13 Andrew H. Miller and Charles L. Raison, "The Role of Inflammation in Depression: From Evolutionary Imperative to Modern Treatment Target," *Nature Reviews Immunology* 16, no. 1 (January 2016): 22–34, doi.org/10.1038/nri.2015.5.

14 Jerrod A. Nelms and Liana Castel, "A Systematic Review and Meta-Analysis of Randomized and Non-Randomized Trials of Clinical Emotional Freedom Techniques (EFT) for the Treatment of Depression," *Explore: The Journal of Science and Healing* 12, no. 6 (November–December 2016): 416–26, doi.org/10.1016/j.explore.2016.08.001.

15 Fred P. Gallo, *Energy Psychology: Explorations at the Interface of Energy, Cognition, Behavior, and Health* (Boca Raton, FL: CRC Press, 1998).

16 "How to Work with the Patterns That Sustain Depression" was organized by Ruth Buczynski, PhD, bringing together leading experts in working with depression. The 16 faculty, in alphabetical order, included Joan Borysenko, PhD; Rick Hanson, PhD; Shelly Harrell, PhD; Marsha Linehan, PhD, Lynn Lyons, LICSW; Kelly McGonigal, PhD; Pat Ogden, PhD; Bill O'Hanlon, MS, LMFT; Christine Padesky, PhD; Terry Real, LICSW; Richard Schwartz, PhD; Dan Siegel, MD; Ron Siegel, PsyD; Stan Tatkin, PsyD, MFT; Bessel van der Kolk, MD; and Michael Yapko, PhD. It was sponsored by the National Institute for the Clinical Application of Behavioral Medicine (NICABM), 2018, nicabm.com.

17 Christopher Peterson, Steven F. Maier, and Martin E. P. Seligman, *Learned Helplessness: A Theory for the Age of Personal Control* (New York: Oxford University Press, 1993).

18 Dennis Greenberger and Christine A. Padesky, *Mind Over Mood: Change How You Feel by Changing the Way You Think*, 2nd ed. (New York: Guilford, 2015).

19 Greenberger and Padesky, *Mind Over Mood*, 37.

20 Wray, "Genome-Wide Association Analyses," 668–81.

21 Meri Levy, "Can Depression Be Cured without Medication?" GoodTherapy, November 17, 2014, goodtherapy.org /blog/can-depression-be-cured -without-medication-1117144.

22 Jean M. Twenge et al., "Increases in Depressive Symptoms, Suicide-Related Outcomes, and Suicide Rates Among U.S. Adolescents After 2010 and Links to Increased New Media Screen Time," *Clinical Psychological Science* 6, no. 1 (2018): 3–17, doi.org/10 .1177/2167702617723376.

23 *Amistad*, directed by Steven Spielberg (Universal City, CA: DreamWorks Pictures, 1997).

24 Marian Sandmaier, "In the Shadow of Depression: How Can We Manage to Stay Well?" *Psychotherapy Networker*, July/August 2018, psychotherapynetworker.org/article /shadow-depression.

25 Sandmaier, "In the Shadow."

26 Sandmaier, "In the Shadow."

CHAPTER 6: HABITS AND ADDICTIONS

1 Adapted from Mary T. Sise and Sheila S. Bender, *The Energy of Belief: Simple Proven Techniques to Release Limiting Beliefs & Transform Your Life*, 2nd ed. (York, PA: Capucia, 2022); paraphrased by Mary Sise.

2 Steven Stosny, "Blue-Collar Therapy: The Nitty-Gritty of Lasting Change," *Psychotherapy Networker*, November/December 2013, psychotherapynetworker.org/article /blue-collar-therapy.

3 Jay Van Bavel and Dominic Packer, "Sick of Failing at Your New Year's Resolutions? There Is a Better Way," *Time*, December 29, 2022, time.com /6243642/how-to-keep-new-years -resolutions-2.

4 Charles Duhigg, *The Power of Habit: Why We Do What We Do in Life and Business* (New York: Random House, 2014); B. J. Fogg, *Tiny Habits: The Small Changes That Change Everything* (Boston: Houghton Mifflin Harcourt, 2000); Stephen R. Covey, *The 7 Habits of Highly Effective People*, 30th ann. ed. (New York: Simon & Schuster, 2020).

5 James Clear, *Atomic Habits: An Easy & Proven Way to Build Good Habits & Break Bad Ones* (New York: Avery, 2018).

6 Clear, *Atomic Habits*, 46.

7 Clear, 45.

8 Clear, 48.

9 Clear, 86.

10 Clear, 189.

11 Clear, 131–32.

12 Clear, 105.

13 Clear, 106.

14 Trevor Haynes, "Dopamine, Smartphones, and You: A Battle for Your Time," *Science in the News* (blog), Harvard University, May 1, 2018. sitn.hms.harvard.edu/flash /2018/dopamine-smartphones-battle -time/.

15 Clear, *Atomic Habits*, 149.
16 Clear, 144.
17 Clear, 170.
18 Clear, 151.
19 Clear, 198.
20 Clear, 197.
21 Clear, 216.
22 Clear, 204.
23 Clear, 92–93.
24 Clear, 94.
25 Clear, 127.
26 Clear, 129.
27 Clear, 172.
28 Clear, 175.
29 Clear, 213.
30 Clear, 198.
31 Adriana Popescu, "Trauma-Based Energy Psychology Treatment Is Associated with Client Rehabilitation at an Addiction Clinic," *Energy Psychology: Theory, Research, and Treatment* 13, no. 1 (2021): 12, doi.org /10.9769/EPJ.2021.13.1.AP.
32 Carl Jung, *Memories, Dreams, Reflections* (New York: Vintage, 1989), 329.
33 Margaret Wehrenberg, "Habits vs. Addictions: What's the Difference?" *Psychotherapy Networker*, November/December 2013, psychotherapynetworker.org/article /habits-vs-addictions.
34 Francesca Mapua Filbey, *The Neuroscience of Addiction* (Cambridge: Cambridge University Press, 2019).
35 Anna Lembke, *Dopamine Nation: Finding Balance in the Age of Indulgence* (New York: Penguin Putnam, 2021).
36 David Feinstein, "Energy Psychology in the Treatment of Substance Use Disorders," in *Complementary and Integrative Approaches to Substance Use Disorders*, ed. Rita Carroll (New York: Nova Science Publishers, 2021), 69–106.
37 A. Thomas Horvath, *Sex, Drugs, Gambling & Chocolate: A Workbook for Overcoming Addictions*, 2nd ed. (Atascadero, CA: Impact Publishers, 2004).
38 Horvath, *Sex, Drugs*, 210.
39 Paul Krebs et al., "Stages of Change and Psychotherapy Outcomes: A Review and Meta-Analysis," *Journal of Clinical Psychology* 74, no. 11 (2018): 1964–79, doi.org/10.1002/jclp .22683.
40 Horvath, *Sex, Drugs*, 40.
41 Horvath, 83.
42 Horvath, 211.
43 Horvath, 23.
44 Selwan Mahmoud, Omima Abo-Baker, and Sahar Mahmoud, "Effect of Emotional Freedom Techniques on Psychological Symptoms and Cravings among Patients with Substance Related Disorders," *International Journal of Novel Research in Healthcare and Nursing* 7, no. 2 (2020): 30–45.
45 Peta Stapleton et al., "An Initial Investigation of Neural Changes in Overweight Adults with Food Cravings after Emotional Freedom

Techniques," *OBM Integrative and Complementary Medicine* 4, no. 1 (2019): 010, doi.org/10.21926/obm.icm .1901010.

46 Horvath, *Sex, Drugs*, 211.

47 "Drug Overdose: Death Rate Maps and Graphs," Centers for Disease Control and Prevention, last reviewed June 2, 2022, cdc.gov /drugoverdose/deaths/index.html.

48 John McDonald and Stephen Janz, *The Acupuncture Evidence Project: A Comparative Literature Review*, rev. ed. (Brisbane: Australian Acupuncture and Chinese Medicine Association, 2017); asacu.org /wp-content/uploads/2017/09 /Acupuncture-Evidence-Project-The .pdf.

49 Nick Ortner, *The Tapping Solution for Pain Relief: A Step-by-Step Guide to Reducing and Eliminating Chronic Pain* (Carlsbad, CA: Hay House, 2016).

50 Robin Bilazarian and Margaret Hux, "Rapid Group Treatment of Pain and Upsets with the Brief Energy Correction," *International Journal of Healing and Caring* 20, no. 3 (2020), ijhc.org/wp-content/uploads/2022 /07/Bilazarian-Hux20-3b.pdf.

51 Morgan Clond, "Emotional Freedom Techniques for Anxiety: A Systematic Review with Meta- Analysis," *Journal of Nervous and Mental Disease* 204, no. 5 (May 2016): 388–95, doi.org/10.1097/NMD .0000000000000483.

52 Amy H. Gaesser, "Emotional Freedom Techniques: Stress and Anxiety Management for Students and Staff in School Settings," in *Applying Psychology in the Schools: Interventions for Mental Health Professionals*, ed. Cheryl Maykel and Melissa A. Bray (Washington, DC: American Psychological Association, 2020), 283–97, doi.org/10.1037 /0000157-020.

53 Dawson Church, Peta Stapleton, and Debbie Sabot, "App-Based Delivery of Clinical Emotional Freedom Techniques: Cross-Sectional Study of App User Self-Ratings," *JMIR mHealth & uHealth* 8, no. 10 (October 2020): e18545, doi.org/10 .2196/18545.

54 Horvath, *Sex, Drugs*, 197.

55 Horvath, 201.

56 Horvath, 23.

CHAPTER 7: PEAK PERFORMANCE

1 Patricia Carrington, *Try It on Everything: Discover the Power of EFT* (Bethel, CT: Try It Productions, 2008), 91.

2 Greg Warburton, *Warburton's Winning System: Tapping and Other Transformational Mental Training Tools for Athletes* (Denver, CO: Outskirts Press, 2013).

3 Discussions and email exchanges with Warburton, along with his book, are the sources for his

stories, techniques, and principles recounted throughout this chapter.

4   Gary Craig, *EFT for Sports Performance* (Fulton, CA: Energy Psychology Press, 2010).

5   Tim Woodman et al., "Self-Confidence and Performance: A Little Self-Doubt Helps," *Psychology of Sport and Exercise* 11, no. 6 (November 2010): 467–70. doi.org/10.1016/j.psychsport.2010.05.009.

6   Dawson Church and Darlene Downs, "Sports Confidence and Critical Incident Intensity After a Brief Application of Emotional Freedom Techniques: A Pilot Study," *Sport Journal* 15, no. 1 (2012), thesportjournal.org/article/sports-confidence-and-critical-incident-intensity-after-a-brief-application-of-emotional-freedom-techniques-a-pilot-study/.

7   Denise Wall, "Sports EFT for Children," in *EFT for Sports Performance*, 2nd ed., by Jessica A. Howard (Fulton, CA: Energy Psychology Press, 2014), 220.

8   Jean M. Williams and Vikki Krane, *Applied Sport Psychology: Personal Growth to Peak Performance*, 8th ed. (New York: McGraw-Hill, 2021).

9   Speech at Rice University Stadium in Houston, Texas, on September 12, 1962. Neil Armstrong stepped onto the moon on July 21, 1969.

10 Dr. Weiss' diagnostic and surgical skills were life-saving when he performed emergency open-heart surgery on Donna. After the operation, a member of the surgical team confided to Donna's family, "We thought we were going to lose her." Apparently sensing that Donna was picking up on this concern, Dr. Weiss looked into her eyes just before the surgery and said, "I don't kill people!" Donna felt his confidence, relaxed completely, and is still here to tell about it!

11 Jessica Höpfner and Nina Keith, "Goal Missed, Self Hit: Goal-Setting, Goal-Failure, and Their Affective, Motivational, and Behavioral Consequences," *Frontiers in Psychology* 12 (2021): 704790, doi.org/10.3389/fpsyg.2021.704790.

12 Steven Ungerleider, *Mental Training for Peak Performance: Top Athletes Reveal the Mind Exercises They Use to Excel* (Emmaus, PA: Rodale, 2005), 24.

13 Quoted in Ungerleider, *Mental Training*, 21.

14 Yogi Berra, *The Yogi Book* (New York: Workman, 2010), 89.

15 Ungerleider, *Mental Training*, 44.

16 Ungerleider, 42.

17 Quoted in Ungerleider, 37.

18 Variations of this research design have been used many times and produced similar outcomes. See, for instance, Kathleen A. Martin, Sandra E. Moritz, and Craig R. Hall, "Imagery Use in Sport: A Literature Review and Applied Model," *Sport Psychologist* 13, no. 3 (1999): 245–68.

19 Ungerleider, *Mental Training*, 4.

20   Ungerleider, 39–41.

21   Ungerleider, 63.

22   T. Llewellyn-Edwards and M. Llewellyn-Edwards, "The Effect of EFT (Emotional Freedom Techniques) on Soccer Performance," *Fidelity: Journal for the National Council of Psychotherapy* 47 (Spring 2012): 14–19.

CHAPTER 8: RELATIONSHIPS

1   Adapted from Fred P. Gallo, *The Amazing Couples Course Manual* (Hermitage, PA: Gallo & Associates, 2013); paraphrased by Dr. Gallo.

2   Jean Houston, introduction to *The Energies of Love: Invisible Keys to a Fulfilling Partnership*, by Donna Eden and David Feinstein (New York: Penguin Random House, 2016), xiii.

3   *APA Dictionary of Psychology*, s.v. "companionate love," accessed May 12, 2023, dictionary.apa.org/companionate-love.

4   Richard B. Slatcher and Emre Selcuk, "A Social Psychological Perspective on the Links Between Close Relationships and Health," *Current Directions in Psychological Science* 26, no. 1 (2017): 16–21, doi.org/10.1177/0963721416667444.

5   Robert Kegan, *The Emerging Self: Problem and Process in Human Development* (Cambridge, MA: Harvard University Press, 1982).

6   Daniel Goleman, *Emotional Intelligence: Why It Can Matter More than IQ*, 25th ann. ed. (London: Bloomsbury, 2020).

7   Daniel J. Siegel and Mary Hartzell, *Parenting from the Inside Out: How a Deeper Self-Understanding Can Help You Raise Children Who Thrive* (New York: Tarcher/Penguin, 2004), 173.

8   Siegel and Hartzell, *Parenting from the Inside Out*, 155.

9   To learn more about Havening, visit havening.org/.

10 Dawson Church, *EFT for Love Relationships* (Fulton, CA: Energy Psychology Press, 2015), 204–5.

11 Diane Poole Heller, *The Power of Attachment: How to Create Deep and Lasting Intimate Relationships* (Boulder, CO: Sounds True, 2019).

12 Eden and Feinstein, *Energies of Love*, 221–24.

13 Robert Plutchik, *Emotions and Life: Perspectives from Psychology, Biology, and Evolution* (Washington, DC: American Psychological Association, 2002).

14 Daniel J. Siegel, *The Developing Mind: How Relationships and the Brain Interact to Shape Who We Are*, 2nd ed. (New York: Guilford Press, 2012), 150.

15 Church, *EFT for Love Relationships*, 247.

16 Eden and Feinstein, *Energies of Love*, 179–82.

CHAPTER 9: WHEN DISASTER STRIKES

1   From correspondence between David Feinstein and Dr. Charles Figley.

2   This chapter includes excerpts from David Feinstein's "Uses of Energy Psychology Following Catastrophic Events," *Frontiers in Psychology* 13 (2022), doi.org/10.3389/fpsyg.2022.856209.

3   Centre for Research on the Epidemiology of Disasters, *The Human Cost of Disasters: An Overview of the Last 20 Years 2000–2019* (New York: United Nations Office for Disaster Risk Reduction, 2020), 1.

4   Les Coleman, "Frequency of Man-Made Disasters in the 20th Century," *Journal of Contingencies and Crisis Management* 14, no. 1 (March 2006): 3–11, doi.org/10.1111/j.1468–5973.2006.00476.x.

5   Mahtab Kouhirostamkolaei, "Integrating Mental Health Support in Emergency Planning and Disaster Risk Mitigation Strategies," *Qeios*, May 8, 2023, doi.org/10.32388/02RTJC.

6   Nikunj Makwana, "Disaster and Its Impact on Mental Health: A Narrative Review," *Journal of Family Medicine and Primary Care* 8, no. 10 (2019): 3090–95, doi.org/10.4103/jfmpc.jfmpc_893_19.

7   Among these are Capacitar International, the Peaceful Heart Network, Create Global Healing, and the Mind Heart Connect Foundation, along with, as you might expect, the humanitarian relief efforts of energy psychology groups such as the Thought Field Therapy Foundation, EFT International, and the Association for Comprehensive Energy Psychology.

8   The Tapping Solution, thetappingsolution.com.

9   Create Global Healing, drlorileyden.com/create-global-healing.

10 N. Ortner, L. Leyden, and S. Lewis, *Newtown Trauma Relief Collaboration Project* (Newtown: Newtown Trauma Relief Collaboration Project, n.d.).

11 Giulia Turrini et al., "Common Mental Disorders in Asylum Seekers and Refugees: Umbrella Review of Prevalence and Intervention Studies," *International Journal of Mental Health Systems* 11 (2017): 51, doi.org/10.1186/s13033-017-0156-0.

12 The World Bank, *Migrants, Refugees, and Society* (Washington, DC: International Bank for Reconstruction and Development / The World Bank, 2023), worldbank.org/en/publication/wdr2023.

13 Turrini, "Common Mental Disorders."

14 Peta Stapleton et al., "Emotional Freedom Techniques for Treating Post Traumatic Stress Disorder: An Updated Systematic Review and Meta-Analysis," *Frontiers in Psychology*, 14 (2023): 1195286, doi.org/10.3389/fpsyg.2023.1195286.

15 Suzanne Connolly and Caroline Sakai, "Brief Trauma Intervention with Rwandan Genocide-Survivors Using Thought Field Therapy,"

International Journal of Emergency Mental Health 13, no. 3 (2011): 161–72.

16   E. Boath, T. Stewart, and C. Rolling, "The Impact of EFT and Matrix Reimprinting on the Civilian Survivors of War in Bosnia: A Pilot Study," *Current Research in Psychology* 5, no. 1 (2014): 64–72, doi .org/10.3844/crpsp.2014.64.72.

17   Jean-Michel Gurret et al., "Post-Earthquake Rehabilitation of Clinical PTSD in Haitian Seminarians," *Energy Psychology: Theory, Research, and Treatment* 4, no. 2 (2012): 33–40, doi.org/10.9769/EPJ.2012.4.2.JPH.

18   David Feinstein, "Uses of Energy Psychology Following Catastrophic Events," *Frontiers in Psychology* 13 (April 2022): 856209, doi.org/10.3389 /fpsyg.2022.856209.

19   R. C. Brown et al., "Psychosocial Interventions for Children and Adolescents after Man-Made and Natural Disasters: A Meta-Analysis and Systematic Review," *Psychological Medicine*, 47, no. 11 (2017): 1893–1905, doi.org/10.1017 /S0033291717000496.

20   Ifigeneia Mavranezouli et al., "Psychological and Psychosocial Treatments for Children and Young People with Post-Traumatic Stress Disorder: A Network Meta-Analysis," *Journal of Child Psychology and Psychiatry* 61, no. 1 (January 2020): 18–29, doi.org/10.1111/jcpp.13094.

21   Bessel van der Kolk, *The Body Keeps the Score: Brain, Mind, and Body in the Healing of Trauma* (New York: Penguin Random House, 2015).

22   Eranda Jayawickreme and Laura E. Blackie, "Post-Traumatic Growth as Positive Personality Change: Evidence, Controversies, and Future Directions," *European Journal of Personality* 28, no. 4 (2014): 312–31, doi.org/10.1002/per.1963.

23   David Feinstein, "Perceptions, Reflections, and Guidelines for Using Energy Psychology: A Distillation of 800+ Surveys and Interviews with Practitioners and Clients," *Energy Psychology: Theory, Research, and Treatment* 13, no. 1 (2021): 13–46, doi .org/10.9769/EPJ.2021.13.1.DF.

CHAPTER 10: BRINGING ENERGY PSYCHOLOGY TO A WORLD IN DISTRESS

1   Adapted from Eric Leskowitz, *The Many Faces of Life Energy: From Biofield Healing to Global Consciousness* (Rochester, VT: Inner Traditions, in press); paraphrased by Dr. Leskowitz.

2   David Feinstein, "Six Empirically-Supported Premises about Energy Psychology: Mounting Evidence for a Controversial Therapy," *Advances in Mind-Body Medicine*, 35, no. 2 (2021): 17–32, how-it-works .energytapping.com.

3   Gabriëlle Rutten and Gary Craig, *Official EFT from A to Z* (Des Moines, IA, 2023), xi.

4 Joseph Campbell, *The Inner Reaches of Outer Space: Metaphor as Myth and as Religion* (New York: Alfred Van Der Marck, 1986), 16.

5 Jean Houston, "Harnessing the Energies of *Politeia*," Eden Method website, accessed April 29, 2023, edenmethod.com/political /harnessing-the-energies-of -politeia/.

6 Anneloes Smitsman and Jean Houston, Future Humans Trilogy website, accessed April 29, 2023, futurehumans.world/.

7 Claude Swanson, *Life Force, the Scientific Basis: Breakthrough Physics of Energy Medicine, Healing, Chi and Quantum Consciousness* (Tucson, AZ: Poseidia, 2009).

8 John White and Stanley Krippner, *Future Science: Life Energies and the Physics of Paranormal Phenomena* (New York: Anchor, 1977).

9 Wayne B. Jonas, editor's introduction to "Qigong: Basic Science Studies in Biology," in *Healing, Intention and Energy Medicine: Science, Research Methods and Clinical Implications,* ed. Wayne B. Jonas and Cindy C. Crawford (Philadelphia: Churchill Livingstone, 2003), 103.

10 Yury Kronn, *The Science of Subtle Energy: The Healing Power of Dark Matter* (Rochester, VT: Park Street Press, 2022).

11 Claire Sylvia, *A Change of Heart: A Memoir* (New York: Little, Brown, 1997).

12 Paul Pearsall, "In Awe of the Heart," *Alternative Therapies in Health and Medicine,* 13, no. 4 (2007): 16–19.

13 Paul Pearsall, *The Heart's Code: Tapping the Wisdom and Power of Our Heart Energy* (New York: Broadway Books, 1998), 7.

14 Thomas S. Kuhn, *The Structure of Scientific Revolutions,* 4th ed. (Chicago: University of Chicago Press, 2012).

15 Rollin McCraty, "The Energetic Heart: Bioelectromagnetic Interactions Within and Between People," *Neuropsychotherapist* 6, no. 1 (2003): 22–43, doi.org/10.12744/tnpt (6)022-043.

16 Bernard Grad, "The 'Laying on of Hands': Implications for Psychotherapy, Gentling, and the Placebo Effect," *Journal of the American Society for Psychical Research* 61, no. 4 (1967): 286–305.

17 Peter Tompkins and Christopher Bird, *The Secret Life of Plants: A Fascinating Account of the Physical, Emotional, and Spiritual Relations between Plants and Man* (New York: Harper & Row, 1973); Yung-Jong Shiah et al., "Effects of Intentionally Treated Water and Seeds on the Growth of Arabidopsis thaliana," *Explore* 17, no. 1 (January–February 2021): 55–9, doi.org /10.1016/j.explore.2020.04.006.

18 Dawson Church, "Measuring the Effect of Emotional Freedom Techniques (EFT) Treatment for Depression using a Seed Bioassay:

A Randomized Controlled Trial," *Psychology* 14, no. 11 (November 2023): 1687-169, doi.org/10.4236/psych.2023.1411098

19 Dawson Church et al., "Clinical EFT as an Evidence-Based Practice for the Treatment of Psychological and Physiological Conditions: A Systematic Review," *Frontiers in Psychology* 13 (November 2022): 951451, doi.org/10.3389/fpsyg.2022.951451.

20 Feinstein, "Six Empirically-Supported Premises."

21 Beverly Rubik et al., "Biofield Science and Healing: History, Terminology, and Concepts," *Global Advances in Health and Medicine* 4, supplement (2015): 8-14, doi.org/10.7453/gahmj.2015.038.suppl.

22 Timur Saliev et al., "Therapeutic Potential of Electromagnetic Fields for Tissue Engineering and Wound Healing," *Cell Proliferation* 47, no. 6 (December 2014), 485-93, doi.org/10.1111/cpr.12142.

23 James L. Oschman, *Energy Medicine: The Scientific Basis* (Edinburgh, UK: Churchill Livingstone/Harcourt, 2000), 94.

24 Hans J. H. Geesink, and Dirk K. F. Meijer, "Quantum Wave Information of Life Revealed: An Algorithm for EM Frequencies that Create Stability of Biological Order, with Implications for Brain Function and Consciousness," *NeuroQuantology* 14, no. 1 (2016): 106-25, doi.org/10.14704/nq.2016.14.1.911.

25 John M. Opitz, "The Developmental Field Concept in Clinical Genetics," *Journal of Pediatrics* 101, no. 5 (1982): 805-09, doi.org/10.1016/s0022-3476(82)80337-5.

26 Harold Saxton Burr, *The Fields of Life* (New York: Ballantine, 1972).

27 Harold Saxton Burr and Filmer Stuart Cuckow Northrup, "The Electro-Dynamic Theory of Life," *Quarterly Review of Biology* 10, no. 3 (1935): 322-33, jstor.org/stable/2808474.

28 Sally Adee, *We Are Electric: Inside the 200-Year Hunt for Our Body's Bioelectric Code, and What the Future Holds* (New York: Hachette, 2023), 194.

29 Knight Kalimah Redd and Patrick Collins, "The Face of a Frog: Time-Lapse Video Reveals Never-Before-Seen Bioelectric Pattern," Tufts Now, July 18, 2011, now.tufts.edu/2011/07/18/face-frog-time-lapse-video-reveals-never-seen-bioelectric-pattern.

30 Adee, *We Are Electric*, 197.

31 Dawson Church, *Mind to Matter: The Astonishing Science of How Your Brain Creates Material Reality* (Carlsbad, CA: Hay House, 2019), 44.

32 Jed Brody, *Quantum Entanglement* (Cambridge, MA: MIT Press, 2020).

33 From a 1947 letter to Max Born, as documented in B. M. Walker, ed., *The Born-Einstein Letters: Correspondence between Albert Einstein and Max and Hedwig Born from 1916-1955, with Commentaries*

by Max Born (New York: Macmillan, 1971), 158.

34   Daniel Salart et al., "Testing the Speed of 'Spooky Action at a Distance,'" *Nature* 454 (2008): 861–64, doi.org/10.1038/nature07121.

35   Jean Bricmont, *Quantum Sense and Nonsense* (Cham, Switzerland: Springer International, 2017).

36   Dean Radin, *Entangled Minds: Extrasensory Experiences in a Quantum Reality* (New York: Paraview, 2006).

37   Vlatko Vedral, "Quantifying Entanglement in Macroscopic Systems," *Nature* 453 (2008): 1004–7, doi.org/10.1038/nature07124.

38   Dean I. Radin, "Event-Related Electroencephalographic Correlations Between Isolated Human Subjects," *Journal of Alternative and Complementary Medicine* 10, no. 2 (2004): 315–23, doi .org/10.1089/107555304323062301.

39   Larry Dossey, *Healing Words: The Power of Prayer and the Practice of Medicine* (New York: HarperCollins, 1995).

40   C. N. Shealy, "Clairvoyant Diagnosis," in *Energy Medicine Around the World*, ed. T. M. Srinivasan (Phoenix, AZ: Gabriel Press, 1988), 291–303.

41   Yan X, Lu PY, and Kiang JG. "Qigong: basic science studies in biology," in *Healing Intention, and Energy Medicine: Science, Research Methods and Clinical Implications*, ed. Wayne B. Jonas and Cindy C. Crawford

(Philadelphia: Churchill Livingstone, 2003), 103–37.

42   Kronn, *Science of Subtle Energy*.

43   Church, *Mind to Matter*.

44   Swanson, *Life Force*, 32.

45   Kronn, *Science of Subtle Energy*, 40.

46   David Feinstein, "Energy Psychology Treatments Over a Distance: The Curious Phenomenon of 'Surrogate Tapping,'" *Energy Psychology: Theory, Research and Treatment* 5, no. 1 (2013), doi.org/10.9769/EPJ.2013.5 .1.DF.

47   Rollin McCraty, *Science of the Heart: Exploring the Role of the Heart in Human Performance*, vol. 2 (Boulder Creek, CA: HeartMath Institute, 2015).

48   Al Gore, *Assault on Reason* (New York: Penguin Press, 2007), 33.

49   Gore, *Assault on Reason*, 22.

50   William A. Tiller, Walter F. Dibble, and Michael J. Kohane, "Exploring Robust Interactions between Human Intention and Inanimate/Animate Systems," *Subtle Energies and Energy Medicine* 11, no. 3 (2000): 265–91.

51   R. G. Jahn et al., "Correlations of Random Binary Sequences with Pre-Stated Operator Intention: A Review of a 12-Year Program," *Explore* 3, no. 3 (May 2007): 244–53, doi.org/10.1016/j .explore.2007.03.009.

52   John S. Hagelin et al., "Effects of Group Practice of the Transcendental Meditation Program on Preventing Violent Crime in

Washington, D.C.: Results of the National Demonstration Project, June–July 1993," *Social Indicators Research* 47 (1999): 153–201, doi.org/10.1023/A:1006978911496.

53 Michael C. Dillbeck and Kenneth L. Cavanaugh, "Societal Violence and Collective Consciousness: Reduction of U.S. Homicide and Urban Violent Crime Rates," *SAGE Open* 6, no. 2 (2016), doi.org/10.1177/2158244016637891.

54 Eric Leskowitz, *The Joy of Sox: Weird Science and the Power of Intention* (Charleston, SC: CreateSpace, 2010), iv.

55 To learn more about the Intention Experiment, visit lynnemctaggart.com/intention-experiments/the-intention-experiment/ or see Lynne McTaggart's book, *The Power of Eight* (New York: Atria, 2018).

56 Jean Houston, "Consciousness Is the Quantum Field of the Cosmos," in *What Is Consciousness? Three Sages Look Behind the Veil*, by Ervin Laszlo, Jean Houston, and Larry Dossey (New York: SelectBooks, 2016), 3–32.

57 Caspar Henderson, *A New Map of Wonders: A Journey in Search of Modern Marvels* (Chicago: University of Chicago Press, 2017), 239.

APPENDIX

1 Dorothea Hover-Kramer, *Creating Healing Relationships: Professional Standards for Energy Therapy Practitioners* (Fulton, CA: Energy Psychology Press, 2011), 151.

2 With thanks to the inspirational Rick Hanson, author of *Hardwiring Happiness* (New York: Harmony Books, 2013).

3 Marty Becker, *The Healing Power of Pets* (New York: Hyperion, 2002).

4 Daniel Lieberman, *Exercised: The Science of Physical Activity, Rest, and Health* (New York, Penguin, 2021).

Index

About the Authors

DAVID FEINSTEIN, PHD, has written a dozen of the most frequently cited scientific papers on energy psychology. He is a pioneer in developing innovative therapeutic approaches, leading to nine national awards for his books on consciousness and healing. A licensed psychologist, he has served as an Instructor in Psychiatry at the Johns Hopkins University School of Medicine and as an Associate Professor of Psychology at Antioch College. He is a recipient of the *USA Book News* Best Psychology/Mental Health Book Award of 2007, the Association for Comprehensive Energy Psychology (ACEP) Outstanding Contribution Award (2002, 2012), the Canadian Association for Integrative and Energy Therapies' 2015 Outstanding Leadership Award, the Energy Medicine Research Institute award for "Innovative Energy Medicine Research," and the *Marquis Who's Who* Lifetime Achievement Award. His most recent book, *The Energies of Love,* coauthored with Donna, reached bestseller status on the *New York Times* Relationship List.

DONNA EDEN is among the world's most sought after, most joyous, and most authoritative spokespersons for energy medicine. She has been able to clairvoyantly "see" the body's energies her entire life, and her abilities as a healer are legendary. From this ability to see the body's energies, she has developed a system for teaching others who do not have this gift to nonetheless work effectively with their own energies. Her "Energy Medicine Mindvalley Masterclass" has had more than six million views. She has presented her work at numerous universities and hospitals, including giving grand rounds at the Cleveland Clinic. She has received Lifetime Achievement Awards for her distinguished career from the Energy Medicine Research Institute and the Association for Comprehensive Energy Psychology. Her classic book, *Energy Medicine,* is the textbook in hundreds of healing classes, with more than a half million sales. Available in 21 languages, it won golds in both the *USA Book News* and Nautilus competitions.

Donna's invigorating presentations are rich with audience participation and stunning demonstrations of simple methods for shifting the body's energies for health and vitality.

TOGETHER, David and Donna have built one of the world's largest and most vibrant organizations teaching the hands-on use of energy medicine. Their 1,600 certified practitioners are serving tens of thousands of clients and teaching hundreds of classes in the US, Canada, Latin America, Europe, Asia, and Australia. They jointly have been honored by the Infinity Foundation as the first couple to receive its annual Spirit Award for their contribution to "the evolution of consciousness" and its "impact on society," and they have also jointly received the Pioneer Award for Energy Healing Leadership.

About Sounds True

SOUNDS TRUE WAS FOUNDED in 1985 by Tami Simon with a clear mission: to disseminate spiritual wisdom. Since starting out as a project with one woman and her tape recorder, we have grown into a multimedia publishing company with a catalog of more than 3,000 titles by some of the leading teachers and visionaries of our time, and an ever-expanding family of beloved customers from across the world.

In more than three decades of evolution, Sounds True has maintained our focus on our overriding purpose and mission: to wake up the world. We offer books, audio programs, online learning experiences, and in-person events to support your personal growth and awakening, and to unlock our greatest human capacities to love and serve.

At SoundsTrue.com you'll find a wealth of resources to enrich your journey, including our weekly *Insights at the Edge* podcast, free downloads, and information about our nonprofit Sounds True Foundation, where we strive to remove financial barriers to the materials we publish through scholarships and donations worldwide.

To learn more, please visit SoundsTrue .com/freegifts or call us toll-free at 800.333.9185.

Together, we can wake up the world.

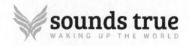